WHAT I DID FOR SEX

[And What It Can Do For You]

Schahrzad Morgan

Copyright © 2017 Schahrzad Morgan
All rights reserved.
ISBN-13: 9781542449397
ISBN-10: 1542449391

DEDICATION AND THANKS

I'm dedicating this book to people who encouraged me on my sexual journey and those who were against it. Both were needed, because if everyone already agreed that a sexually expressed woman is a powerful woman, there would be no need for this book.
I thank the men and women who made their way into this book. Their names and details were changed to protect their anonymity.
I thank you for reading my story.

CONTENTS

Preface		xiii
	Dreams	xiii
Chapter 1	**Desire**	1
Chapter 2	**Childhood**	4
	Germany	4
	Nebraska	8
Chapter 3	**Puberty**	12
	My First Orgasm	12
	"Get Your Education"	14
Chapter 4	**Curiosity**	18
	Intercourse	18
	The Line Cook	22
	Sex With Women	26
	Vibrators	30
	Porn And The Missing Clitoris	32
	"I'm Gonna Marry That Girl"	34
	A Crush On Zoe	38
	Call Girl	39
	Cocaine	42
Chapter 5	**A Good Girl**	47
	Sobriety	47
	B.S. Computer Science	49

		Engaged	51
		Compromise	52
Chapter 6		**Marriage And Raising A Family**	62
		Counseling	63
		Children	64
		Little Yellow Pills	76
		Avoidance	77
		Sequencing	83
		Coldness	85
		Love	88
		Dreams	91
		Indifference	94
		Hope	103
		Addiction Is A Choice	105
Chapter 7		**My Open Marriage**	109
		Swinging, Or The Lifestyle	110
		Lost In His Cock	115
		Threesomes With Other Couples	126
		He Watched Me Masturbate	130
		Lesbians	133
		An Older Woman	133
		Sex In My Minivan	133
		Her Skilled Tongue	139
		Our Couple Swap	142
		"If You Won't Fuck Me, I'll Find Someone Who Will"	147
		"I Am So Tired Of Being Told No"	149
		Jenna: She Finger Fucked Me Like A Guy	151
		Jenna: "What Do You Like About Men?"	162
		The Guestroom (March)	165
		A Previously Scheduled Vacation (April)	171
		Andrea: "Don't Make Any Noise"	171
		Shannon: "I Feel You"	174

Chapter 8	**Broken Dreams**		179
	Marriage Counseling		179
	Can I Afford To Leave Him?		184
	My Own Place (May)		184
Chapter 9	**Freedom**		186
	Kegels		187
	My Type Of Man		189
	"Let's Get Drunk"		190
	"Your Candor Is Refreshing"		192
	His Very High Libido		193
	Filing For Divorce		194
	"I'm Hard Because You Make Me So Hard"		195
	A Condom On My Nightstand		195
	His Sister Fetish		199
Chapter 10	**Lesbian Hookups**		206
	Her Leather Strap-On (July)		206
	Empty Nest		210
	Telling My Dad About My Divorce		211
	Noelle		212
	Fisting Felt So Good		215
	"Include Me In Your Fantasy When You're With Me"		217
	My Male Energy And Mens' Clothes		219
	Noelle: "Let Me See How Wet You Are"		222
	A 23 Year Old Marine		224
	Social Norms Around Women And Casual Sex		232
	Kris: She Excelled At Oral Sex		234
	Abstinence		234
	Snuggle Party		235
	Ashley: "Are You Sure Your Kids Don't Mind?"		239

Chapter 11	Younger Men	243
	Justin, 20: "I Love Older Women"	244
	My Ex Came For Dinner (October)	251
	Polyamory Retreat	253
	Cunnilingus: Can He Make Me Come?	260
	"I Love How Open You Are About Sex"	260
	"I Don't Go Down On Girls"	262
	"I Love Going Down On A Girl"	263
	Tommy, 21: The Connection Between My Heart And My Pussy And His Open Eye Orgasm	264
	I Paid For A Room	269
	The Fuck List (November)	270
	Two Men On The Same Day	272
	Nate, 23: "Your Pussy Is So Tight"	273
	Kevin, 28: He Was A Stud	277
	Bored And Distracted At Work	278
	Lonely, Yet Unavailable	279
	Kevin, 28: Rail And Bail Office Sex	282
	"He's Always Onlne"	283
	Female Condom	285
	Two Men In One Day Again	286
	Justin, 20: Trying Out Taboos	286
	Billy, 19: Professional Skateboarder	289
	Two Men In One Evening	290
	Caden, 19: He Did Not Make A Sound	290
	Rick, 24: He Loved Rimming Me	292
	Can A Woman Ask A Man Out? (December)	293
	Ghosting	295
	Co-Parenting And My Ex	296
	"You Should Be Satisfied"	296

	Porn Caused His Erection Problem	298
	"Spit On My Cock"	300
	Jackson, 22: "I Love Facesitting"	302
	Inner Peace	306
	"Are You A Sex Addict?"	308
	Danny, 28: Falling For A Man I Never Met	309
	"The Key For Schahrzad Is To Seek Connection With Herself"	310
Chapter 12	**I Want A Relationship**	313
	Bill, 49: It Was Just Physical	314
	His Limp Dick: "I Masturbate Too Much"	315
	Why Are Men Always Leaving In The Morning?	316
	He Liked Me	317
	Booty Call	318
	Christopher: A Family Life Fantasy	318
	Walter, 35: Comfort	320
	Girlfriend Advice	322
	My Divorce (January)	324
	A Cancelled Date	325
	He Met All My Sexual Needs	325
	Squirting Was A Disappointment	327
	Pegging	329
	Orgasm During Penetration And Ladies First	331
	Power Parting	337
	Bedroom Persona	339
	The Bar Fly And Whiskey Dick	345
	I Love Anal	346
	The Bad Girl Myth	348
	My Neediness	349
	Dwight, 53: "I Have Such A Headache"	350
	"Leaving The Office For Sex Makes A Bad Impression"	352

	Dick Pics And My Relationship To My Pussy	353
	"Mommy, What Is Sex?"	356
	Steve: "We Need To End This" (March)	357
	The Man I Fell For Online	359
	Dominating A Woman	360
	"I Realized I Want A Wife And Children"	360
Chapter 13	**Purpose And Mission**	363
	Mormons Don't Masturbate (May, One Year Single)	364
	Sex Education, Government, Church, Auras, And Lots Of Fear	366
	A Black Man	367
	David, 32: Inspiration	368
	Abstinence	376
	"You Should Write A Book"	378
	What If I Never Find A Man?	379
	Tinder	381
	Lingering	382
	He Had A Girlfriend (October)	383
	The Clitoris Is A Large Organ, Mostly Internal	384
	"I Don't Use Lube"	385
	Many Of Today's Young Men Rock In Bed	387
	I Orgasmed While Masturbating During Penetration	387
	His First Time Doing Oral And I Had An Orgasm	387
Chapter 14	**Finding My Groove**	388
	My Career (May, Two Years Single)	388
	Sexual Harassment	388
	Quitting My Job	389
	My Sex Memoir	389
	A Nude Strip Club	390

Escort	392
A Relationship Prospect :	
He Wore His Pajamas	394
He Led Me On	397
A Relationship With Myself	
(May, Three Years Single)	399
The Softness And Mystery Of	
Us Women	400
Public Speaker And Consultant	400
Falling In Love	401
Relationship Coaches	402

Epilogue 405
Dreams 405
About the Author 406

PREFACE

DREAMS

As a young woman, I dreamed of college, a loving husband, a beautiful home, and staying home to raise my children. I got all that.

I didn't dream about sex. I figured sex was something that would keep happening and if two people loved each other and liked sex, the sex would be good…at least for the first two years while it was new and exciting. So when it became boring, I thought that was normal.

I didn't dream about the kind of woman I would be for my husband, and whether he would be pleased with me and look forward to coming home. By the time he came home to the kids and not to me, I no longer cared if he came home at all.

I didn't dream that when the kids were older I would find a renewed interest in my husband, a surging sexual desire for him, and a readiness on my part for intimacy, vulnerability, and connection of which I was not capable before. I thought husbands liked sex and closeness with their wives and that he would be happy with the new me.

I didn't dream about divorce.

CHAPTER 1
DESIRE

I heard his car pull into the driveway and smiled.
"Hi honey, I'm home!" Brad bantered into the kitchen and gave me a hug.

He looked so handsome in his collared shirt and tie. I loved how his eyes twinkled and his dimples showed when he smiled at me. I had baked lasagna, his favorite dish. The smell of garlic wafted from the oven. I tossed olive oil on the arugula salad.

We heaped the fresh food on our plates and took them to our dining room. Our long table had once seated our family of five. Now it was just the two of us. Brad sat at the head of the table and lit the candles.

"Hmmmm...honey, this is delicious!" he beamed at me.

"Thank you." I felt appreciated.

"How was your day?" he asked.

"My boss invited me to a conference in Sacramento," I told him excitedly.

"Well, it's no surprise, I knew they would see how smart you are!"

"Awww...thank you honey."

I told him about my beach run that morning, and something I had heard on the news.

"I love listening to you talk," he said.

He told me that often. I liked listening to him too. I was glad our kids were gone. I loved being alone with my husband. It wasn't always that way. For most of our 24-year marriage, I resented him and we slept in separate bedrooms. A few years earlier we had rediscovered each other during a family vacation. Lately, we took walks in the morning where we held hands, met for coffee after work, and cuddled at night. I felt "in love". I couldn't get enough of him, especially sexually. Our marriage was not perfect, but the areas that were not so good were moving in the right direction.

After dinner, I cleaned up the kitchen, while he washed the dishes. Then we went to bed so we could be alone. It was only 9 pm.

"Do you want a foot massage?" he asked.

"Yes!"

I sank back into the pillow while he massaged my feet. I felt grateful for the pleasurable touch and our closeness. When he finished, he picked up Smithsonian Magazine on his nightstand. He lay back and got absorbed in his reading. I wanted to be close, so I snuggled up against him. He smiled at me, so I took it as a sign it was okay to get closer.

I reached over to rub his stomach. That always turned me on, so I started grinding a little against him. It felt good to be close like that, just a little turned on. I wished he would want to make love to me. I knew he wouldn't. We had sex yesterday and he liked to wait a few days in between.

Brad turned the page. I felt a little aroused, so I ground up more against him and moaned softly.

"Not. Tonight. I. Don't. Want. Sex. Tonight!" he exclaimed.

His voice was loud, filled with disdain. He enunciated every word. He kept his eyes on the magazine. He was probably annoyed with me, wanting sex again. He waited a few seconds, and then reached over and turned off the light.

I had heard "no" to sex so many times before. Each time, I felt hurt in my heart for not being able to express my love and desire for him, and sexually frustrated because I was horny. I did not feel rejected. Brad loved my body and me, and I knew I turned him on. The problem with "no" was not rejection; the problem was I felt like a surging volcano of desire, and he kept pushing the lava down.

Over the years, I tried various coping strategies to deal with his no: telling him how I felt and what I wanted, forcing myself to be okay with it, pushing my desire aside, turning my desires to women, letting myself feel my sadness and longing in the hopes the acknowledgement would make it pass, and finally self pity. I talked it all out with my friends and often I cried. Brad didn't like when I cried, especially when the crying was about him.

For some reason, that night, it was no longer acceptable to push me away, not care how I felt, and squash my self-expression. *No! No more. I'll never again make him the object of my arousal, and subject myself to being so easily cast aside. I need take care of myself. I need to get away from him.*

I let go of my arm around his stomach and moved to my side of the bed. *Wow, I can't believe I'm doing this.*

I lay down to sleep. Then I had a profound realization: *To avoid getting turned on by him, I have to stay on my side forever.* What was the point of being there at all?

I grabbed my pillow and jumped out of bed.

"I'm sleeping in the guest room."

I stormed out of our bedroom, and slammed the door behind me. I went into the bedroom of our daughter Chandi who was away at college. I lay in her soft comfortable queen size bed. I fell asleep right away.

CHAPTER 2
CHILDHOOD

GERMANY

Baba, my dad, left Iran to study medicine in Germany, and that's where he met Mama, my mom. They married at the justice of the peace when my mom was eight months pregnant with me.

I was born in Düsseldorf, Germany, in 1961. My parents named me Schahrzad Pour-Mohammedian. My sister, Sarina, was born 17 months later, and my brother 16 months after that.

We lived in small towns, as Baba worked in the city and climbed the career ladder as a pathologist. Mama stayed home to raise us. She was the embodiment of classic soft motherhood, the most beautiful woman I had ever seen. She devoted herself to being a housewife and pleasing my dad, even though no matter what she did, he didn't seem to appreciate it too much.

Baba didn't like the noises or inconveniences of little children, especially after work, so he made sure Mama had us in bed before he got home from work. On weekends, we acted out his home movie scripts until the scene was just right, while Mama held the clapperboard and heavy lights. Later we recorded the dialogue. "One day you'll be glad we have these films," Baba often said.

My parents believed childhood was for play and education. We didn't have chores, but we had many toys and were often sent outdoors to play. I rode my bicycle and Kettcar much farther from home than I was allowed to go. I don't recall if my mother ever got mad at me for just wanting to explore the world and be free.

Mama taught me to read long before I started school. The tales of the Children's Bible, Grimm Brothers, and Arabian Nights amused me. I wasn't sure if the bible's talking snake and parting sea were real, or if they were imaginary like flying carpets, genies in bottles, and wolves who swallowed girls in red petticoats. Were women really so helpless as in these tales?

My idol was *Pippi Longstocking*, the independent self-expressed girl who created adventure because there was no other way she could be. I wanted to be just like her, minus the aloof part. I didn't believe anyone could really be happy not needing anyone at all. I yearned to be an adult so I could be free like Pippi...free to go to bed when I wanted, free to stay home alone and not have to go on those boring picnics and fishing trips with Baba in the hot sun which always gave me a headache, free to give my opinions without being yelled at, and free to do what I wanted without being punished.

Soon I was school age. I ran all the way, because I loved running as much as I loved school. School was a place for more satisfaction in learning and more attention for being smart. My 2nd grade teacher was getting a large stomach, so one day I asked Mama about it.

"Mama, how did she get that big belly?" in German of course.

"There's a baby growing inside."

"How did it get in there?"

I wasn't going to buy the stork story, but I thought that's where she would go. She leaned down and looked at me sweetly.

"When a man and woman love each other very much, a man puts his penis inside the woman's vagina, and sperm comes out to fertilize the egg, and a baby is made. The baby grows and when it's done growing, it comes out."

That sounded super gross. I was incapable of such a love as that. Maybe I didn't want children after all.

My parents sometimes invited guests for dinner. We children curtsied and shook their hands. Then the women cooked in the kitchen while the men talked in the living room. The kitchen was hot and boring. I would never be shut away in a kitchen. I usually went into the living room and sat on the sofa, absorbed in the exciting conversations of adults. Sometimes I sat on my dad's lap while he stroked my leg. After dinner, we played Persian music and the adults danced.

"Every man wants a virgin," my father said one evening, while he and his friends danced.

His friends laughed. I struggled to understand. My dad was always talking about the value of education. Why was the opposite preferred when it came to sex? Maybe this would make sense when I was older.

One afternoon, when my mom had a friend over for coffee, she said, "My husband said a woman's vagina is just an ejaculation vessel for men."

"Really?" the woman replied.

The word "vessel" reminded me of dark antique vases and cremation urns from my geography books. How could my dad reduce beautiful beings to hollow, lifeless objects? When would I become an ejaculation vessel for men?

My early childhood messages about sex were that men wanted only sex from women, and women should never give it to them because it made them tainted and less desirable to men.

Sex seemed like a bad thing people could only do if they were married, and bad enough to never be discussed at all.

When my parents went on vacation to Italy, Spain, France, Greece, Turkey, or Iran, they left us with Mama's parents. This was a great joy for me. I did not know until I was older that other parents took their kids along on vacations.

Mama's parents, Opa and Oma, still lived in her childhood home in Recklinghausen, a city with cobblestone streets and soot-covered buildings in the coal-mining region of Germany. During World War II, American soldiers had taken over the house and lived in it, leaving it ransacked. My grandparents had rebuilt it. The backyard bunker served as a reminder that bombs sometimes fell from the sky.

I was fascinated exploring their house: the empty bedrooms, the attic with musty smells of books, the stereo console and 45rpm records, the mealtime gong in the foyer, the food storage room with its thick concrete walls, and the bookcase of novels in the living room. I loved holding the books with the older German fonts, smelling each page as I devoured *East of Eden* and *Désirée*.

Maria, the live-in housekeeper who helped raise my mother, still lived with my grandparents. She told stories about our grandparents and spoiled us with chocolate when Mama wasn't looking. She rose every morning at 5 am and immediately started cleaning. She opened windows for fresh air, cleaned all the toilets, and mopped floors. I was surprised a clean house required such rigorous daily scrubbing. Maria served lunch exactly at noon, and then cleaned up while my grandparents retreated to the living room with its recessed lighting and large windows to the backyard. They put on their reading glasses, smoked cigarettes, and worked crossword puzzles. I learned to work the crossword puzzles. Mostly I just sat and watched them in awe. My grandmother smiled a lot and smelled good and wore pretty jewelry.

On Sunday mornings, Opa and I walked to church. I loved walking with him, admiring his suits and cane. I was awed with the beautiful architecture of the Catholic Church, its holy silence, and moving hymns. There was kneeling and standing and more kneeling, repeating words the priest said, and going up to the front to eat wafers and drink wine. They said it was Jesus' body and blood, and we ate it out of love. The holy ritual had an ironic resemblance to cannibalism.

"Mama, why don't we go to church?" I asked her after I returned home.

"We want you kids to decide which religion you like," she replied.

"What religion are you?"

"Catholic."

"What religion is Baba?"

"He is Muslim."

I had never heard that word. I recalled a big book called a Koran in our bookcase, although I had never seen him read it. If religion was optional, why did adults take it so seriously?

Our parents thought we were wise and interested enough to study all the world religions, and then choose one we liked? It seemed like a lot to figure out, and maybe I'd never get around to it.

NEBRASKA

When I was nine years old, my parents began to talk about something that had them excited. One day they shared it with us.

"We're moving to America," my mom said.

America. I heard that word when I watched the western Bonanza. I wasn't sure why my parents would take us to a desert with cowboys, pistols, horses, saloons, and no cars, but I trusted them and figured it would all work out. Mama bought german-english audiotapes and books, and taught us children to speak, read, and write English.

We landed in Omaha, Nebraska. It was 1971. I joined the third grade class in the middle of the spring semester, and became the popular "girl from Germany". Mama remained a housewife, and Baba started a job in cancer research.

We had barely settled into our new apartment, when my dad stopped coming home at night.

"I was so tired, so I slept at work," he said without looking at us.

Where at work? It didn't make much sense, and Mama didn't buy it either. Shortly thereafter, Mama said our dad was having an affair. Mama started crying a lot. She signed up for a night class in computer programming, and came home from class with her stack of punch cards. She graduated with an A+. But the class wasn't enough to still her crying heart.

She finally found solace in Transcendental Meditation (TM). Twice each day she went into her bedroom, and 20 minutes later she emerged with a glowing smile and hugs for us children. I wanted this meditation that made my mom so happy. Mama took me to the Omaha TM Center for instruction in the children's walking mantra. It didn't do much for me and I couldn't wait to be old enough to get my sitting mantra.

That fall, my parents bought a house on one acre, in an area of Omaha with good schools. I don't know why they bought a house when their marriage was falling apart.

"The fruit trees remind me of Iran," Baba said, in Farsi of course.

The property became a family affair. In summer, our family pulled weeds, and in winter we shoveled the long driveway. The muggy summers and cold winters made this all horrid, and eventually my parents also realized this all sucked, so they hired a gardener and a snow shoveling service. That put an end to me doing any kind of work around the house.

One morning, on my walk to elementary school, I noticed magazines with pictures of naked people tossed in a vacant lot. I walked over to have a closer look. A naked woman with round perky breasts and a gorgeous mane of blond hair graced the cover of a magazine titled Playboy. I flipped through the magazine. Inside was a foldout of the woman, displaying her dark blond pubic hair and her legs spread wide open, showing her pink fleshy lips and crevices. It was the most gorgeous sight I had ever seen. I wondered if I was normal, to be aroused by a woman. I considered taking the magazine home, but was afraid my parents might find it and get mad at me or think I was gay, so I left them.

My dad was still having the affair and coming home less, and eventually he didn't even come home for Christmas, a holiday he had always despised. The only sign that we even had a dad were his clothes left in the closet, our paid bills, and an occasional phone call asking us to go to dinner with him. Mama said he was a bad, evil, and dirty man for cheating on her, taking up hunting, and drinking a lot of beer. I believed her, and had not been close to him anyway, so whenever he asked to spend time together, I refused.

I still didn't like being around Baba anyway. First, I hated him for his authoritarian parenting style, which consisted of him lecturing and telling us what to do, without ever asking what we wanted or how we felt. He said we had to listen to him because he was older and that meant he was wiser, and things had always been done a certain way which was tradition, and that meant it was good. It all felt confining and constricting.

Second, I could not communicate with him because of the language barrier. He required us to speak Farsi, a language he taught us to the vocabulary of a 5-year-old. Therefore, as we children grew older and had more complex thoughts, which we could not say in Farsi, we often spoke to him in German or English. He always said he didn't understand, "Man hichi nimi-famam" ("I don't understand a word"). Or he would get mad, "Farsi hafbesan!" he scolded. Yet he never taught us new words or enrolled us in lessons.

I had just started the 6th grade, when my uncle called from Germany. Oma had died of a heart attack. I wasn't sad, because I had forgot about my German family after we moved to the USA, aside from the letters we were forced to write. Besides, old people were supposed to die. Mama said Oma's soul would live in eternity until she was reborn. She flew to Germany to attend the funeral. She probably needed her family too, at a time she was devastated over the end of her marriage.

When Mama returned from Germany, she said her family would watch us children while she attended a 9-month-long TM teacher-training course, which was available only in Switzerland.

CHAPTER 3
PUBERTY

I spent my 7th grade school year with Opa and Maria, and attended the gymnasium. My sister and brother stayed with my uncle's family.

I gained 20 pounds that year. My once lanky girl body grew rounder, especially in my butt and breasts. I did not know it was a normal part of puberty.

My dad came to Germany and took me to lunch. We had just finished eating, when I felt a wetness on my leg. I went to the bathroom, and saw my vulva and panties were soaked in blood. I cried for a minute. Was this menstruation or did I have an injury? I did not feel any pain., so I composed myself, stuffed my pants with toilet paper, and came back out to Baba. I hoped nobody would see the red stains on my pants. I couldn't wait to get back to Maria. After Baba dropped me off at Opa's house, I told Maria everything. She gave me a hug and then she went upstairs to get maxi pads. The pads were bulky in my pants. I did not like this part of being an adult.

MY FIRST ORGASM

Opa's house had only one full bathroom. It had a bathtub with a handheld shower attachment. The menstruation had made me curious about my body, so the next time I took a bath, I looked at my body closely. I was rinsing off the soap in my pubic area, when I noticed an intense pleasurable tingling. I liked the tingling, so I continued letting the water spray on my vulva. The sensation grew in intensity, and then I had a most wonderful rolling wave of pleasure between my legs. It was my first orgasm. I took baths several times a day after that, and wondered if everyone in the house knew what I was doing, and if they also gave themselves orgasms in the bathtub.

After completing her teacher-training course, Mama returned to Germany and instructed us children in the practice of TM. I liked the deep silence of my meditation, and the joy I started to feel for no reason.

About two months later, our school year ended, and we returned to Omaha. I masturbated with the water from the bathtub faucet. I scooted all the way forward and let the warm water gush down on my vulva and clitoris. I orgasmed within minutes.

My dad stopped by the house occasionally to get some clothes or see us children. I didn't like it when he came home, because I did not enjoy his company. One afternoon, my dad came home and my parents yelled so much, I hid under my bed. After Baba left, Mama said she was filing for divorce. I thought I was supposed to be sad about the divorce, but I was happy, because the fighting would end and we would be rid of my dad.

That summer, my parents put the house up for sale. Baba helped Mama purchase a new, smaller, 3-bedroom house in the suburbs. For the first time, I had my own bedroom, and I had privacy. I wanted orgasms without a bathtub. I learned to masturbate with my fingers while I looked at the clitoris of a Playboy centerfold. Other times, I looked at my own clitoris with a magnifying mirror between my legs. I watched my finger slide next to my clitoris, and got more and more aroused. My clitoris became engorged and swollen. Eventually, I got so turned on looking at myself, I didn't need the magazines anymore.

"GET YOUR EDUCATION"

That fall, I started the 8th grade. Compared to my German school, the curriculum was so easy, in the second week of class I skipped my grade and started the 9th grade.

I took home economics and I sewed my own dresses. I liked the dresses, but I did not like my body. My bowlegs stuck out under the dresses. I yearned for straight legs. My nose was too big, my hair too thin, my fingers too short. I looked best in the baggy corduroys, which hid my big butt. And I was too short, just over 5'2". I hoped I would continue growing and then maybe my legs would straighten out too.

My Algebra III teacher was hot. He often had his back to the class while he stood at the chalkboard, impressing me with complicated formulas and his gorgeous ass. Did he wear those tight pants to turn us girls on? Did other 13-year-old girls get turned on by adult men, or was there something wrong with me?

My dad called often and asked to see us. He paid his alimony and child support, and even though I was his favorite child and he had many pet names for me and hugged me sweetly, I still did not like him. He used our visits as lecture opportunities.

"Discipline is very important. Discipline. Discipline and respect."

"Always keep learning. Education is very important."

"Get your Ph.D., not just your bachelor's degree."

"Pediatrics is a good field for women because you have time for a family."

Mama also talked to me about education. She made sure I took English and math every semester even when it wasn't required. She said it all in German.

"Don't ever give up your education for a man like I did."

"Get your education so you can provide for yourself and never have to depend on a man. A man can leave you for a younger woman, so make sure you can provide for yourself."

"Your education is one thing nobody can ever take from you."

I believed everything they said. I loved books and learning anyway. I devoured books about juicing, fasting, vegetarianism, and meditation. I was at Baba's house reading a book when he and his girlfriend came in.

"We have something to tell you," Baba said, in Farsi of course.

"What?" I put down my book.

"We got married."

"When?"

"Three months ago."

He did all the talking. I fought back tears, so they would not mistake them for sadness over their marriage. I liked his girlfriend, and had hoped to be part of the marriage celebration. Instead, he left me out and blindsided me after the fact. I wasn't about to tell him my feelings when he had never cared about them before.

I swallowed my sadness, so I could speak. "Oh, that's good."

I looked at her hand. She was wearing a diamond ring.

When I got home, Mama was making dinner. She had not been on one date since her divorce. Although I was glad she wasn't one of those divorcees who ignored her children to run amok with men, it seemed odd she had no interest in men at all.

"Why don't you date, Mom?"

"I don't like men," and she kept her eyes on cutting vegetables.

"There are nice men out there, " I said.

"I'm not interested in men. I am interested in enlightenment."

"Do you ever get lonely?"

"No. People should not need other people. "

"Do you ever think about sex?"

"No, I have no interest in physical union anymore."

Was she secretly a lesbian? I didn't know, but it sounded final.

I vowed to never hate men. The part about not needing people made sense though, because the goal of life was seeking God and letting go of our desires. Besides, people could leave me. I imagined I could have sex and love men without opening to them fully. That way it wouldn't matter when they dismissed my feelings and it wouldn't hurt so much if they left me.

I loved meditating. When I meditated, I felt the deep inner peace written about by poets. My mind was awake while my body was so relaxed, my breathing almost stopped. I started feeling a connection to what I called The Universe, or God, and experienced "support of nature", a state of living where life flowed effortlessly, and my actions felt supported.

That fall, when my classmates started the 10th grade, I used the insurance money from a car accident to spend three months at Maharishi University of Management (MUM) in Fairfield, Iowa to complete the first phase of the TM teacher-training course. When I returned to Omaha in early December, I started my high school year. I had to work hard to catch up.

By then, puberty had transformed my lanky figure into a voluptuous woman with a DD bra size. I was 20 pounds overweight and felt uncomfortable and embarrassed carrying the extra weight. My periods were so heavy, that on my highest flow days, I changed my maxi pads between every class. Still, blood often leaked out onto my clothes. At night, it leaked onto my sheets and stained them with blood.

I hated my womanhood, vagina, and uterus for the mess, cramps, back pain, and bloating they caused. I read books about celebrating the "moon flow", in hopes I could love my womanly rhythms, but it didn't change anything. I wanted freedom from the mess, like the women in TV ads who wore white pants and jogged while they bled. I was done with pads. I needed tampons.

I rode my bicycle to the store and purchased OB tampons (no plastic applicator). I locked myself in the bathroom and used a handheld mirror to look for my vagina. I fumbled around, looking for the opening. It took a while and then I found it. I pushed the tampon past the pain and it felt like a lump lodged in my body all through dinner. Eventually the menstrual blood soaked it and made it wet, and then I could push it deeper in, and no longer feel it.

CHAPTER 4
CURIOSITY

I was in high school and curious about men and relationships and sex, so I asked my parents about dating. There wasn't a single boy I was interested in at the time, but maybe one day there would be.

"You can't date until you're in college," Mama said.

"You can't date until you are 32 years old," Baba said.

Were men that bad, that I could not even date them? Was it because they thought men would want sex from me? Was sex really that bad? I was embarrassed to ask my dad, so I asked my mom.

"Mama, what do you think about sex?"

"That's for earthly people. Spiritual people don't have sex," she replied.

Priests, monks, and nuns were the only spiritual people I knew, and none of them had sex, so maybe she was right. I didn't want to be enlightened from my meditation before I was old enough to experience sex. I didn't care if I experienced dating, but I definitely wanted to try sex.

INTERCOURSE

At the age of 16, I set out to experience sex before it was too late. I used the first boy who showed interest in me in high school.

Bill was in my human physiology class and lived a few blocks away. He was a runner, lean and fit, about 5'10". I invited him over after school while my mom was out. We were both sober. We went into my bedroom, took off our clothes, and lay on my bed. Our nakedness was not too awkward. I don't think we ever kissed. His penis was beautiful, quite hard, just like in the pictures I saw in a friend's Playgirl. He lay on top of me and pushed his hard penis around looking for my opening. It reminded me of inserting my first tampon.

"Ouch, that hurts!"

"Yeah, we just have to keep trying," and he gently pushed on.

"Okay, but why does it hurt?"

"I'm not sure," and he kept pushing.

I spread my legs and allowed him to push his way inside, past the pain. Then he stopped moving and just lay on me. He felt heavy. It didn't feel amazing like in the books and movies. He should know what to do. He was the man.

"What are we supposed to do?" I asked.

"I think we just lay here."

"We do?"

"Yeah, and your vagina will start contracting."

I didn't like this guy, and I especially did not like him laying on me. I wasn't contracting and his penis inside me was painful.

"Let's stop," I suggested.

"Good idea," he agreed.

Bill got dressed and went home. I washed off my disappointment in a long hot shower. Why had it hurt? Why did they call it 'losing' virginity, when I had not lost anything at all, not even a hymen, judging by the lack of blood on my sheet? Did I remove my hymen when I inserted my first tampon, or were hymens fictional like tooth fairies and flying carpets? Why didn't I feel any passion?

Bill invited me over a few days later when his parents were out. He took me to his room and showed me his racing ribbons.

I liked the warm feeling when he stood close to me. Maybe we could go out sometime.

My reverie was interrupted by the sound of the garage door. It opened and I heard a car pull inside. Bill dropped the ribbons, and frantically yelled at me to climb out the back window. Bill didn't seem so hot anymore. I didn't know he snuck me in. I thought boys were allowed to have girls over.

He practically pushed me out. I climbed out his parent's bedroom window, and ran the three blocks to my home. I was no longer impressed with the boy who invited me over and then threw me out, instead of taking a stand for me in front of his mom, introducing me properly, and seeing me to the front door or even walking me home.

The next day at school Bill explained his parents were religious and wanted him to be a virgin until he got married, and he wasn't allowed to date or have girls over when his parents were out. He must have told his friends about me, because a few days later, a popular boy from school called and asked to come over. I had never talked with him before.

The boy pulled up and honked. I didn't like being honked at, but there he was, waiting outside, so I came out and got in his car. The boy's face was full of acne, and I didn't want him near me. He drove around the dirt roads adjacent to my neighborhood and parked in a secluded spot. What did he want? He kissed me and I kissed him back. I was really grossed out by his sloppy kisses and acne. He undressed and touched me and I went along with it all because I didn't have the confidence to tell him I didn't want any of it, and I wasn't going to be a frigid girl who withheld sex from men. And I had my curiosity about sex. Maybe this boy would know what to do. The boy fumbled around and put on a condom. He stuck his hard penis into my dry vagina, and since it was painful, I was glad it was over quickly.

I didn't like sex with this boy, and I hated having it in the car because it felt demeaning, it wasn't private, and I was squished in the seat. A boy who cared about a girl would take her to a bed. After he had his orgasm in the condom, he drove me home. I was glad to get away from him. I took a long shower to wash off his yuckiness. Then I ran downstairs and had dinner with my mom who thought I was still a virgin.

I had sex with other boys after that. I made sure I liked the boys going forward. Sometimes my best friend Chelli was with me, and we took turns having sex with a guy. I liked sex, even though socially I would be considered a "bad girl". The free love era was over and we were a civilized society with morals. Girls like me, who had sex for fun, were called easy and slutty. Magazine articles said we came from bad homes, were rebelling against our parents, or seeking attention from men to make up for an absent father figure. None of the articles said a young woman's sexual exploration was cause for celebration. Maybe the problem was with the girls who didn't have sex, because they were bowing to social mores and afraid to discover that part of themselves.

I liked my sexual adventurous side, although I didn't enjoy the sex so much. The men always had an orgasm at my expense. I did not fake orgasms, so the men could not say I climaxed. What was wrong with them or with me? And why did the men always want it in the car?

I read newspaper articles about women and orgasms to understand. The article said 30% of women orgasmed from intercourse, the other 70% needed clitoral stimulation to orgasm, some women never had an orgasm, and many women faked their orgasms. I hated my vagina for being in the 70%. I wanted orgasms from intercourse, just like the men.

I watched a couple porn movies to learn more about sex. The porn women seemed to love sex. They didn't kiss or have foreplay, which proved foreplay was for frigid women who couldn't get turned on without it. The action revolved around the man and his penis. It reinforced that what was happening in the cars was normal, and there was something wrong with me for not loving it.

I was thrilled when a popular handsome boy from school asked me out. I asked him to pick me up while Mama was out, because I wasn't allowed to date. He picked me up in his sports car, and drove to the church parking lot next to our school. We kissed and fondled and had oral sex. I asked him for intercourse and he refused, because he was saving sex for marriage. When he dropped me off, he asked if we could go on a date. That evening, when Mama came home, I asked her again about dating, and again she told me no. I could have sex in a car, but I couldn't go out with a boy. It seemed fucking was all I could ever get from a man.

THE LINE COOK

That fall, I turned 16 and was finally old enough to work. I got a job at a local steakhouse. The 21-year-old line cook, Griffin, caught my eye. He cooked the steaks, talked with the customers and was good friends with the owner, while I only served drinks and salads. I was impressed with his confidence and abilities.

Griffin noticed me too. He asked me out and picked me up from school. In the car, he pulled out a small pipe and took a deep breath from it. He said it was weed (marijuana). I was frightened, because I remembered the drug education movies from 6th grade, where people on drugs jumped out a window thinking they could fly, or touched a gas burner thinking the flame was a flower. The teachers said marijuana killed brain cells and was a gateway drug that led to heroin and death. Was I safe with Griffin, or should I open the car door and make a run for it?

Griffin took another hit and handed me the pipe. "You want to try this?"

"No."

I didn't want to hallucinate or enter the gateway to heroin. He took another hit. He wasn't jumping out the car window to fly or doing anything strange and he wasn't looking for heroin. The teachers lied. Damn them.

"I want to try it." I took the pipe from him.

I took a hit and coughed. About a minute later, my entire body tingled and the world seemed woozy and far away. I wasn't sure I liked it. Griffin took me home to his apartment, and offered me beer and more weed. He put on fabulous music I had never heard like the Outlaws and the Allman Brothers.

He leaned over to kiss me and it was awkward because I was high, but I went along with it, because I didn't want to be frigid. It wasn't much better than being in a car and I did not have an orgasm. He was 21. He should know how to please a woman. Afterward, he drove me home and asked when he could see me again. We set a date for that weekend. I went to my bedroom and masturbated. I was angry with him for not knowing I could have orgasms too, and using his penis to get off at my expense. I went to my desk calendar and put a G for sex with Griffin, and O for my solo orgasm.

I came across a book on sexual fantasies, and thought something was wrong with me for not having them. I began fantasizing during masturbation, a habit that turned out to be difficult to undo later in life. I imagined a man watched my swollen clitoris for the entire 15-30 minutes it took me to climax. I was proud of my clit and wanted men to admire it, just like men wanted women to worship their cocks. I was too embarrassed to tell Griffin any of this.

Griffin became my boyfriend and I his girlfriend. I didn't go out with other boys or have sex with them anymore, because I wasn't going to be a cheater like Baba. It wasn't because I loved him. He bored me and rarely took me out. We stayed in his apartment, listening to music and smoking weed. He wasn't suitable long term either, because he was blue collar. For marriage I wanted a man with a college degree who meditated, could provide for our family, and didn't do drugs.

I liked Griffin because he gave me freedom and a footstep into the adult world. He had his own place, alcohol, and weed. I loved cleaning his apartment, with the music blasting and a drink in my hand, and no parents or teachers telling me what to do. At work, he aroused me, with his tight jeans and nice ass, and the respect he got from our boss and customers.

That Christmas my dad gave me a red VW super beetle. It was a stick shift, and only a few years old. My dad had lovingly cleaned and waxed it. I was astounded. I had not even asked for it. Finally I was free to go places without borrowing Mama's car.

I spent more time with Griffin after that. I had a curfew, which I ignored. Sometimes I spent the night. I lied and told Mama I was with Chelli. She figured it out, and a few times she came to Griffin's apartment late at night to get me, presumably to avoid us having sex, which we had already done, so it made no sense. I was angry that she made me come home, when I wanted to be with him. Griffin was nice to me and all her efforts just prevented us from cuddling at night. When I did spend the night, she stewed silently and gave me the silent treatment when I came home. I still couldn't see what was so bad about being with my boyfriend.

I went to Planned Parenthood to get birth control pills, because I didn't want to get pregnant. Baba found out. He brought it up when we were standing on his patio looking out over the fruit trees.

"You're like a dog, having sex. Sex is for animals," he yelled.

It was super awkward. Was he a dog too when he had sex? Why wasn't he glad I was on the pill? Should I be ashamed of liking sex and having a boyfriend? I wanted to get away from Baba's anger. I walked to the house, and just after I passed him, he turned around and slapped me. He was mean to attack me from behind.

Sometimes I forgot to take a pill. I missed a period and by the time I realized it, I was over two months pregnant. I didn't want children until I graduated from college. Griffin and I didn't have money for an abortion.

"Mama, I'm pregnant," I finally admitted, hoping for money for an abortion.

"You need to get an abortion. I'll lend you the money. I am not raising any babies."

She was so nonchalant about the abortion. She wasn't even mad I had sex. She wanted me to get a college degree and support myself before I had a husband or children, and she didn't want to be stuck with babies while I got my education. I tried to make myself feel sad over the abortion, but despite looking at pictures of aborted fetuses at books in the school library, I could see no wrong. Any soul planning to enter my uterus could do it later in life when I was ready. I went to Planned Parenthood and had a D&C abortion. A few weeks later, Griffin paid my mom back for half the abortion. The second time I got pregnant with Griffin, I was not as far along, so I had a suction abortion.

I kept seeing Griffin, although I wasn't satisfied in the relationship. I didn't enjoy intercourse that much, and sexually I was not impressed. He never gave me an orgasm or sexual pleasure of any kind, and I was too shy to masturbate in front of him, even after our threesome with Chelli. I had my secret sex life away from him, my private place where orgasms happened, alone in my bedroom at home.

Griffin and I mostly had missionary or girl on top intercourse and I often gave him blowjobs. Sometimes I pushed my large breasts together and stroked his cock between them. I don't recall him ever going down on me. Over a year into the relationship, Griffin asked me to get into a new position: doggy style. I felt ashamed, as if I was a dog for being in a dog position, which seemed degrading. Yet I wasn't going to be one of those girls who said no to everything so I endured being fucked like a dog, and convinced myself it was okay. I was glad when he was done.

Eventually, his adult world could no longer compensate for the lifestyle differences between us, and since I did not have any feelings for him even after two years together, I ended it.

SEX WITH WOMEN

I was intensely curious about sex with a woman, especially because I was so turned on watching those playboy centerfolds. A gay bar would be a place to find women for sex. I used my fake ID to get into the only gay bar in Omaha, *The Stage Door*. Strobe lights beamed down over the large dance floor, and loud disco music blared over the speakers. I was mesmerized by the sexy vibe of men grinding on each other, women kissing, and performances by glamorous drag queens.

One night at the club, I noticed a blonde at the adjacent table, smiling at me and holding long eye contact. She walked over and sat down next to me. She leaned close and I smelled her fragrance, like a flower. She was Eve, a 35-year-old lesbian. Her age was intimidating because she was twice my age, a real adult, and what would I talk about with her? She leaned even closer and put her soft lips on mine. I'd never kissed lips like that. Her lips were softer than the lips of any man I ever kissed. I was curious about touching her body and clit, so I invited her over to Baba's house, which is where we kids were staying (and having parties) while he and his girlfriend were on vacation.

Eve and I walked hand in hand, to the master bedroom. We filled the Jacuzzi tub, added bubbles, and played and kissed in the water. I wasn't turned on by any of it. I couldn't wait to get to the good part. We wrapped ourselves in towels, and went in the guest room. She lay on top of me, and we kissed. She ground her pelvis on top of mine. She did it so long, I got bored. Is that how girls did it? Did she like my kisses? Should I just let her grind on me? Was it okay to touch her clitoris or would that be rude? Would she get mad? Was I allowed to be dominant the way men were with me, or did I need to be slow and passive like she was? I had no idea what to do with a woman.

Just then, the bedroom door opened. It was my brother. He saw us in bed together and quickly shut the door. We laughed at getting caught. Eve asked if she should leave. I told her it was fine to stay, so we went back to grinding and kissing. She went down on me for a few minutes. I liked how her tongue felt on my clit. She gave me an orgasm. I couldn't wait to have my turn. Her vulva smelled sweet and musky, like corn tacos. I started licking her clit and I liked it.

"Here, put your fingers in me," she said, and placed my fingers inside her vagina.

I licked her clit again and she stopped me. She pushed down on my fingers. If she liked penetration, why wasn't she with a man? I did what she wanted.

The inside of her body felt warm and moist, and her vaginal walls felt strong and muscular, with ridges. Did my vagina have ridges too? I did not like fingering her. I wanted to play with her clit. I moved my fingers in and out of her vagina. My wrists hurt from it, and it didn't turn me on. She leaned her head back and moaned. She pushed down harder on my finger, so I moved my fingers deeper, faster, and harder. My wrist was really hurting, and I couldn't wait for it to be over. How could men enjoy being with women, when women were so much work in the bedroom?

She moaned louder, and then she had an orgasm. The books were right. Women could orgasm from penetration. She apparently did not mind I was sexually broken, because she was a woman and could overlook such things.

I didn't like our encounter. I was disappointed I didn't get to play with her clitoris, jealous about her vaginal orgasm, and mad because she knew how to have vaginal orgasms yet had not bothered to give one to me. She was 35 years old and a lesbian - she should know what to do.

The next day, Eve sent flowers to my home. Not just any flowers, but an enormous bouquet of long white expensive looking flowers.

"Why is a woman sending you flowers?" Mama asked.

How did she know it was from a woman? My brother must have told her.

"I don't know," I said, because I was embarrassed to tell her.

Mama smiled and walked back into the kitchen. Maybe she was glad I had sex with a woman and not a man, because men were bad and women evolved.

Eve and I hooked up again the following week and a few times after. I had an orgasm each time. That was different from how it was with men. With Eve, I felt like the sex was about us, not just about getting off the man. Shortly after we met, Eve left for India to live in an ashram. When she returned a few months later, she and her new girlfriend stopped by my work. They said they were celibate.

After my first girl-on-girl with Eve, I continued going to the gay bar. I was attracted to pretty butch lesbians. A slender brunette with a hip short haircut and pretty makeup, caught my eye. She dressed like a man. An undershirt peeked out underneath her man's shirt, and she wore jeans and boots. I liked how she moved on the dance floor. I went over to her table. Her name was Tina, and she was also 18 years old. We wanted to hookup.

She lived at home and couldn't have me over, so I invited her to my house. I figured Mama wouldn't know, or wouldn't mind. My brother was away that weekend, so we went into his bedroom in the basement.

Tina asked me to turn off the lights, which seemed odd because I liked seeing our bodies. Didn't she want to see mine? She lay on the bed and I climbed on top. I liked kissing her soft lips and feeling her soft face against mine. I noticed the absence of a hard bulge to grind on.

I slid my hand into her jeans and she didn't stop me. I was glad. She wasn't saying anything or making any noises so I wasn't sure if she liked what I did. I moved my hand into her damp panties and felt my way around. Her vulva lips felt full, soft, and warm. She allowed everything I did. I moved past her outer labia and reached inside to a treasure trove of slippery wetness. She was soaking wet. I grasped finally how aroused she was, and it was because of me. I took off her pants and fumbled around her inner lips and folds to find her clitoris, but I didn't know where it was in the dark. I thought I should know my way around a woman's body.

I finally found a hard spot which seemed like her clit, but I did not know how hard she wanted it touched, and how to move my fingers. Would she like to be touched in the same way and places I liked? She didn't make any sounds, and she didn't say anything. She seemed as inexperienced as I was. I moved my fingers around in that slippery wetness and eventually she started to breathe heavily and then she stopped and I think she had an orgasm but I really didn't know. I lay down, and Tina slid her fingers on my clitoris but it didn't feel good. She had no idea what she was doing, so I stopped her and masturbated while she held and kissed me.

I saw Tina once after that, but since we had nothing to talk about, it all felt awkward and we never see each other again.

I got fired from the restaurant job for calling in sick when I wasn't. I found a better job as a nurse aid in a nursing home attached to a major hospital. Out training taught that old people were not just ugly wrinkled bodies; rather they were lonely and needed love and affection. My job included perineal care, which meant washing women's vulvas and everyone's rectum with a soapy washcloth. I changed bedpans filled with urine, wiped feces off bottoms, and transferred seniors locked in fetal positions into chairs so they wouldn't get bed sores. The nursing homes were severely understaffed and we could not stop our duties to talk to the people. I gave them backrubs at the end of the shift when I had time and they thanked me over and over. Most residents had no visitors the entire two years I worked there. I hoped I would never end up in a place like that.

At the nursing home a fellow nurse aid caught my eye. His good looks, kindness, and energetic personality were appealing. He asked me out and after a few dates we were official. He adored me and loved going down on me, but I was always uncomfortable with it. I don't recall if I had orgasms from his oral. He talked too much about the awesome relationship with his old girlfriend, and I felt like I could never compete. Also he was too needy and his career ambitions were not high enough. I didn't like these things about him, so after six months, I ended it.

VIBRATORS

I heard many women used vibrators. I was curious how a vibrator would enhance my masturbation. I drove to an adult store in downtown Omaha. I used all my courage to go in. The store was stocked with dildos, lubes, vibrators, pornography videos, and lingerie. I browsed through the videos and selected two for purchase.

I went to the front to ask for help with the vibrators. Many of them looked way too big and had dildo parts. Some were discreet and looked like a lipstick case. I needed something that felt good and could be easily hidden.

The retailer showed me several vibrators and turned them on to show they functioned. Did he feel aroused holding those vibrators, imagining I could be holding it on my clit when I got home?

All his vibrators were loud. It was ridiculous to make vibrators with so much noise. How could I relax enough to orgasm, when I everyone in my house could hear my vibrator and knew I was masturbating?

"Do you have any quiet vibrators?"

"No, they all work by vibrating and the vibrations make noise."

The vibrator designers were idiots.

"What's the most quiet vibrator you have?" I asked.

"If you want less noise, choose a smaller vibrator that uses only one AA battery."

He took a tiny vibrator out of its packaging, put a battery inside, and turned on the switch. It made a whirring sound.

"This works, Ma'am."

"Ok, I'll take that one. And I'll buy these videos."

He put my vibrator back in the packaging, pulled out a black plastic bag, and put my vibrator and the videos inside. I was a little stunned. The unmarked black plastic bag was not pretty like the clothing store bags boldly labeled with the name of the merchant and colorful graphics. His plastic bag reminded me of paper sacks used by alcoholics to hide their beer. Were adult items equally shameful, that they had to be hidden in dark bags? Was the store ashamed, were the other customers ashamed, and should I be ashamed too?

I drove straight home, eager to try it. I turned it on. The whirring sound was even louder in my quiet home, too loud for me to use in my bedroom with my sister and mother in adjacent bedrooms. I waited until everyone was out of the house and then

I turned it on. I put on some music to play over the whirring sound. I held the vibrator on my clit and within a few minutes, I had an orgasm. It wasn't any better than the orgasm I had with my fingers, but it was less work.

PORN AND THE MISSING CLITORIS

The next time my family was out, I put the porn videos into our home VHS player. The videos made me cringe, because the acts looked painful and violent for the women. The women looked high on drugs and made fake moans. I was sure they were not wet and had to use lube. The action revolved around penises and cum shots and blatantly missing was kissing, sensuality, men ejaculating inside vaginas, and orgasms for women. I found a few clips where men went down on women, but they always stopped after a few licks, making it appear like a clitoris was just not worth the bother.

My friends said porn was made for men, and the men imagined being the male actor, fucking the women. That proved to me conclusively that men did not enjoy giving oral sex or pleasing the woman. Still, I couldn't understand why the women did not complain about the bad sex, and why their orgasms didn't matter.

I graduated from high school. It was 1979.

That fall, I enrolled as a freshman at the University of Nebraska at Omaha. I debated majors in premed, biology, and engineering. I didn't know what I wanted for a career and I envied people who had that figured out. I skipped classes when I didn't feel like going. Sometimes I went out at night and hooked up with guys I met at the bars. The men were nice, but they didn't care if I had an orgasm. I felt used because it seemed they got all the pleasure out of sex. Men were useless when it came to orgasms. I had my orgasms from masturbating in the privacy of my room. Sometimes I used my vibrator under my covers so it would be quiet. Usually I used my fingers.

I naturally lost my puberty weight. I no longer felt awkward about my big body, and my breasts were down to a C size.

That summer, I took a 6 weeklong meditation course at MUM and obtained more mantras, which deepened my experience during mediation.

That fall, I enrolled as a sophomore at MUM. I liked the curriculum, because we studied each subject for one month at a time, and all knowledge was tied back to the unified field, the same field of silence we experienced in meditation.

In college, I no longer let my orgasms slide. After the man had his orgasm from penetration, I expected him to get me off. I taught my lover to use his fingers to rub my clitoris. That's when I started a bad habit: performance moans, to reassure my partner I liked his touch and keep him entertained so he wouldn't get bored bringing me to orgasm. I wished I could just lay in perfect silence and say, "that feels soooo good and I want to lay here and just enjoy it", but I was too embarrassed to talk in bed. So I moaned in short heavy breaths. If the man took a long time to bring me to orgasm, the quick breathing often made me lightheaded and my fingertips became numb. Then I would tell the man I had moaned too much, again a testament to his prowess, and I needed time to catch my breath. When he started rubbing my clit again, I usually had my orgasm before I got lightheaded again. The whole thing sucked. And when I had been drinking, it took me even longer to orgasm because my body was numbed.

I liked the curriculum at MUM, but not the attendance rules and living in a small Midwest town. I wanted to be free. One week into the spring semester I called Mama, and said I was coming home for good.

"I'M GONNA MARRY THAT GIRL"

I enrolled again at the University of Nebraska-Omaha. I was 19 years old. My second week at school, he came into chemistry class and sat next to me.

"Hi, I'm Brad," he smiled at me.

He was 5'10", athletic, with curly blond hair. I had no interest in him at all. The next day, he sat next to me again. He said something funny and I noticed his dimples and I laughed. The following day, he sat next to me again. He told me he was 24 years old, and studying for his B.S in Engineering. He had served two years in the army, and loved cycling, running, and the outdoors. I loved his whole story, so when he asked me out after class, I eagerly agreed.

Brad picked me up in his MGB convertible, and we went to a matinee movie. When he dropped me off, I invited him in. He noticed the photo albums in the family room, and asked to see them. I liked that he wanted to know me. While I showed him childhood photos, he scooted closer and kissed me. I wasn't interested in him enough to kiss him, but I didn't want him to think I didn't like him, so I kissed him back.

Brad lay me down on the carpet, and got on top. I didn't like being mounted in my family room in broad daylight. Mama would be home soon, and I wanted a bed and privacy so I could feel safe and let go. His weight was heavy on my chest. Why didn't he know how to touch a woman? He was 24 years old. He should know what to do.

I felt a wetness on my leg. He quickly sat up and looked sheepish. I was furious that once again a man had an orgasm at my expense. I wanted an orgasm too, but not in my family room in broad daylight. I said nothing, because talking about what happened was embarrassing, and I judged myself for not speaking up, stopping it, or having an orgasm also from the rubbing.

Brad asked if he could stay. He seemed to regret the rubbing incident, and I liked him, so I agreed. We sat on the living room sofa to talk. I wanted to find out if he was worthy of dating.

"What's the purpose of life?" I asked.

He had to give the right answer. He had to show me he was spiritual.

"It is to gain experiences," he said.

Wrong. I debated whether to just end it right then and ask him to leave.

"No, the purpose of life is to get enlightened," I corrected him.

Maybe he could stay, even if he didn't know these things. Maybe he would understand all of this once I explained it better. We talked more and he made me laugh. Mama came home, and I introduced him, and he stayed for dinner. Before he left, he asked when he could see me again.

A few days later, he invited me to dinner to meet his parents. They seemed nice enough. After dinner, Brad invited me to his room in the basement. He pulled out a graph paper notebook and showed me his engineering drawings for designs he wanted to build. He showed me his books on earth homes and I imagined being his wife and making dinner for our children in a home that merged with mother earth. He lit candles. His face glowed in the flickering light as he strummed his guitar and tenderly sang "Vincent" for me. This was really romantic.

The next time we went out, we had sex in a bed, in private. He couldn't get hard. I tried to get him hard, and he tried too. We thought that maybe he could only get hard for women he fucked, not women he cared about. I was the first woman for whom he had strong feelings. I hoped he would say, "I care about my erections. I will research this at the library or go to counseling." He didn't say anything. I offered to go to the library and do some research on why men couldn't get an erection. I was disappointed he didn't at least want to go with me.

The third time we had sex, Brad was hard. He was hard every time after that. He had a large girthy cock and the head was so large, I could barely get it in my mouth. I had really scored with this guy. We had sex every chance we could. We both lived at home, so we often splurged on a hotel room, or we had sex quietly in our basements while our parents were asleep. Our sex was mostly about experimenting with intercourse positions, me giving him blowjobs, and him giving me hand jobs.

Brad was everything I wanted in a man. We studied together for hours everyday at the library. He always said I was better at math and he loved when I helped him study. That summer, we took Calculus V together, and since I was retaking the class, I could explain the assignments. He often told me I was beautiful. We went out for drinks and talked about life and our futures. He was financially responsible and had a savings account. I felt protected and loved when he pulled out his wallet to pay for us. I loved his fit strong body, his love of the outdoors, and that he was an avid runner and skier. I admired that he was mechanically inclined and could work on cars. We drove around with the top down on his MGB. He showed me off to his friends and he learned to meditate because that was important to me. My parents liked him. I wasn't so sure his parents felt the same, mostly because I didn't go to church and I had an eastern meditation practice.

One day, when I called his house, his mom answered the phone.

"Brad isn't home now, but I'll tell him you called."

"Thank you. I'm at school now so I'll try again later."

"Schaz, I want to tell you something. Yesterday Brad told me, 'Mom, I'm gonna marry that girl!'"

I was elated. I didn't know he loved me so much.

That summer he took me on a vacation to Key West, Florida. He introduced me to his friends. That was the first time I remembered our sex was boring. When he thrusted in me, I lay on my back and looked at the ceiling and wondered why it didn't feel good. My mind wandered to other couples and whether they enjoyed their sex. Maybe it was normal to become sexually bored after a few months, and that's why my dad always cheated.

That fall, we transferred to the University of Nebraska-Lincoln, known for its engineering program. We looked for apartments and signed a lease. I cleaned our home and learned to cook. I had a part-time job as a nurse aid caring for elderly people in their homes.

Our sex life was good when we experimented with positions. We didn't connect emotionally during sex, and I didn't know that mattered, so once again the sex got boring and I yearned for novelty. I wanted to have threesomes with a woman, go to strip clubs and sex shops, watch porn together, wear sexy lingerie, and take a sex class. Anything I suggested that was sexual, he answered with "no". I was mad, yet I was glad he wasn't sexual, because it meant he would never cheat on me. Since I wasn't satisfied with him, I masturbated alone, usually while he was in class.

Brad's priority was studying, and mine was having fun. I still enjoyed drinking alcohol and staying out late at bars. When I got tipsy, I got moody and started fights. We had many unnecessary arguments late at night about how to spend our time, whose turn it was to clean up, or how loud I could play my music.

I thought he was boring to stay home and study all the time, and not be more sexually exciting, so after two semesters I left him and moved back in with Mama. In Omaha, I changed my major to premed and got a job as a nurse aid on the surgery floor of the hospital. I was pretty much abstinent from then on, except for an occasional hookup with Brad. Sometimes when I drank, I got horny and made the 45-minute drive to Lincoln late at night so we could have sex.

One day after I got home from school, there was a phone call from Germany. It was my uncle. Opa died of a heart attack. Mama cried. She had been closer to him the past years, and they had talked on the phone every week. She said there was no point in flying to Germany to look at his lifeless body, when his soul had already moved on to another plane and he knew she loved him. She said dead people don't care if you're at their funeral.

A CRUSH ON ZOE

That year I met Zoe at a party. I was 19 years old, and she was 18. I was immediately attracted to her blond hair, flawless skin, thin lips and turned-up nose, her curvy body and small breasts, the way she moved and talked, her love for home decorating and cooking, and her sexual energy. I wanted to be close to her, and it wasn't just sexual. I had a huge crush. I asked her over, and she refused all my invitations. The reason was usually her boyfriend, Tom.

Finally, Zoe asked me to join her and Tom for a threesome. I put up with him so I could be with her. I had never kissed lips so soft. I went down on her and gave her an orgasm, and then she did it too while her boyfriend watched. He saw how much we were into each other, and she told me later that made him jealous.

Sometimes we spent the night together. For some reason, although our kissing had been tender and sweet, she wouldn't kiss me anymore. She said she didn't like kissing. Sadly, we only had sex when she decided we would. She never wanted to have sex at night when we went to bed.

"Let's wait until morning," she would say.

"Let's wash up," she said when we woke up.

We both washed up and went back to bed. Then she went down on me until I came. That turned her on a lot, and she came quickly when I went down on her. I loved licking her clit and pussy. One time when I was licking her clit, I licked her asshole and put my finger in her pussy and her ass. She moaned harder and then she came.

"Wow, that felt so good! You were doing so many things to me," she said.

Zoe was the only person who could give me an orgasm every time. No man had ever done that. With them, I had to masturbate to come. She probably just did to me what felt good to her. Her technique was amazing, and since I could tell she loved it, I could fully relax and let go. Being with Zoe led me to believe that a woman wanted to lick another woman's clit, while a man was doing it out of duty or as a favor (if he even bothered at all).

My biggest problem with Zoe was that I had feelings for her and she avoided me. Many times when I called and asked to see her, she said she was with her boyfriend. I couldn't understand why she would choose him over me. I knew she liked me, because on her living room wall she hung a framed poster of two women, a blond and a brunette. She told everyone who came over, "that's me and Schaz."

CALL GIRL

I was pretty much abstinent from. I wasn't sexually attracted to most men. Also, I didn't feel sexual about ten days out of the month because of bloating, cramping, and menstruation. I was concerned about pregnancy, and birth control was a pain in the ass. I used the sponge after I got tired of the diaphragm. Sex was not always pleasurable, because I was often dry and got frequent urinary tract infections, and it seemed unfair that men came so easily and I did not. However, all that changed when I went out to bars.

When I drank, I picked up men. I must have been more promiscuous than other girls, because my sister's friend made a comment about it one night.

"You have sex with so many men, you might as well get paid for it," she said.

My mouth dropped open. "Oh my god, you are brilliant!"

I felt she was connected to the universe because she spoke of something that resonated deep inside me and felt right. That is exactly what needed to be done.

I became a call girl. It was the early 80's, and I was about 21 years old. I worked for an escort service that sent me to service businessmen in hotels. A married couple ran the escort service from their home. They required us girls to be available at nights (daytime optional) and take our outbound phone calls from their home. We had to be sober and drug free. We had beepers so they could reach us after hours.

The wife was also an escort. She gave me some advice.

"Lick their balls to death before you suck their cocks. It makes them come faster," she instructed.

I started licking men's balls from that day forward. Sometimes I ventured lower, to their assholes, a technique called rimming. The men liked it and I vowed to rim every day from then forward.

"Use a warm washcloth to wash off their penis after they come," she said.

I did it, and the men liked it.

"On the nights you work, you must be sober and at our house. If you drink or do drugs while you're on call, you're fired," the husband told us.

We girls sat around, smoked cigarettes, played cards, and talked, and waited for calls to come in. The husband answered the phone, verified the client's identity, sent us out on calls, and handled the credit cards and payments to us. We used a portable credit card swiper, and a business name of T&S Advertising.

The clients paid us $180 for 20 minutes, and $250 for 30 minutes. We gave the agency $50 and kept the rest. I made about $8,000 per month. The year was 1982.

I quickly had enough money to move out of my Mama's house. I took my cat and rented a nice 2-bedroom townhome. I quit my day job as a hostess at a restaurant. I was still taking college classes.

I didn't have a boyfriend, but I was experimenting sexually. I had sex with some of the girls from work, and twice I had orgies. I found the orgies boring, because we were just bodies moving, with no feelings between us. I had enjoyable intercourse for the first time that year, with two men who were interested in me for dating. They let me ride on top, while they grabbed my ass and moved me up and down on their cocks. With those men, I felt the passion I had seen in movies, but I wasn't attracted to them for a relationship and they were not worth quitting my good paying job.

Most of my clients were businessmen staying at nice hotels. They dressed in suits, which was a huge turn on. I liked that the men paid me for sex. I was in power and got attention. I couldn't understand why prostitution was illegal, but I was glad because it meant we could charge more.

In the year I worked for the escort service, I had sober sex with many strangers. That was easy for me, because I loved sex, kissing, showing off my body, and pleasing men. In my mind, I was the beautiful madam who gave them love and sex and affection they craved and didn't get at home. I didn't have orgasms with them. I was there just to provide a service. The men mostly wanted blowjobs. I used a condom every time for intercourse. The men were so horny by the time they called for an escort, they usually climaxed in just a couple minutes. The married men said their wives no longer had sex with them, or would not give them blowjobs. I decided that when I got married, I would please my man so he didn't need to seek sex and blowjobs elsewhere.

My family kept talking to me during this time, except my dad, because he couldn't handle his beautiful intelligent daughter in such unbecoming behavior. In Iran they probably stoned women like me to death.

Brad called me one evening when he was in Omaha. I invited him over, even though Zoe was there. We talked him into a threesome, which took a while because he did not like them. After a couple drinks, he finally agreed. He could not get an erection, so I was done with this boring Brad guy for good.

I liked my job, but the problem was, I kept getting arrested. We had been told to ask clients if they were police officers. The men always said no. It turns out, police officers were allowed to lie. The officers would solicit prostitution, and when I agreed to it, I was the one who got arrested. There was always a recording device and another officer as a witness in the adjacent hotel room. They took me away in handcuffs. After my second arrest, I vowed to be more careful with my words, and not be entrapped again.

COCAINE

One of my clients, a 45-year-old successful regional sales manager named Drew, snorted a white powdery substance during our appointments. He said it was cocaine and he asked me to try it. Initially I refused. He kept offering it to me. I remembered the teachers had lied about marijuana, so they had probably lied about cocaine too. I decided to try it. I liked the cocaine high as much as Drew's company. Drew would call me to service him, but be too high to want sex, so we sat in his indoor hot tub and snorted cocaine. Once when he was high he suggested that I shave my pubic hair. We used a razor and shaved it off. I shaved my pubic hair from that day forward.

Drew and I became friends, and he started coming over to my place. Once when we had barely started fucking, he said he had to go to the bathroom. He was gone quite a while, so I went looking for him. I found him in my bathroom snorting cocaine. He noticed me, and asked if I wanted some. He never came back to bed.

A few weeks later when I went to his house, Drew was injecting the cocaine. He prepared his spoon, pulled the liquid into his syringe, tied a tourniquet around his arm, inserted the needle into a vein, drew it back with the blood swirling inside, and then pushed the liquid into his bloodstream. Then he sat there like a zombie and said he heard voices and acted strange. I didn't see the point. I would never put a needle in my arm. I would just snort it.

Drew and I took cocaine constantly. The cocaine killed my appetite and I went days without eating, and lost weight. I needed to do it every ten to fifteen minutes to avoid the discomfort of coming down. Drew showed me how to pinch my skin so I knew when I was dehydrated. When the skin didn't snap back, I had to drink water.

Drew began cooking the cocaine with ammonia, to prepare it into a pure solid called freebase. Since freebase didn't burn efficiently with the low heat of a lighter, we used a blowtorch to it. We both freebased and often he injected.

One morning when I woke up, Drew's face was ashen white. He told me he had almost died of an overdose during the night. He managed to get himself in the shower and lay for hours under the stream of cold water. Maybe I shouldn't date this guy.

"Make sure I never inject cocaine again," he requested. "I only want to snort or smoke it."

"Okay," I agreed. It seemed easy enough.

My cocaine habit was interfering with school and my prostitution job. I was paranoid and afraid to leave the house. I stopped going to school and failed my classes that semester. It was harder to look men in the eye, and my tongue was numb and it was harder to give blowjobs. I wondered if the men's' penises got numb too, but I was afraid to ask.

At one of my appointments at a Best Western hotel in Omaha, a man gave me $150 and asked if he could get a blowjob for the money. I thought it was safe to say yes, since he was the one who broke the law by asking for sex in exchange for money. I agreed to his solicitation of prostitution. Seconds later, several men stormed into our hotel room. They pulled out handcuffs, and took me to jail. Drew bailed me out. That time, the police raided our agency's home and the owners left the state.

My next arrest would be a felony, and I knew I had to stop prostituting. I considered going back to school or getting another job. But I had that cocaine problem. So when Drew asked me to move with him to Wichita, Kansas, I agreed. We put all my furniture into a U-Haul van and I moved in with Drew.

One morning I came home from the grocery store, and I saw Drew and his friend in the living room, preparing an injection.

"Drew, you asked me to not let you do that," I reminded him.

Drew and his friend kept whispering, hovered over their paraphernalia. I repeated it louder, and Drew ignored me. His attention was laser focused on his lover on the spoon. I was furious. I was going to show him, so I bought some vodka and got drunk and picked a fight. It didn't get Drew's attention because he was too high to care.

Drew and his buddy asked me to go to the pharmacy to get syringes. They said they looked like druggies and wouldn't get them. Drew and his buddy always had trouble injecting because their veins were scarred, collapsed, or otherwise too injured for a needle to enter. Sometimes they injected in their hands, feet, or neck. Drew wore long sleeves to hide the long tracks (scars) on his arms.

"I can't get the drugs into my body," Drew would lament, as he searched for a working vein.

"I can't get high anymore, no matter how much I inject," he would say.

After weeks of watching Drew and his friend inject for hours, I asked to try it. Drew tied a tourniquet around my arm. He found my vein easily. He pushed the needle into my vein, but it wouldn't go in, because the tip was blunt from so many uses. That was in the early 80's, before anyone had heard of AIDs.

Eventually the needle went in. Drew pulled back and my blood swirled in the cylinder. Then he pushed in and released the tourniquet. I felt an immediate warm rush in my body, the taste of cocaine on my tongue, and a sense of emotional rigidity and paranoia. I sat in a dark corner in the bedroom. Drew and his friend sat on the floor in the dark next to me. We were all high, but we were separated from each other, and from ourselves. It was the complete opposite of what I felt in meditation.

Drew kept injecting cocaine, and we also freebased together. We smoked cigarettes and stayed up for days without eating or drinking, because the cocaine killed our appetite. I was so thin, I borrowed a belt from Drew to hold up my pants. When we ran out of cocaine I pawned my jewelry and Persian rugs and we bought more cocaine. I stole checks from Drew's mom and wrote out $200 in checks to myself and we bought more. The only thing keeping us from being street junkies, was Drew's paid-off house, and his mom who brought us groceries. I felt embarrassed that an elderly woman delivered groceries to her 45-year-old son, and that I was not working or going to school. My life felt like it was closing in, instead of moving forward.

A few days later, Drew gave me a pill called a Quaalude. He said it was illegal in the U.S. I felt fine, so I drove to get some alcohol. My car hit a pole on the wrong side of the road. The jolt woke me up. I backed up, drove back over the grassy median, and continued driving.

My next memory was laying in an ambulance, and then I woke up in the emergency room. The nurses said I hit a pole, my car was completely damaged and likely totaled, and I was lucky to be alive. I escaped from the hospital when the nurses were not looking and hitchhiked back to Drew's house.

Drew didn't open the door, so I broke the bedroom window and climbed in. Drew was walking around the house with a loaded gun. He said people were coming to get him. It seemed dangerous. I had a totaled car, no job, and a boyfriend who heard voices and walked around with a loaded gun. Everything was just getting too weird.

That day, I called Mama and asked to move back home. My brother came two days later. We got my belongings out of the pawnshop. My brother loaded my furniture and clothes into a U-Haul van and drove it back to Omaha. I would drove his car back.

CHAPTER 5

A GOOD GIRL

SOBRIETY

On my drive back to Omaha, the police pulled me over on the freeway. They said I was driving 105 miles per hour, and the speed limit then was 55 mph. The police searched my car, found my open container of beer, put me in handcuffs, and transported me to county jail. I waited three days in the jail cell to see the judge. In my cell, I went into withdrawals and got sober for the first time in years. Baba hired one of Wichita's well-known attorneys.

"Are you addicted to cocaine?" the attorney asked.

"No." I lied, because I was embarrassed to be seen as weak and not in control of my life.

"Your father wants you to go to rehab."

"I don't want to go to rehab."

I wanted to get out, so I could be free.

Two days later, the judge sentenced me to drug rehabilitation (rehab) and one year of probation. My parents came the next day from Omaha, and drove me to rehab.

In rehab they told me I was an alcoholic because I was addicted to cocaine and someone addicted to one drug was addicted to them all, because it was a disease and everyone was helpless and powerless to do anything about it. I had to write a lot and make a list of everything that was wrong with me, called character defects. We were never asked to make a list of everything that was right. Our families came to visit and we talked to each other in a session with one of the counselors.

In group therapy we took turns sitting in the "hot seat", a chair in the center of the circle. The poor soul on the chair was told his or her deficiencies according to us. During my turn, the other patients told me everything that was wrong with me, including how I acted helpless so people would do things for me. I decided to never act helpless again.

A new patient was put into a bed near the nurse's station so she could be monitored during her alcohol detox. I learned that both alcohol and benzodiazepine withdrawals could lead to seizures and death. She was on sedatives so she wouldn't have seizures. She cried and screamed intermittently for days from hallucinations that were part of the withdrawal, or delirium tremens (DTs).

When the woman felt better, she joined our group. She was constantly crying into her crumpled Kleenexes, and said she drank so much because she was heartbroken. She was in love with her married boss, who would not leave his wife. Alcohol soothed her pain. She had frequent blackouts and had done dangerous things, which people told her about, but she couldn't recall. I was fascinated by her story. I had never met an alcoholic.

After rehab, I returned to Wichita to start my probation, which included six months in a sober living house. My probation officer was a kind woman. At each monthly appointment, I provided a urine sample and the attendance record from my court-mandated 12-step meetings. Sometimes I went to Alcoholics Anonymous (AA), but usually I attended Narcotics Anonymous (NA). In NA, I entered the world of reformed heroin junkies, outlaws, and motorcycle riders with tattoos. These people, who had struggled deeply with their humanity, admitted their defeats and talked about their feelings honestly. It was easy to like them.

I was hired as a full-time administrative assistant at Wichita State University. I got my own apartment, a kitten, and a new car. I started meditating again, stopped smoking cigarettes, and began exercising. I became toned, and I felt a new joy and vitality from my new habits. I was not interested in dating.. I masturbated when I was horny. I made amends, which included paying Drew's mom for the forged checks and paying off all my debts, including unpaid utility bills from my townhouse. These things made me feel good about myself.

Drew called. He said he was in rehab. He was in a program based on love and acceptance, not confrontation and hot seats like mine. He invited his mom and me for a family weekend. It was good to see him, but there was no way I wanted to date him.

I liked my job at the university. That January, I enrolled in night classes. I took a 300-level Biology course and Introduction to Programming. The night classes rekindled my interest in getting a degree. I needed to go back to school full-time, and was willing to give up my freedom to do it. When the semester ended, I called Mama and asked to move back home.

B.S. COMPUTER SCIENCE

My desk and ruffled bedspread with the roses were just like I left them a few years before. It felt good to be home. I enrolled full-time at the University of Nebraska at Omaha in the Computer Science program. Mama said she wanted to go back to school for her degree. She was 50 years old, and wanted a bachelor's degree in philosophy. I was proud of my smart mother who went after what she wanted. We took some elective classes together. She felt like a friend, which was better than her former role as an authority figure constantly scrutinizing my actions to make sure they would lead to enlightenment.

I loved school, and got A's in every class. I wasn't having sex or dating, and that proved I could be happy alone. I worked part-time in the medical records department of one of our hospitals, attended NA and AA and did my 12 step service work, paid off the rest of my debts, and went to court for my third prostitution charge. My week in county jail served as a reminder that judges didn't like women taking money for blowjobs.

I liked living with Mama, but I didn't feel the same about Omaha. I hated everything about the hot humid summers, which made my clothes stick to my body even when I was just sitting, and the bone-chilling winters which made my teeth chatter and numbed my fingers and toes, no matter how many clothes I layered. I had to make sure my future career would be a ticket out of Omaha.

Maybe it was fate. A friend from school said he was interested in earth homes. I remembered Brad knew about them, and I wanted to help my friend. It had been four years since I talked to Brad. I looked in the phone book, and thankfully Brad's parents were still in Omaha. I called his mom. She said he lived in Phoenix, and gave me his number. Brad was happy to hear from me. He said he would be in Omaha soon to visit his parents, and would love to see me.

A month later, he came to pick my up for our date. I opened the door, and when I saw him, a warm feeling flooded my heart. Maybe there was something inside letting me know he was right for me. Being together felt like old times, but better because we were more mature. Over drinks, he asked me to visit him over spring break, and said he would cover the airfare. I liked how he pursued and paid for me.

A few weeks later, I landed in Phoenix, in an oasis of palm trees, sunshine, and love. I felt happy with him. I was smitten by his discipline and beautiful body, especially his gorgeous cock.

"What are you looking at?" he joked in bed one night.

"Your body is so perfect. You look just like the statue David by Michelangelo."

"Thanks honey," he smiled at me. "You have a beautiful body too."

I thought my ass was too big, but maybe he liked all the other parts. He took me on a weekend trip to Las Vegas.

"Will you marry me," he asked one afternoon after we had sex.

"Yes!" I immediately replied.

I was pleased he asked me spontaneously, right after sex. It seemed a tribute to my sexual prowess. I looked around for a ring. He didn't have one. He didn't know he was going to propose.

ENGAGED

A few weeks later, Brad visited me in Omaha and we went to the jeweler and bought my ring. Our engagement felt official. I was happier than I had been in a long time. I had a purpose. A man I loved wanted me badly enough to marry me.

That May, Mama graduated from college and I moved to Phoenix. Brad and I were finally together. That night when I unpacked in the apartment we shared with a roommate, he came up from behind and hugged me. I leaned back into the safety of his strong arms.

"I'm so glad you're here," he said.

"I love you," I whispered.

He didn't say anything. I wished he would say "I love you" back, but I understood why he didn't. He told me years before that you show love, you don't say it.

"Here, come here," and he took me on the bed.

I giggled. He took off his pants and slid his penis inside me. I was a little dry, so I got out some lube. He moved me into various positions and I liked how he took charge. He came in about

90 seconds, and then he rubbed my clit until I came. I didn't like the sex so much but at least we were together.

I got a part-time job. We talked about work and ran on the canal by our apartment. It was good, but I wasn't satisfied sexually. I pondered the sex lives of other couples, wondering whether any of them felt the passion I had seen in movies, if the women had vaginal orgasms, and if the man ever went down on the woman.

COMPROMISE

That summer we went to an Open House. The realtor said we could afford a house with Brad's income and his down payment. I wanted a new townhouse with a modern kitchen. Brad said he saw a cute older home while driving through a historic neighborhood near work. He asked the realtor to show it to us. The house was a 2-bedroom/1bath fixer upper from 1937, and was probably charming at one time. It was in dire need of maintenance.

"Wow, I love this!" Brad's eyes lit up.

"You do?" I asked in disbelief, hoping he would come to his senses.

"I can really increase the value of this house," and he walked through it, looking around. I followed right behind.

"I'll tear out this carpeting. There are probably wood floors underneath….I'll replace this old tile on the kitchen counter. We'll wash down and prime and repaint the interior, and we can repair the masonry. Oh, and I'll refinish these old doors and window frames. Come here – check out the backyard. We can cut down all these overgrown oleanders….."

"How long will it take you to do all that?"

"Oh, years. It will be ongoing," and he kept walking around, pointing at things.

I didn't like the word "ongoing". I had never seen such a run-down house except in the movies and I couldn't imagine living there "ongoing".

"Look – check out this old gas furnace in the floor," and he pointed at an ornate grate on the living room floor.

"What? That's our heater? It looks dangerous."

"It's no longer functional. We can have it removed. The house has a heat pump, which both heats and cools."

Although I didn't want to live in that rundown house, I was turned on by Brad's vision, knowledge, and boyish enthusiasm. I had no idea he knew so much about houses. On the drive home, he said he wanted to make an offer on the house. We argued about it for several days. I wanted a move-in-ready home near families with children. He wouldn't back down, and since it was his money paying for it, and the realtor said a detached house was a better investment than a townhouse, I agreed. It was compromise, and marriage was compromise.

That summer, we closed escrow on the fixer. We had no furniture. We slept on the badly stained mattress the owner left, and sat on the floor to eat. I put my Krishna and Maharishi pictures in our bedroom.

"Oh, I don't want those pictures in my house. I don't like them," and he handed them back.

My heart felt heavy. Those pictures were not just objects. They represented my spiritual beliefs and gave me comfort. But it was his house too and he let me have my way on other things, so I put them away.

On weekends, we ran together on the canal just a few blocks from our house. The wide dirt banks were perfect for jogging. Brad often sang an army cadence song and I laughed. I had never heard him sing that before, because I wasn't a runner the last time we dated. I liked the discovery part of my relationship.

"….2,4,6,8 who do we appreciate…" he sang out, looking all strong and sexy.

"…One mile, no sweat…" and I laughed and sang it after him.

"You're such a fast runner!" he usually told me.

We sprinted together, and I kept up, which surprised him. Afterward, we made a bountiful breakfast at home or went to our favorite brunch spot. Then I read the Wall Street Journal while he read the politics and sports, and we worked on the house.

In the first rain, in the summer "monsoon", the roof leaked in several places. We used large buckets to catch the water. Home inspectors did not go on roofs back then, so we didn't know about the leak and the realtor and inspector had done nothing wrong. We borrowed from Brad's retirement fund to pay for the roof.

That fall, I started my final year of school and Brad had a raise and promotion. Our life seemed good, but we were not connected. My sex life was boring and we were not even married yet. I had sex anyway because I wasn't going to be one of those women who didn't give her man sex so he had to cheat or get prostitutes.

Our sex was predictable. Brad woke up with an erection and reached for me. It was the only time he ever touched me. We didn't kiss or have foreplay, which was fine, because foreplay was for weak people who couldn't get turned on without it. I started out wet, so he slipped in easily. He didn't like me on top, so I lay on the bottom in the missionary position and looked at the ceiling while he thrusted. He kept his eyes closed and neither of us talked. Sometimes I was dry and needed KY Jelly. Brad always came quickly, in a few seconds or 2 minutes. When I asked him about it, he said we could try the squeeze technique, but after a few times he lost interest. I didn't know it was called premature ejaculation. Since I didn't enjoy penetration that much, I didn't push the issue.

On rare occasion, he put a pillow under my hips and gave me oral sex. But he didn't look at my pussy or say it was beautiful or tight or wet or anything at all.

I went down on him almost every time we had sex, and gave him high-quality call girl blowjobs and swallowed his cum. Men had once paid for my blowjobs, and he was getting them for free. He should go down on me too. Besides, he was my husband and should know I want. Maybe he thought my pussy was ugly. My inner labia were long, and the color was different from what I had seen in magazines. And if he did not like it, I didn't want to make him go there.

After his orgasm, he lay next to me with his eyes closed, reached over, and rubbed my clit. I felt like a project he despised working on, and was determined to see to completion. He seemed so bored doing it, that I wasn't aroused at all, and it took longer and longer for me to come. Eventually it took too long and I could tell he didn't like giving me the hand jobs anymore. Sometimes I masturbated lying next to him, but it took much longer to climax when he was there.

I preferred masturbating when Brad was away. I used my makeup mirror and watched my fingers rubbing my clit. I used the magnifying side so I could see better. My pussy was beautiful and it turned me on to watch. Sometimes I used objects, like rocks or a toothbrush. I bought a vibrator and sometimes used it, but preferred my fingers. A few times I used the bathtub faucet for my orgasm. Once I asked Brad if he wanted to see me do that, and he did, so I showed him. He said it turned him on, but he never asked me to do it again.

After work and on weekends, we worked on the house and it was fun. We pulled up the musty carpet and curtains, washed the smoke stains off the walls, cut overgrown oleanders, and took it all to the dump. A few paychecks later, we bought a folding table and folding chairs so we no longer ate on the floor. We bought a new mattress with a box spring, and a frame and tossed out the old stained mattress. His brother gave us a used TV, and his mom gave us her old piano and I got some piano books and played again. Brad designed and built a dining room table and a futon frame. I bought some aprons and a bread machine, and when I baked I made extra loaves for our neighbors. We had a home and invited our family for Christmas.

We got a German shepherd. I took the dog to obedience classes and taught him to sit, stay, and roll over. Our dog became a source of shared pride, and he slept in our bed.

We loved reading so we got library cards. We went to the library together. Brad got his home improvement books and westerns, and I got my nonfiction books on investing and money management.

One day I went alone and returned with books on vegetarian cooking, relationships, and self-improvement. I wanted to discover what was possible in our relationship, and surely Brad would want to know this also.

"I got some relationships books at the library. Do you want to see?"

"Not really. You read them, and tell me the highlights."

I looked at his morning newspaper, still on the table. Why would he prefer news and the sports section to learning how to communicate and be closer? Maybe he would change his mind after I told him some of the highlights.

"Oh, it's 4 o'clock. My game is on!" he said, excitedly.

He went into the living room and turned on the TV. He cheered for his team. I hated sports. I hoped he wouldn't be one of those guys who spent all weekend glued to the TV. I closed the bedroom door and fantasized I had the kind of man who was vegetarian, meditated, and read relationship books.

"Good play!" Brad cheered out.

Hmmm...that was hot. His enthusiasm and sports knowledge turned me on. Maybe it was okay to expand myself by being with this man who didn't have that much in common with me. In the ways that mattered he was good for me, and anyway, no relationship could be perfect. I got absorbed in my books.

That evening, I told him some of the highlights and he still didn't want to read my books, so with tears in my eyes, I put them away. What was the point of learning about relationships and trying new ways to communicate, when my partner wasn't going to participate? It was better to just forget about it. I drove to the store and bought a pack of Marlboros and a bottle of wine. It had been years since I smoked. I lit my cigarette on the back porch. Brad saw me smoke and he didn't mind. He said he liked the smell of cigarettes. I was glad I didn't have to hide it from him. The cigarettes made up for not having the relationship I wanted.

After that, I smoked a cigarette whenever I was upset with him. When I smoked, I felt wild and free, and that was better than feeling sad.

Sometimes we argued. Each of us would say something meaner to the other. Sometimes I threw dishes at the floor to let him know how mad I was. The dishes broke. I didn't like my part in escalating the arguments, but I wasn't going to admit I was wrong. A few times I was so angry, I started packing boxes, but I didn't have a plan about where to go and I was broke. Wanting to leave came from my feeling of dissatisfaction. Heeding its call would have required too much of me. Where would I go - back to horrid Omaha? How would I support myself if I stayed in Phoenix? I was a student and dependent on him. What if I never found anyone better? What if I did find someone better, but was too old to have children? Besides, Brad always looked sad when I packed. He wanted me, and I wanted his stability, optimism for life, and family man energy. I ignored my dissatisfaction because it was easier to stay.

We often slept on opposite sides of the bed, and when he was angry with me he slept in the guestroom. When we were mad at each other, we could go an entire day without talking. And then, we fell back into our familiar roles, and never spoke of the thing that caused the argument.

I had been using the cervical sponge for birth control. It was messy and I didn't like having to insert it right before we had sex. I switched to the natural family planning method. Ovulation could be predicted by a slight rise in morning temperature and a slippery cervical mucus. I took my temperature every morning before arising, and charted the results. Around my ovulation, I inserted my fingers deep into my vagina, squeezed my cervix to get a sample, and examined its consistency. During fertile days, a woman's cervical mucus changed from cottage cheese-like, to stretchy and slippery like egg whites. On those days, we were either abstinent or I used a cervical sponge. I liked this natural method that brought me closer to my body. Yet it almost felt embarrassing to go to all that trouble, when our sex was so boring.

One Sunday morning while we drank our coffee, I found something in the newspaper that could help.

"Brad, look, I found a tantra class."

"That doesn't interest me. I'm going to Home Depot to look at flooring."

"I really want to go to this."

"Well, ok, but how much does it cost?"

"The introduction is free. Here, look at the topics they cover."

Brad finally agreed to attend the introduction. The couple leading the class said there would be no nudity or sex in class. Some of the exercises, like the prolonged eye contact and sexual exercises in which we lay in bed with our partner for hours, seemed confronting. During the break, I asked Brad if we could sign up.

"I don't want to take this class," he said.

"Come on, I want to do this."

"No. It costs too much and I'm really not that interested. We still need to pay back the loan on the roof and our house needs a lot of work."

It was final. I sulked all the way home and wouldn't talk to him for the rest of the day. That afternoon, he got out his sketchpad and drew plans for a porch cover. I felt envious of the house that excited him more than our sex.

I had another idea. Maybe if we did some fun activities together, we would feel closer, and then the sex would get better.

"Let's take a ballroom dancing class," I asked one Sunday morning over coffee.

"No, I don't like dancing," he said.

"I want us to do something together."

"We live together. We're together all the time."

I decided if I really liked dancing that much, I would go on my own. Brad loved the outdoors: hiking, camping, skiing, and I didn't like any of that either, and he wasn't pushing me to do those things. So we each pursued our separate interests. I started going to the TM Center and made new friends. He joined a basketball league and played golf. I flew to Omaha to visit my parents. He went backpacking in Colorado with his friends from high school. I was glad he took time for himself and that I was a woman who let her man be free and do what he wanted. Besides, men who ventured into the outdoors were sexy. I was glad we could take separate trips. It proved our confidence, independence, and trust in each other.

Brad didn't like dealing with money, while I loved everything about it. He set up his paycheck to be automatically deposited into my checking account. I paid the bills and put our money into index funds and mutual funds.

We removed the carpet in our house and refinished the wood floors. We replaced the kitchen counter tiles with Formica. We got estimates for an addition to our house. Brad built the front porch cover and it was charming. Everything that Brad said he would do to the house, he did. I liked that he kept his word.

One evening when I felt horny and playful, I suggested we go out.

"Hey Brad, let's go to a strip club."

I figured he would enjoy watching nude women, and consider himself lucky to have a wife who encouraged it.

"No way, I'm not going into one of those places."

"It'll be fun. I really want to go."

"I don't like strip clubs."

It sounded final. I was still playful, so I thought of Plan B. I looked through my closet for my garter belts and stockings from my call girl days. Brad had not liked lingerie when we dated years earlier, but we were engaged. I slipped into my white corset, fishnet stockings, and high heels. I freshened my makeup. I looked stunning, absolutely hot. Hopefully he wouldn't think I was sleazy or slutty or too forward. I was fertile, so I inserted a sponge.

Brad was in the living room, reading a report. When he saw me, he looked up, and smiled.

"I like you better naked."

My heart sank and I felt embarrassed for thinking I was pretty.

"Oh, you don't like this?"

"No, I don't like lingerie. I like you naked. Take that off and come here."

I didn't want to get naked for him anymore. I wanted to be alluring and playful and turn him on, not just get naked and fuck. But he was my fiancée and marriage was about compromise, and I wanted sex, so I did what he asked. Then we went to our bed where he got what he wanted and I felt dissatisfied once again.

There was a guy in my physics class, Tom. He turned me on immensely. Tom was 22 years old, three years younger than I. He was lean, fit, and a cyclist. When I looked at him, my entire body felt warm. I fantasized about him constantly, even when I was in bed with Brad. One morning when I made my lunch for school, I made two sandwiches. Brad asked me about the extra sandwich, and he didn't like it, but I did what I wanted. Tom and I ate lunch and studied together, and soon the warmth in my body became a roaring flame in my groin. I had never in my life been so sexually attracted to anyone. I had vowed to never cheat and I was engaged, yet I wanted to fuck this guy so badly.

Tom had his own apartment near campus. He invited me over one afternoon. He said we should get oiled up and have sex on the bathroom floor. I had really wanted tenderness and closeness in a bed, but I said nothing because I didn't want to be one of those uptight girls who always needed a bed for sex. Besides, what good would he be in bed if he wished he wished for the bathroom floor? We rubbed oil on our torsos and he lay on me and rubbed his penis on my stomach. He was heavy and the tiled bathroom floor was cold and hard. It was worse than the sex at home, and I couldn't wait for it to be over. After he came I just wanted to leave. I never saw him again.

I thought I should feel guilty for going against my values and cheating on my fiancée. I didn't. Brad was not hurt by any of it because he didn't know. Had I not gone through with the cheating, my whole life I might have wondered if Tom would have been a better match.

With Tom out of the way, I focused again on my relationship with Brad and my upcoming graduation. I read about resumes, interviewing, negotiating salaries, and dressing for success. I graduated and started my career as a Quality Assurance Analyst for a software company. My corporate woman wardrobe signaled my career intentions. I made as much money as he did and opened a retirement account.

I decided to overlook the meditation part, the arguments, the lack of affection, the lower attraction, and the boring sex, and made final arrangements for our wedding.

CHAPTER 6

MARRIAGE AND RAISING A FAMILY

I was 26 years old when we married in the presence of our immediate family and two friends. I wanted a bigger wedding, but we were broke and did not want to go into too much debt for a wedding. What mattered was our life together.

I thought our sex life would improve once I was his wife. It didn't. He still used my body to get off, and I still felt defective sexually because he came quickly from the penetration, and I didn't come at all.

Brad was a good husband and provider. He was frugal, took his lunch to work, and was appreciated at work. He was still changing the oil on our cars. I found his car know-how exciting. My old Datsun was giving me problems almost every week. One day after work, I told him about a squealing sound in my Datsun. He went right out to look at it. He opened the hood, and asked me to start the car and then turn it off. He scooted under the car and tugged at a few things, and when he got up again he had grease all over his blue shirt.

"Oh my god, Brad, your nice shirt is all full of grease."

He laughed. "You have a loose fan belt. I can replace it tomorrow after work."

He was so sexy, being so mechanical and knowing how to fix things. I was so feminine, knowing how to bake bread and make a home. I liked our traditional marriage.

COUNSELING

Brad and I still had those escalating arguments over mundane matters. We wanted to get along, so we went to counseling. We told our counselor about our one-upmanship in arguing, where each of us would say something meaner to the other.

The counselor looked at me. "Schahrzad, the next time you both argue, are you willing to just stop?"

I thought about it. "No."

The counselor looked at Brad. "Brad, the next time you both argue, are you willing to stop?"

"Yes," he immediately answered.

And the next time we argued, he stopped. I was impressed! And then he did it again, and the next time I was willing to stop first.

Our arguing stopped but our closeness did not come back. When we talked, we didn't look each other in the eye. When I sought comfort, I didn't go to him. At night after dinner, I drank red wine and talked on the phone to my married girlfriends, while he sat in bed and read. I didn't want to be in there with him. I knew something was missing, but I didn't care and didn't know how to change it. Besides, I had nothing to complain about, because he was a good man, and I felt secure and valued in our relationship.

Work was going well, even though I didn't like trading the freedom of college for being stuck indoors all day. When my boss got a promotion, I applied for her job and got it. My new title was

QA Manager. I enrolled in the MBA program at Arizona State University, and took classes in the evening after work.

We had our degrees, careers, savings, and a house. We were ready for children.

CHILDREN

I flew to Los Angeles for three days of panchakarma, a detoxifying ayurvedic treatment. I meditated more, and started taking vitamins. We had sex on my fertile days and after three months I was pregnant. I started saving for my maternity leave.

Running became uncomfortable in the first trimester, so I joined the YMCA to cycle and swim. I didn't have morning sickness and I loved being pregnant.

"Honey, you're so beautiful and sexy," Brad told me every day.

I was glad he was still turned on by me, because I was getting more horny every day. I masturbated in the YMCA sauna after my morning workouts. When I had an orgasm, my uterus got hard and balled up. I looked for answers in my bestseller pregnancy books. None of them mentioned uterine contractions during orgasm It was well known pregnant women were more horny, so surely other women would have the same question about their hard uterus during orgasm. The only reason to leave it out was sexual repression. Good grief.

I also wanted more sex with Brad. As my stomach got larger, we debated whether it was proper. The pregnancy books recommended talking to our baby, because she could hear us. What if she could hear us fucking, too? We finally agreed it was okay. Having sex during pregnancy reminded me of the first time we had sex when our dog was in the room.

I prepared the baby room, interviewed nannies, and wound down things at work. I told my company I would return part-time, because I didn't want to leave my baby with a nanny all day, and get to know her in an hour after work and between naps on weekends. It meant giving up my manager position and being paid hourly. The cut in pay would be worth it. I had always wanted to be a mom more than a career woman.

I looked through a list of Indian baby names and we chose Chandi. It meant Great Goddess.

Chandi was born by vaginal delivery, after a long labor that began on my due date. She was 7.5 pounds, beautiful and strong, and she latched on easily. We were supposed to wait for intercourse until my 6-week post-delivery doctor visit, but we snuck in a quickie at 2 weeks. I hoped Brad would tell me my vagina was still tight enough, but he did not say anything, and I was embarrassed to ask. Mama came for one month to help me with the housework and the new baby.

I was running again, this time with her in the stroller, and within two months, was back to my pre- pregnancy weight.

My baby girl was charming most of the time. She woke up in a glowing smile from her naps, and cooed for us. At night, I took her to our bed, so I could sleep while nursing. I bought her cute outfits and sent videos and pictures to my family. I took her places so she could see the world, and spoke to her in German.

Baba paid for our airfare to Omaha every few months. It warmed my heart to see my father doting on my little baby, holding her, cooing to her in baby talk, feeding her, and taking her on walks. My "daddy issues", or any anger remaining over him not being how I wanted, disappeared. Maybe we weren't close and we had the language barrier, but from then on I loved him.

When Chandi was three months old, I returned to work part-time, as I had planned. I brought my breast pump to work and pumped milk in my office. I felt happy providing Chandi with her quiet home and a loving nanny, instead of a noisy daycare with stressed employees.

I was back at work only a few months, when my company called on my day off to say my department and job were eliminated in a layoff. It was Valentine's Day. Was it a sign to be in my heart and stay home with my family? I wrestled with the decision of staying home full-time, and losing my identity of career woman. Anyone could be a mom. It didn't require any brains. Computer science proved I was smart. Besides, I had student loans to pay.

What were my options? A popular term in the early 1990's was sequencing. It meant an educated woman interrupted her career for child rearing. Moms stopped lucrative careers to stay home with kids, and went back to work later in life. My neighbor started her art consulting business after her children were in college. Another friend restarted her career when her kids were in high school; she got a job at a temp agency and within two years she was head of a major department. I would be like them. I would sequence.

I asked Brad if I could stay home with our baby. He said I could, but he also wished I had paid off my student loans first, and he did not like paying for my graduate degree. Nobody had paid for him, and he did not like paying for me. He hoped I would go back to work when I graduated. It all seemed reasonable, except I really liked him paying for me.

I loved being a mom, except my baby wasn't like the baby in the magazines. She cried a lot. I wasn't prepared for the irritation and noise. Silence and solitude had been my foundation, and I had never kept the TV on for 'background noise'. Our baby changed all that. She cried frequently for no reason. I judged myself for being irritated with her, losing my patience, and yelling. Why couldn't I smile like the moms in the magazines?

My baby took off her diaper and smeared poop all over the crib. She had tantrums in the grocery store and screamed in her car seat when she lost her pacifier. Should she even have a pacifier? She wanted to be held a lot and she cried when I put her down to do laundry or make dinner. It was hard to cook with a baby in a baby carrier, and was that even safe? If I stopped everything to comfort her, who would make dinner?

Other times she smiled or did something cute and I felt like the luckiest woman alive. Brad and I fell in love with our baby and became united in our mission of Team Parent. We looked her in the eyes and cooed to her, and it became obvious we were not doing that with each other. Why didn't we want to? Did he notice it too?

Sometimes Brad wanted sex. I was "touched out" from holding a baby all day. I didn't want sex. I wanted to grocery shop alone. Besides, sex with him wasn't that great. I had wondered whether he would become a better lover after I bore his child, because he would perceive me differently and that would bring out new feelings in him. The only thing that changed is that we had sex less frequently, and that was because of me. It wasn't just fatigue. I was unable to relax when I was constantly listening for baby's breathing in the adjacent bedroom and whether she would wake up and need me. Often she slept with us and I didn't want to fuck with a baby in our bed.

When our baby was 9 months old, she and I took another trip to Omaha. Baba and his wife watched her while I attended a weeklong meditation retreat at MUM. It was so good to be back in the golden domes, meditating. I pumped milk several times a day to keep up my milk supply. On the retreat, my sex drive came back with a roar. I couldn't wait to get home to fuck Brad. The night we got back, Brad allowed me to be on top. I felt sexy riding him, and he felt super good. I didn't know I would conceive.

I loved being pregnant. I gained 30 pounds, just like the first time. I birthed our son via vaginal delivery on his due date, within minutes of arriving at the hospital. He was 8 pounds, healthy and beautiful. He latched on easily. Mama came for one month to help me.

Our baby boy slept in our bed, and when he woke at night I put him to my breast, and he drank and suckled himself to sleep. I had waited to name this baby until after his birth. I wanted to meet him and pick a name that fit. I found nothing in the baby name books, so I turned to the Bible. There I saw it and knew it was right: Matthew. Brad liked it and Mama got goose bumps when I told her.

After having another baby come out of my vagina, I thought my vagina was loose and less valuable for fucking. Brad never said a word. He came quickly like he always did.

We had to make a decision on the circumcision. Circumcision seemed like plastic surgery or genital mutilation. Brad and the men in my family had it done. Almost every man I had been with sexually had it done. Our pediatrician said the American Academy of Pediatrics recommended doing it for medical reasons, and they didn't anesthetize babies for the procedure because babies didn't feel pain. I didn't believe that, but I didn't know what to do, so I trusted the doctor and made an appointment for the procedure. I asked Brad to go with me. He said he had work. He always had work. I took my baby for the surgery and I kept telling myself that babies don't feel pain. They took him in another room and I heard a wail that lasted half a minute. And then they brought him back to me and he seemed fine.

Brad was the dad I wanted for my children, the dad I never had, and he loved me. In the mornings, he sang in the shower, and he was funny and made me laugh. He wasn't one of those men running off to bars or cheating. He came home after work and spent his weekends at home, because he enjoyed being there. His boyish enthusiasm and energy, and the way he easily and cheerfully added children to his responsibilities of work and home projects, were attractive. He changed diapers, held crying babies, packed up diaper bags, took the kids on errands, gave baths, told bedtime stories, tumbled and roughhoused, fed them, joked with them, hugged them, and sang with them. Whenever I saw Brad with the kids, I thought to myself, *"this is my perfect life!"* Brad and I weren't fucking, but we were a family.

I was proud of myself as a housewife. Maybe I didn't bring in money, but I kept a clean home, made nutritious vegetarian meals, invested our money, and took care of the children. I worked out and kept myself beautiful. In the morning, I got up early for my 6 a.m. step aerobics class, so I could workout before Brad went to work so someone could be home with the kids, and after six months I lost my pregnancy weight. At night I took my MBA classes. I enrolled Chandi in preschool three mornings a week, so I could get some alone time with Matthew and study while he napped.

I loved cuddling with my children. I got at eye level when I spoke with them and held them tight so they could feel my love. I sang lullabies and felt the warmth in my heart when they smiled. Our children slept with us, and I bought a book called The Family Bed, which said this was healthy. I read parenting books, bought wooden toys from Germany, took them for runs in the double stroller, and cooked fresh meals with mostly organic produce.

There was also the other side, which was rarely mentioned.: feeling unfulfilled. The kids' frequent crying and demands, on top of the sweltering Phoenix heat, often left me feeling irritable and depleted. I wanted an hour alone to meditate or go to a movie, but our parents and relatives were several states away, we didn't have babysitters on our street, and Brad was at work all day. I had my family, but I had lost my freedom.

I often felt lonely at home. The kids were too young to talk. I missed adult interaction. I asked Brad to take me out and he either declined or said we had to take the kids. Young children and one-hour restaurant meals were mutually exclusive. Our kids wanted to move their bodies. Brad always took them outside, while I stayed at the table alone, waiting for our food. Then we took turns eating while the other held our squirming toddlers. How did he even enjoy any of it? Didn't he know I needed a break, and wanted a connection with him?

A few times he relented and we went to dinner, and we always talked about our children.

"Let's not talk about the kids on this date," I suggested.

"That's a great idea!" he agreed, and then we sat silently all through dinner. What had happened to all the conversations we once had about work, investing, exercise, and goals? Our children had changed everything.

I needed friends. I hoped to get my needs met at La Leche League meetings and a mommy's playgroup. I went to quite a few meetings. We brought our nursing babies and toddlers. Our young kids were constantly interrupting our conversations, and created more noise than I had at home. I left feeling more stressed than when I arrived. I knew my meditation would calm me, but I didn't meditate for the same reasons I didn't want sex: I couldn't go inside myself when I was responsible for the safety and nurturing of young children. When the children slept, I did homework.

I envied Brad's life. He was free to move through the world without the chains of children. He didn't have a wife who worked as well, and take turns leaving work early to pick up kids from daycare, or take time off to stay home with a sick child. He could miss well baby visits and preschool orientation. He could stay late, take on extra projects, and travel for work. He wasn't trapped at home. He could climb the corporate ladder, build his career in the free world, and accomplish anything he wanted, knowing his wife took care of everything at home.

I completed my MBA when our kids were 2 and 3 years old. I didn't want to attend my graduation, because it required sitting for hours. Brad insisted that we go.

"Kids, we're going to watch your mom graduate."

I was glad he was proud of me. He held our squirming toddlers through the ceremony.

I had my graduate degree, but I did not want to go back to work and let someone else raise my children. Besides, childcare for two toddlers would take a significant chunk out of my income, so what would be the point of working for a few extra hundred dollars a month? Brad hoped I would go back to work when our children were in elementary school. Brad's checks still went straight into my checking account. I was a faithful steward of the money he earned. We drove our used cars and saved for retirement.

We were a family, but Brad and I were still not a couple. After nursing and holding babies all day, I was tired, and "touched out". Just as after Baby #1, I didn't want any touch at all. I didn't want sex. I wanted to shower alone, cook without interruption, and meditate in quiet. Brad never touched me anyway, except in the mornings when he wanted sex. I knew he wasn't just using me for sex. Brad loved me. Still, I didn't want to give him my vagina when he had not bothered to hold my hand, give me a hug, or take me out on a date.

Our family bed was also a problem with sex. It had started out as a convenience for nighttime nursing and became a ritual we all loved. Eventually we sent the toddlers off to their cribs so they could self-soothe, but they always climbed into our bed in the mornings. Even when I was in the mood for sex, I thought about the kids. I still couldn't relax to have sex, let alone an orgasm, when my children could interrupt me anytime by calling my name, or climbing out of their cribs and into our bed.

We wanted our children to have a spiritual upbringing. We went to the Methodist church where Chandi attended preschool, so our children could learn about the bible and God. The Active Parenting class was offered at our church, and there was free childcare. I asked Brad to take the class with me. He said I could give him the highlights. I wished he would do something together with me. I went alone, like I always did when it came to self-growth. The class transformed me as a parent. I learned the mistaken goals of children's behavior, positive reinforcement, how to increase freedom along with increasing responsibility, logical consequences, communication, and family meetings. After the class, I enjoyed my children much more.

When Matthew turned two years old, life became easier. He could follow instructions, and play alone or with his sister. I started a resale furniture business with my best friend. I painted the interior of our house. Brad and I did a concrete wash on the exterior of our brick house and painted it a sage color that we spent months selecting.

I turned my attention back to my husband and sex. I tried to kick start a connection by asking Brad to do intimate activities with me, such as taking classes or going out with other couples. Several times I asked him to go away with me overnight, for a weekend, or a longer vacation. Each time, he said we had to take the kids. Why did he always want the kids, when I wanted to be alone with him? Brad had his own interests. Sometimes he made priority lists and showed them to me. He wanted to fix our house, watch sports, work out more, start a business, and play more with our children. I was not anywhere on the list.

I yearned for the sexual excitement and escapades of my earlier years, and I missed the sexual intensity he and I had when we met. I was worried that I lost my sex drive, so I made an appointment with the counselor to learn how to get it back.

"Do you masturbate?" he asked.

Of course I did. I did it with a magnifying mirror held up to my vulva and watched myself do it and I had amazing orgasms all by myself.

"Yes!" I proudly answered.

That's when I understood. I *did* have a sex drive. I just didn't like sex with my husband anymore. The counselor said we could recreate the feelings we once had. We just had to sit with our eyes closed and remember how it was when we met. I tried that when I got home. Then Chandi crawled up my leg and it was time to make dinner and I forgot. I thought of it a few more times, but I didn't really remember the feelings I had when we met. It was so long ago.

Sometimes I fantasized about men I knew, but I never considered actually doing anything, because I was committed to fidelity and affairs were messy things leading to divorce and DTs. I fantasized about oral sex with women. I had a huge crush on my lesbian massage therapist and fantasized about her constantly. She had a girlfriend so nothing ever came of it.

I asked Brad if I could have sex with women again, and he encouraged me to do it. He wasn't interested in participating. I went to a gay bar to meet women, but every lesbian I found attractive, did not want sex with a married woman. Out of sexual desperation, I settled for an encounter with a gorgeous bi-curious woman who didn't turn me on. In our encounter, she went down on me until I came. Then she had to leave, and I was glad, because I did not feel aroused by her.

I fantasized about my times with Zoe. It had been years since we spoke. I called her, and invited her for a visit. Zoe came that summer. We drove to Mexico for a sex weekend, while Brad watched our kids. Zoe made me come every time she went down on me. I loved making her come with my tongue. Once I put one finger in her pussy and one in her ass while I licked her to orgasm and she moaned super loud when she came.

"You did so many things to me," she said when we cuddled afterward.

I wished Brad would like me doing so many things to him, and that he would go down on me and make me come.

After my weekend with Zoe, I turned my attention back to my family. Shortly after that, Brad started a consulting job for an out of state firm, expanding in Phoenix. While Matthew napped, I helped with Brad with marketing and technical reports.

One afternoon while walking on our street with the kids, I had a feeling that someone was missing. It was another child. I talked to Brad about it that night. He wanted another child too. On my next ovulation, we had pregnancy sex, which means it was obligatory. I got pregnant the first time. I loved being pregnant.

We wanted a bigger house before our third child was born. I wanted to live in town near people, but Brad wanted acreage outside of town and since he rarely insisted on anything, I let him have his way. I convinced him to buy a house we could afford with a 15-year mortgage, instead of a more expensive house with a 30-year loan.

I was over 8 months pregnant when we moved into our house on the outskirts of town. We removed the old carpet, and Brad worked every night after work and all weekend to smooth the concrete with a sander and install the wood flooring.

I bought a nursing picture book and showed the photos of childbirth and nursing babies to our children. They were excited they would be invited to the baby's birth at the birthing center. Our baby was born on his due date via vaginal delivery and weighed almost 9 pounds. Mama and our other children were there to watch his birth. We consulted a jyotishi, an Indian astrologist, regarding an auspicious name. The Jyotishi said any name starting with the sound "Ahhl" as in "Olive" was good, so we named him Oliver.

I was grateful I had never needed an episiotomy. I did my Kegels to strengthen the entire area and hoped it would suffice. Brad never mentioned my vagina, so I figured it could be loose and he was just too nice to say anything about it. I was too embarrassed to ask.

I had my quiet time alone with Oliver, while Chandi and Matthew were at Montessori school. I lay on my bed, as he nourished himself on my breast and drifted off to sleep. "What a lucky baby to be with his mother, in this peaceful home," I thought. I was grateful to Brad for making this all possible.

I was really enjoying my older children. The parenting classes made all the difference. Other parents were glad when school breaks were over and they got rid of their kids, but I actually enjoyed being with mine. My children were joyous, healthy, helped with the baby and chores, and did their own self care. I was proud to be seen in public with my three beautiful well-behaved children. I was a success, and I felt fulfilled. I probably would have had babies forever, if Brad hadn't said he was done.

"Honey, you know I love children, but there are other things I want out of life."

What things? What was better than being pregnant and nursing babies?

When Oliver was just a few months old, Brad went in for his vasectomy.

I still had some pregnancy weight. I stopped eating chocolate, and soon, I was back to my pre-pregnancy weight. I had born and nursed three children, and I barely had a stretch mark and my breasts were firm. The only proof of my motherhood was the bladder that leaked when I ran or did jumping jacks. I wore maxi pads for running and aerobics, and it was a small price to pay for my children.

That Christmas, Brad bought me a pearl necklace. I felt secure and loved. Why didn't I like fucking him? Was it because when he was home, he was never really with me? Or was I the problem?

Since I was bored sexually, I turned to porn. I heard women had started producing porn. I hoped to find porn catering to female pleasure, including clitoral attention and orgasms.

Unfortunately, female porn directors were making the same hostile porn. They just added some dialogue before the fucking started. All of this substantiated my belief that men used women as sex objects, and what was happening in my bedroom was normal. I didn't have good sex, but I had something else: the family I never had growing up. I decided to forget the entire sex thing, focus on motherhood, and seek solace in the occasional Tylenol #4.

LITTLE YELLOW PILLS

When Oliver was two years old, Brad had a job offer in San Diego. After our move, our older children were in elementary school, and Oliver was in Montessori preschool. I was home alone all day, lonely and bored. A part-time job at a bookstore sounded amazing, but that was beneath me. I considered making new friends, but the moms at school were boring. I researched companies and invested in stocks, but something was missing. Was it my dead end marriage or was I the problem?

We loved cuddling with our kids, but not each other. Our bed was the only place Brad ever touched me, and it was for his orgasm. I often slept on the opposite side of our bed, so he would not think of reaching for my body in the morning.

I had an idea. A few years earlier, I read a Wall Street Journal article about buying hydrocodone online, but I was busy raising kids and it wasn't a good time to take pills. But there, feeling alone in San Diego, I wanted them. I went on the Internet and found many sites offering phone consultation with an out-of-state doctor. The doctor prescribed a pill I hadn't heard about before, called Norcos.

Norcos were not the strongest pain medication available, but they were a controlled substance and addictive. It had the same active ingredient as vicodin: hydrocodone. I liked how the hydrocodone made me feel: warm inside, yet mentally alert. It was much better than alcohol. Initially I took them only before dinner, but within a few weeks I took them earlier in the day and eventually I took two pills when I got up in the morning.

The pills became my lover. They gave me the love I didn't get from Brad. I delighted in their existence and stashed them in my closet so nobody would find and take them from me. I developed a tolerance and became addicted. Within a few months of regular use, I needed to take them every few hours to avoid feeling restless and physically exhausted. I needed them to function. I knew I needed to stop. I called Chelli, my friend from high school. Maybe telling someone would make it easy to forget them.

"I think I'm addicted," I admitted.

"You need to stop," she advised.

But I didn't. I kept taking them.

AVOIDANCE

While Brad was at work, and the kids were at school, I went for my runs, cleaned the apartment, shopped for groceries, did family errands, and looked for a house to purchase. I explored neighborhoods and houses for sale in our school district because it had high test scores. I knew the test scores reflected the parents' emphasis on education and not superior teaching methods. Nonetheless, I wanted our kids to be surrounded by students who also valued studying.

We finally found a small manufactured house on 5 acres outside of town. On our final walk-through, we planned where we would put our furniture. I dreaded sharing a bed with Brad and being on alert for his groping hands. I was done being touched just for sex, especially when the sex was so bad. I had an idea.

"Why don't you take the guest bedroom, and I'll sleep in the master bedroom with the kids?"

He agreed without hesitation. Maybe he wanted his man cave so he could stay up late to read or watch TV in bed, without feeling guilty for keeping me awake. Or maybe he didn't want to be in bed with me either.

We had our family dinners on the patio, attended our kids' soccer games, and went on family runs on the trails by our house. We did home improvement projects. We had a dog, cats, and dirt bikes for the boys. I drove our kids to their activities, volunteered at school, and kept up the home. I exercised regularly and felt fit and attractive for myself and for him. I picked up his dry cleaning, made his dinner, and ordered his newspaper. All day long I had my pills. At night, we retreated into our separate bedrooms.

Brad worked long hours, wrote tedious reports he did not enjoy, and dealt with annoying clients. He had gone as far as he could in his field. Earning more money required moving into sales or management, roles he did not love. He dreamed of quitting it all and pursuing his design work, but felt trapped by the financial obligations of a family. Taking risks was for other men who dared such things. He resented me for not contributing to the income, but since he didn't take a stand for it and I wanted to be home with the kids, I did not go back to work.

Life in southern California was more expensive, and the kids cost more as they grew. I enrolled our children in too many activities, so they could have "all the advantages". Brad didn't think our kids needed so many classes, and we fought about it. He usually let me have my way with the kids, but that didn't mean he agreed. Sometimes I bought things we did not need and brought them into the house when he was at work. At night, Brad tucked in the kids while I sat outside, high on pills, smoking cigarettes and reading the Wall Street Journal. Maybe Brad and the kids would have been better off with a woman who worked and did not take pills.

I compared myself to other moms at the school, whose lives were presumably happier. They had large houses and new cars. I felt inferior to them. I wanted to love the manufactured house which embarrassed me. My self-worth should not depend on my house or which material objects I owned. The dads at the school looked attractive and dressed well. Why couldn't I have a husband like that? Brad drove an older car and wore his clothes a long time. He had gone up a pant size and wore the cheapest glasses they had at Walmart. He no longer looked hot. Instead of penny pinching, why didn't he just step it up and increase his income? He was the breadwinner. He should know what to do.

"I hate looking for work," he said whenever I brought it up. "I can't get any higher up in my field," he said. I lost respect for him when he did not grow his career, take me on about my spending or the pills, or handle his resentments against me. I wished I had a man who was not afraid of me or that I could appreciate this man who was providing for our family and let me be a stay at home mom in southern California.

Brad was actually good at his job. He was smart and worked hard. His company and clients loved him. He knocked it out on presentations and proposals, and his designs. These things kept me interested and respecting him, but mostly I couldn't stand him.

Sometimes I got glimpses of the attraction I still had for him, buried under years of neglect. The school offered family portraits at a discount. We signed up. Brad and I bickered all morning getting ready and making sure we wore matching whites. I couldn't stand him. At our photo session, we stood apart and put the kids between us. The photographer moved us next to each other, with our kids off to the side. Brad put his arm around me, and I liked it. I couldn't remember the last time I felt happy like that and I wanted it to last forever. And then the picture was done and all I could see were his unattractive glasses, bulging waistline, and annoying mannerisms.

Mama came to visit. She initiated our older children into TM. I was taking pills, but I was still exercising and meditating.

"Are you addicted to pills?" she asked.

"No, I'm not," I lied, knowing she couldn't prove it.

When she and Brad were alone, she asked him about it. "You need to talk to Schahrzad about the pills."

He looked at her and changed the subject.

I liked my pills. When I ran low, I felt listless. The pills gave me energy for trail runs and cleaning our house and picking up the kids after school. Yes, I liked my pills. I fantasized about an endless supply of pills. If I could get all the pills I wanted, my life would be perfect.

The pills were hard to get because they required a prescription. Sometimes I inadvertently filled my script at a pharmacy linked to another pharmacy's computer system, and my prescription was denied. The pills had side effects. They numbed my connection to myself. They made me want to smoke cigarettes. I was smoking an entire pack of red carton Marlboros a day. I only ate when I was very hungry, and I had lost 10 pounds and was down to 118 pounds. The senna herbs I took for constipation often caused intestinal cramping. My eyes, toes and fingers were puffy. I knew this wasn't good, and a few times I stopped taking them. Within a few hours I grew restless and listless, so I took them again.

I liked my healthy beautiful well-behaved children, but was I a bad mom because I was disconnected from myself and therefore could not give them all of me? I thought back to the Feelings diagram I had posted on the refrigerator when my kids were toddlers, so they could learn their feelings. But I was not feeling my feelings, and a poster would no longer suffice, and I knew I was letting them down. I got out my cookbook and made my grocery list and pushed the entire parenting matter aside.

In October 2003, our house burned in the largest wildfire in California history. We rented a nice house in town while our house was rebuilt. I worked with our insurance company, architect, and contractors to build our dream house, and held my ground with our mortgage company that delayed payments. I started a website on the housing bubble. This all proved the pills didn't interfere with my life.

That winter, we went on a family reunion ski trip with Brad's side of the family. While we were on that trip, a large amount of blood gushed out of my vagina. Upon our return to san Diego, I went to the doctor. He told me I had uterine fibroids. The fibroids grew, and within months, my uterus was the size of a three-month pregnancy and I could no longer zip up my pants. After much deliberation, I agreed to a partial hysterectomy. The doctor removed my uterus. I kept my cervix and ovaries. I was 43 years old.

We bought a baby grand piano, and I took piano lessons with the kids. I drove them to their activities and oversaw the construction. We got another dog and two cats.

"Mom is addicted to pills," the kids said to Brad one night.

My heart raced and I felt light headed. I needed those pills.

"No, I'm not," I lied.

Brad didn't say anything about the pills. He asked the kids about school.

Our newly built home was beautiful. Our entire family had been involved in its design. It had been exactly two years since the fire. I felt a sense of doom as I unpacked the boxes in our master bedroom. What would it hold - our sexless marriage? Maybe there was an excuse for not having sex in the other houses, but this was our dream home. If we didn't have sex in there, where would we ever have it? Then all kinds of realizations went through my head. It been years since we had sex, and Brad had not asked for it. Had he lost his drive too, or was he getting sex elsewhere? What had happened to my once hot sex drive and masturbating in front of my mirror? It been years since I masturbated. That night, I masturbated to see how it would feel, and I couldn't orgasm. The pills had numbed my body. I wasn't going to give up my beloved pills or go through horrid withdrawals for an occasional orgasm. I pushed the entire matter out of my mind.

We moved into our dream house and shared a bed, and Brad did not touch me. I liked our house, but I saw a financial opportunity. Our house had tripled in price in the 6 years since we had bought it. Prices had grown at a much faster rate than incomes and were made possible by loans based on wishful thinking. Even the Federal Reserve was in on allowing it all to happen. But one day it would pop. I begged Brad to sell the house. After prices plunged, we could buy another house for a fraction of the price. Brad refused. He loved the house and had plans for doing more improvements. Besides, he hated renting.

We had lived in our new house for about two months. After dinner one night, when I was in the living room, Brad called to me.

"Schahrzad, we need to talk."

His voice was serious. My heart raced. He obviously found out about the pills, and I would need to stop. My life felt like it was over.

"Come into the bedroom," he called out.

I took a deep breath and went into the bedroom. Brad was sitting on the bed. He looked serious.

"Things are not going well at work. We need to sell the house."

I didn't think about how he felt, or of comforting him. I thought about myself. I was elated because he did not know about the pills and we could sell the house and make the profit.

Two weeks later we put our house on the market, and two months later the sale was complete. We stashed our profits in CDs and gold and silver coins.

We found a home to rent in town, near the kids' school. Chandi and Matthew were teenagers, and I had not talked to them about intercourse, masturbation, the clitoris, or birth control. I still could not bring myself to talk about it, because sex talk turned me on, and it felt wrong to be aroused in front of my children.

I went to the bookstore. I bought a book, What's Going On Down There? Matthew bookmarked the pages, and then Chandi read it too. Finally, Oliver took it to school, and the teacher said it was inappropriate. All the kids thought I was the cool mom for teaching my kids about sex. I knew I failed because I gave them a book, and not a conversation.

SEQUENCING

The kids were older, and I was done building the house, and there was no longer a reason to be a stay-at-home mom. Other women at my kids' schools were also still at home except they had bigger houses and cleaning ladies. They had stopped their successful careers when they bore children, and then their kids were in high school and they were still stopped. What did they do all day while their children developed their brains at school, and their husbands created ideas and income at work? What was our purpose in life and could we take care of ourselves without a husband to pay our way?

I knew Brad resented me for being home, while he worked 60-hour weeks at a job that wasn't going anywhere. What was it all for - so one day we could retire? And then what? I would be a woman who was provided for her entire life and whose only accomplishment was raising kids, something that working moms did too.

Brad started saying he wanted me to work again. He didn't like the pressure of being the sole provider, and he wanted my help to build our financial future. He said when he met me in college, he saw an ambitious woman who would work. He didn't know I planned to raise children and let him earn all the money. But since he didn't like confrontation, he had kept quiet and let his resentments build. And since I wanted to stay home and he did not bring it up, I ignored him.

I could no longer handle the guilt over doing almost nothing while the kids were at school all day, and raiding our savings to spend on the kids' activities and my pills. I also needed to face a basic question: Could I support and provide for myself? I did it once when I was in college, but that was only for one year. Could I do it on an ongoing basis? Who was I without Brad, and what would I do if he died?

It was time to sequence. I became a real estate agent. I bought a new wardrobe to go with my new job, and worked part-time so I could be home with the kids after school. The job excited me and boosted my confidence.

Getting clients was not easy like the realtor courses made it seem. My high commission checks were followed by months of no sales, so after expenses I earned less than minimum wage. I took sales courses, boosted my marketing, learned about SEO, went door knocking, promoted my research and housing bubble reports, and held seminars at local libraries, yet my income did not increase. I was still using our savings to pay for the kids' activities and my pills. Brad trusted me so he did not look at our accounts. I vowed to work harder and make up the money but it never happened. I hated myself for it, and then brushed my remorse away with more pills.

I liked my gorgeous body. I had lost 10 pounds because of the pills and I noticed I had stretch marks. My big butt was no longer bothersome, I was lean, and all the muscle I had built up with exercising made my legs look strong. They no longer looked bow legged. I longed to show off my body in a bikini, but what about my stretch marks?

One day at the community pool I spotted a mom from the school in a bikini. She looked good. I could do that too. I went to the local surf shop and bought a bikini made by Roxy. I looked good. My breasts were firm, even though I nursed three babies. My body was toned. My shoulders were strong and I stood straight. I had some stretch marks, but so what? I was a mom, and moms were supposed to have stretch marks.

The next day, I wore my bikini to the pool. I was a little nervous, but I did it anyway. Within a few weeks, I had a tan and my stretch marks were less visible. I looked fantastic. I wished Brad had a hot body to match my bikini body.

I started waking up in the middle of the night, soaked in sweat. My sheets and clothing were drenched. It went on for months. Was it menopause? Since I had my uterus removed a few years earlier and had stopped menstruating, I wasn't sure.

COLDNESS

The kids were getting older, and spent more time with friends or alone in their rooms. There were fewer dinners together and no more tucking in at bedtime. I knew they needed autonomy, but I didn't like us drifting apart. Also, I was not that interested in their lives. I had my pills, my real estate business, and my Wall Street Journal.

Brad asked his boss to telecommute. Three days a week, he was home all day. He got up and went right to his desk and worked until evening. He was no longer wearing ties and cologne, and his eyes looked lifeless and he wore those old T-shirts. I hated looking at him and resented him for existing. Maybe I would be better off single, but I wasn't sure if the source of my discontent was him or me. If it was me, leaving would not solve anything. At the very least, I needed to get off Norcos first, so I could handle life on my own.

Brad and I argued about trivial things, and then gave each other the silent treatment because neither of us cared if we got along. I ordered his newspaper, picked up his dry cleaning, and had dinner ready, but I didn't eat with my family. When Brad and the kids went on weekend outings or trips, I asked to stay home. I smoked my cigarettes and read my economics books. We hosted several German exchange students and sent our kids to Germany. A friend of our kids who was close to graduation needed a place to live, so we let her live with us for one year. I liked having children in our home. But I wasn't connecting with anyone.

Brad went into the office two days a week, and then he came home to Oliver, not to me. The garage would open, he called our son's name, and then the two laughed and joked and watched a comedy on TV. I heard this all from other rooms in the house. If I were more loving and a proper wife, my husband would look forward to coming home to me. I didn't blame him for wanting Oliver, our happy child who adored him. Nobody wants to come home to a wife who is a bitch. After all the years he had pushed me away, I didn't have it in me to want him anymore. I had found my happiness in pills, and he found his in work and children.

Brad avoided dealing with our distance. He had always avoided confrontation, yet he also liked being in a relationship. He did not say one thing about his resentments, personal development, or going to counseling to work on our relationship. He wasn't on pills. He was sober. What was his excuse?

One night, when I was up late watching TV, Brad came downstairs. He asked if I wanted to have sex. I couldn't remember the last time he wanted sex. "No," I said softly, because I hated myself for refusing him. He worked hard and deserved the closeness. I hoped he was getting sex elsewhere. He went quietly back to bed.

A few weeks later, when we were both awake in the middle of the night, he asked again. I had been low on pills the past day, so I was actually feeling aroused, and I said yes. His penis was hard, but not rock hard. Still, I was very wet and enjoyed it more than I had in a very long time!

The next day he asked me out. That weekend, we went on our first date in over four years. The next day, I got mad at him for something minor and we stayed angry and we didn't talk for three days. Why did I always have to ruin it?

A few weeks later we had sex again and it was super hot, and I wanted more. I enjoyed penetration more than I ever had, and I felt closer after sex. If only Brad's penis would be harder! Was this part of ageing and how long had this been going on? I was glad Brad didn't try getting me to orgasm, because the pills made that impossible.

The Norcos were easy to take while the kids were little and one day melted into the next. But Matthew was a senior, and I couldn't stand it anymore. I wanted to take him to visit colleges, something I had not done with Chandi. My need for constant access to doctors and pharmacies kept me trapped from traveling or even planning my calendar more than two days out. Worse, I felt guilty for all the money I was spending, and helpless for having a dependence on a substance for my well-being. When would I stop? At 70 years of age? At 80 years? If I didn't stop in this life, would I be born addicted in my next life and have to face it then? I might as well deal with it now.

The pills were no longer a friend. They were the glass wall that kept me separated from life. But if I stopped, how would I have energy to clean the house and exercise? I felt listless every time I stopped, so I thought the pills gave me energy. I was desperate. I needed to reconnect with the world. *Maybe I can live without pills. Maybe my life will be better without them.* I didn't know anyone addicted, so I had nobody to ask how to stop, or what to expect from my new life. I was too embarrassed to go to my family or friends. I had to figure this out on my own.

I had recently heard ads on the radio for a medication to help with opiate withdrawal: suboxone. I went to a psychiatrist to get the medication. My doctor ran lab work to check my liver, kidney, and thyroid function, and fortunately my test results were in the normal range. I weaned myself off the laxatives. I did all this on my own, without telling my family or going to meetings. My doctor encouraged me in my new life and said I should tell Brad everything. I told her I couldn't, because I wanted to make everything better, not worse.

LOVE

I was on the suboxone and gradually, my body and my heart woke up. I felt more alive. Colors appeared brighter. My family appeared loveable. I started going places with Brad and the kids again, and I made better dinners and I was nicer. All that time I had spent going to doctors and pharmacies, I could spend at home, and I felt free. I started hugging people, even the dental hygienist. Instead of listening to talk radio, I blasted soulful music in my car and sang along. It had been years since I listened to music. TV shows and people were funnier.

I started to laugh, from deep in my belly.

"I love your laugh!" Brad often said.

That July, Brad and I took our kids on a family reunion vacation with my side of the family. Our destination: a houseboat on Lake Powell. I was happy to be around my family, and off Norcos for the first time in years. Our houseboat moved slowly through the beautiful serene canyons. I cooked and talked with my family.

"Where is Brad?" my dad often asked.

I went to look. Every time, I found him sitting alone in a chair on the top deck, kicked back, his legs spread wide, and his mouth in a half smile. He always loved the outdoors, the sun, and his solitude. The stress of work had washed away. His face had softened as he relaxed, and he was handsome again, like when we first met.

"Hey, how are you doing?" I asked.

"Happy," he smiled at me.

I smiled and went back downstairs and cooked his favorite dinner: chilaquiles with mushrooms.

The next night I played on the shore, and I looked up and saw him sitting on a chair on the front of the houseboat. He looked sexy in his baseball cap. I noticed his muscular body and strong shoulders. I wanted him again, for the first time in decades. I walked over.

"Can I sit in your lap?" I flirted.

"Yeah, sure," he smiled.

I sat on his lap and he wrapped his arms around me. I pressed into his strong chest and a moan escaped my lips. I couldn't remember the last time I moaned just from the way a man held me. I buried my face in his neck. I liked his scent: sweet, with a hint of sweat. I turned my face to kiss him, and he kissed me back. It had been years since we kissed; we didn't even kiss during sex. This kiss melted my heart and my panties felt moist. My pussy throbbed and ached to be filled with his cock. I longed for him to hold me tight, his naked body pressed against mine. I had not felt that much desire and lust in years. I thought quickly of where we could be alone. The boat had one bedroom, and our kids were using it. We could easily take it.

"Let's go in the bedroom," I invited him.

"Let's go," he took me by the hand and led me into the bedroom. "Kids, mom and I are using this room tonight."

We made love. It was passionate, lusty, and filled with love and desire. He was on top of me in the missionary position, and I was lost in a cocoon of his strength and passion. Even though it lasted only three minutes, I was emotionally completely fulfilled.

I woke up, turned on and excited to have more sex. I reached over and put my arms around Brad. I rubbed against him.

"No, I want to get my day going," he said, and got up.

I was surprised and disappointed. Didn't men want sex 24/7? Wasn't he thrilled to be offered sex first thing in the morning? He had sensed my lack of interest all those years and left me alone, but I was back. Maybe he would want sex later that day.

That afternoon when I went on the top deck, he sat in the chair facing the back of the boat, looking at the water and canyon walls.

"Hi Brad. It's so beautiful out here," I said.

"Hi," he turned around and smiled at me.

I stood behind his chair and wrapped my arms around him.

"Here, listen to this," he said softly and handed me his earphones.

The song "Songbird" by Fleetwood Mac played softly in my ear. My heart felt warm as I hugged him from behind, looked out at the beautiful canyons, and listened to the sensuous music in my ear. I had romance again. It seemed that anything was possible in that new life without pills.

He turned around and brought me in front of him.

"Come here, lift your skirt and ride me," and he pulled me gently toward him.

"What about the kids?"

"Just sit on me. Quick. Nobody will know," he said calmly and lifted my skirt.

"What about my parents or sister? They're downstairs."

"Come. Sit on me," he coaxed and put his hands firmly around my hips.

I trusted him. I gave in to our mutual desire. I used my legs, while he pushed me up and down by my hips. His cock was rock hard and he felt good. After 30 seconds it was done and his warm liquid dripped down my inner thigh. I felt mischievous for fucking my husband of 23 years in broad daylight in public. I gave him a hug and went downstairs to have breakfast with my family. Coffee had never tasted so good.

We slept together that night on the front deck of our houseboat, and I liked being close to him. And early the next morning, while everyone slept, we made love out there in the open. I was ecstatic. I believed a whole new world of sex, lust, and passion had opened to us. Best of all, I finally had the marriage I had always wanted. We weren't just a family anymore. Brad and I were a couple.

DREAMS

"What a beautiful morning," Brad said as he put our suitcases in the car.

"Yes, it sure is." I felt grateful for my family.

"Dad, can we stop at Starbucks?" Chandi asked.

"You got it!" I loved how his dimples showed when he smiled.

"I'll drive," Matthew offered.

We got our coffee and Matthew drove, while we enjoyed the beautiful Arizona scenery. The open road was a good place to relax and let my mind wander. Getting off pills was even better than I imagined. I had a roaring sex drive, I felt happy and laughed a lot, and I was in love with my husband again.

I dreamed of relationship classes, sharing our deepest secrets, and the intimacy and vulnerability I had read about in books. We would make love and I would let him open me to God because now I wanted it and would let him. There would be camping trips in the woods where he built a fire and I cooked our meals followed by lots of hot sex in the tent, and romantic dinners at upscale restaurants followed by a rush home where we ripped off each other's clothes. We could try new sexual things we had not done before, like slipping my panties in his pocket when we were out at dinner, kissing passionately in public to demonstrate our lust to the world, browsing sex toy catalogs and choosing fun toys, and whispering sexy words to each other in the heat of the moment instead of having sex quietly because we were afraid to speak these things out loud. Maybe I could even have a vaginal orgasm or get over wanting it at all. Men liked sex and Brad loved me, so naturally he would be thrilled with all of this.

Brad sat in the backseat, absorbed in the newspaper. Unbeknownst to me, he was thinking about getting back to work, his over-50 soccer league, and the news at bedtime. He wanted a wife who cooked more and contributed to the family income. Sex was not anywhere on the list. Sex was just something that gave him orgasms when he was horny. The extra sex on the boat was just vacation sex. He didn't know I woke up to life and would want a lot of sex, sex that he probably didn't want because he had never complained all those years when it wasn't happening.

It was dusk when we got home. The kids helped us unpack, and we did the laundry and fell into our familiar beds. Brad and I lay next to each other watching the evening news. My vagina was tingly from arousal. I snuggled up closer against him.

"Honey, I'm tired," he said and turned out the light.

Damn, I was tired too and I still wanted to fuck. What was wrong with him? Didn't all men want sex 24/7, and it was the women who were saying no and complaining about headaches? He probably would want sex in the morning. I wanted to masturbate, but I did not want to share my arousal with him, when he had just said no to sex. I snuggled into his arms and we drifted off to sleep.

It was still pitch black out when his alarm went off. I longed for his cock. Brad jumped out of bed. Damn it. I fell back asleep. Brad came in the bedroom, dressed in his business clothes and looking so hot, I wanted to fuck him even more. He gave me a kiss on the cheek, and then he was gone.

That night in bed, I gave him a massage. He turned over and his penis was hard. I slipped him inside me, and he felt so good. He flipped me over and ejaculated in less than two minutes. I was barely warmed up. He lay down to sleep. I reached my hand down to caress my engorged hard clit. Brad's breathing got heavier and then he snored. I rubbed myself in my slippery warmth. I held back my orgasm moans so I wouldn't wake him, because he did not deserve to be a part of it.

Brad was the same after the vacation, but I was much different. First, I resumed my hunger for personal growth. I yearned to spend more time with our children, develop my career, save for our future, and transform my marriage.

Second, my sex drive was stronger than any other time in my life. My clitoris tingled, my vagina ached to be filled and I was constantly wet. I masturbated several times a day, making up for years of neglecting my sexuality. When Brad fucked me, I no longer stared at the ceiling in boredom. I felt passion and surrender like the people in movies. He was the same in bed he had always been. But I was different. I was shocked at how much that changed everything.

Third, I felt love in my heart for other people and especially for Brad. I no longer criticized him. I showered him with compliments, laughed at his jokes, and freshened up before he came home from work. I learned his likes and habits, such as what time he got up and the TV shows he liked. I was amazed I had never paid attention to any of that before. We watched comedies at night in bed and laughed together. We took walks by our house and on the beach and he spoke to me of his goals. When he snored, I no longer hated him. Instead, I was happy he lay next to me. We gave each other long hugs lasting at least 30 seconds where we melted into each other's arms.

And because I was so loving and fun, he changed how he felt about me. He no longer came home to the kids. He came home to me. I concluded he shared my dream of an expanding relationship. I never considered he had his own dreams.

INDIFFERENCE

It was late August, and the kids were back in school. I had two new real estate clients, and was cutting back on my suboxone so I could get off it within six months. I was happy in our relationship, except for the bedroom where I felt completely unfulfilled.

The worst was his erectile dysfunction, because I could barely feel him. My one finger inside me could send shivers up my spine, but his wide soft penis did nothing. I had no idea when it started, because we spent so many years abstinent. His erections were never rock hard anymore. Even if he started hard, he went soft within a few minutes into sex, and once he was soft, he could not get hard again. He never mentioned doing anything about it.

He still had premature ejaculation, no kissing, no cunnilingus, quickie sex, closed eyes, and no orgasms for me. It wasn't about orgasms though. Many times throughout our marriage, or with other men before him, I didn't want to come. It seemed like too much work or I was tired, or I simply did not want to. However, there were times I definitely wanted an orgasm too. He never mentioned changing any of this.

I delicately asked him if he could go to the doctor for his erections, and he said he would never go. He didn't like doctors. I called the doctor for him, just like I called to schedule his dental appointments, because Brad did not like dealing with these things. I called the doctor's office and said my husband wanted Viagra.

That night, Brad came home and he was mad.

"The doctor called to verify if I wanted Viagra, and I don't!"

"Oh, I thought you would want it."

"Besides, I have to go in for an exam. They don't prescribe that over the phone."

Brad liked sex. He reached for me every two to three days for his orgasms, and then he got up and went to work, leaving me laying there dissatisfied. He couldn't hear me cry over the noise of the shower.

Every time I wanted sex, he pushed me away. He had rejected all my sexual advances since the vacation. One afternoon when we sat on the sofa talking and being close, I thought he wouldn't mind, so I ran my fingers up his legs.

"Don't do that!" he said, frowning, and he pushed my hand away.

After that, I was afraid to initiate anything at all. I waited for his advances. I lay in bed in the mornings quietly for hours, until he awoke. Sometimes it paid off and he reached for me. His cock felt really good, especially when he was close to being very hard. And after a couple minutes, it was all over and he jumped out of bed.

"I have to go to work," he said.

At night he was tired and in the morning he had work. On the weekend he had soccer and projects. He did not have passion, emotional connection, or orgasms for me. I had a huge problem and he had no problem at all.

I was devastated and heartbroken about his complete indifference to how I felt. I often sat on our living room sofa, sobbing or wailing. Other times I did it in my car, or on a trail. Why was he so unwilling to open emotionally? Did he resent me or did he just hate sex? How could I deal with this, without constantly crying? The kids and Brad were puzzled. They had never seen my cry. I googled feelings and talked to my friends, yet I still had no idea how to handle my emotions. Was I allowed to hate him for pushing my sexual expression down, or was I the problem?

Early on a Saturday morning in September, I lay wet and engorged in bed like usual, hoping he would want to have sex with me. When he woke up, he jumped out of bed and went downstairs. I heard the coffee grinder. I was devastated. I went into the kitchen, crying. He was making coffee.

"Did you get up to get away from me?" I sobbed.

"Honey, I'm not going into combat. I'm just going to play soccer. I'll be back soon." He paused and looked concerned. "Are you okay?"

He thought I had flipped out. I couldn't keep my secret. I waited until he was outside drinking his coffee and reading the paper.

"I have to tell you something."

"What is it?"

"Well, I was taking pills for ten years and three months ago I stopped and that's why I am having feelings again." I looked down as I spoke.

He threw the paper down.

"Damn it, Schahrzad."

"I'm really sorry. I was afraid to tell you."

Brad was quiet for a moment. Then he sighed. "Let's take a walk on the beach this afternoon and talk about everything."

That afternoon, we walked on the beach, and then we sat in the sand to talk. He had questions and I answered them. He said he knew I took pills but he did not know I was addicted. I picked up some pebbles.

"How much money did you spend?"

I held a black pebble in my hand. I turned it over and over for reassurance and then I forced out the words.

"$100,000."

He glared at me. He seemed angry. Why couldn't he join me in putting the entire pill thing behind us and be happy to have his wife back?

"I'll work and pay back all of it."

I meant it. I had made amends before and I had paid off debts several times in my life and I knew I could do it again. I intended to work hard, and one day he could retire and I would keep working and support him the way he had supported me.

He slept on the sofa that night. I cried myself to sleep. I wanted him so badly and he didn't want me at all. Brad spent many nights on the sofa after that. He was still doing things with the kids, playing soccer, getting new projects at work, and reading his novels, and at night he sometimes he slept in our bed and sometimes he slept on the sofa.

After I told Brad, I had to tell the kids. Then I told my family, real estate broker, and neighbors. My family already knew, but everyone else was completely surprised about my pill addiction. I took Brad and the kids to a therapy session with our HMO's chemical dependency department, to see if I had damaged the kids. The therapist talked with them and said everyone seemed fine, because I was a functional addict.

It was late October. I had reduced my suboxone dosage and would be off it in a month. I had enough of the crying. I didn't give up pills to cry over a man who avoided sex, slept on the sofa, and wasn't talking about any of it. I wanted a full marriage, where we opened our hearts to each other fully. I called a divorce mediator. The attorney called Brad to verify the appointment. Brad called me right away.

"Honey, I want you. I don't want a divorce. Let's talk tonight," he said.

That night we talked and we got closer and I stayed. And sometimes for no reason at all, he slept on the sofa. He didn't mention any withholding or resentments or ask me to change anything. He seemed the same, except he was on the sofa. I had no idea how to handle myself. Sometimes I wished I could knock myself out with a frying pan, so at least I could sleep at night.

If a divorce was out, we needed counseling. I asked Brad to take time off work for marriage counseling. He agreed to go only because I was so distraught. I told the marriage counselor about the pills, my crying, and Brad on the sofa. I thought she would be sympathetic. Instead, she looked at him.

"How do you feel about your wife taking those pills all those years?"

I looked over at him. Out of the corner of my eye, I saw that Brad had his arms crossed and tapped his foot up and down. That meant he was mad.

"I feel betrayed and foolish for not knowing what was happening."

Wow. Of course. That's why he was on the sofa. He had every right to be mad. I was selfish and out of touch for not realizing his side of it. Why had he not told me any of this? I wondered what else bothered him that he never mentioned.

"Yes, of course you feel betrayed," the counselor said.

I looked at Brad. His face had relaxed. When we left the appointment, Brad took my hand. He asked me to dinner. Over fish tacos, he said he did not like how cold I became over the years. He put up with it because it happened so gradually. He planned to leave me when the kids were grown. He didn't know I was addicted, and he had found his own happiness in life outside of his relationship with me. He didn't cheat on me because sex wasn't that important to him. He wasn't sure how long he would stay angry. He definitely wanted me to repay the $100,000 I spent on pills.

What I Did For Sex

The next morning we took a walk and Brad confided in me some of his dreams and what he thought was holding him back in life. I was aroused and wet and wondered when he would stop talking, so we could go home and fuck. I felt small for wanting his cock when he just wanted to be heard. Was I really a bad person, or had I just married the wrong guy? After our walk, he wanted to have sex. It lasted three minutes and it was done.

Maybe if I could climax faster, he would be happier with me. I bought two electric vibrators and experimented. The vibrators were fun to use. I timed my masturbation for a month, hoping to find a technique to climax in less than 5 minutes. When I was aroused it could take just three minutes, but that was rare. Usually it took 10 to 30 minutes to climax. I kept the vibrator or manual stimulation going to get a second orgasm or achieve the multiple orgasms I had read about in the magazines. Whenever I tried for a second orgasm, it took just as longer or even longer than the first orgasm. I had failed at multiple orgasms and coming quickly. I needed advice.

I made an appointment with a sex therapist that was also trained in addiction. The sex therapist said 20 minutes was not too long for a woman to reach orgasm. Brad went with me to the second appointment, and after that, he compromised on the sex. He went down on me sometimes, and tried several medications for his ED. The Viagra or Cialis made his penis engorged and spongy, but not hard. It I still could barely feel him. They did not create erections either. The TV ads were misleading.

Brad did not enjoy the intimacy of sex or pleasuring his woman. Sex was just an activity he used to reach his orgasm. A week later when I masturbated after his orgasm, he got angry it took me too long, so he got up and left the room. I didn't know he hated me.

I consulted a sex coach from New York City about our sexual problems, as well as my desire to expand sex beyond the physical.

I wanted emotional sex that could open our hearts and explore our sexuality, without constantly being shut down. The sex coach said I needed to ask Brad for what I wanted and it had to be done with a very sweet voice.

I asked Brad when would be a good time to talk about some things and he said on Saturday afternoon. On Saturday afternoon, Brad came up to me while I was doing laundry.

"What did you want to talk about?" he asked.

I turned around and smiled at him. "Brad, I want more sex."

He looked at me with compassion. "Honey, although you are so sexy and beautiful, I am not as turned on by you as when we first met. I need two to three days to recharge."

"Well, can't you go down on me even if you're not in the mood, or hold me while I masturbate?" I asked, sweetly again, showing my desire. I figured he could do it as a favor, the way he did yard work or had once changed the oil on my car.

"I don't want to do that when I'm not in the mood."

He was always washing dishes, although I never asked. Did he love doing dishes more than eating pussy? I brought myself back to sweetness, the way the therapist had suggested.

"Honey, can you go to the doctor to find out why you're not getting hard anymore?"

"No, I'm fine."

My heart sank, yet I persisted…sweetly, so as not to upset him.

"Maybe your testosterone level is low. Can you get your testosterone checked?"

"I am fit, I work out, I'm healthy, and I'm not going to take hormones anyway, because that's not good for my body."

"Well, I really enjoy the penetration and I want you to last longer during sex. It's over way too fast. You feel so good."

"Honey, you just turn me on a lot. That's why I cum fast."

"Can you read some books on how to last longer?"

"I'm not interested in those types of books. Besides, I don't think I can. I tried that once when I was younger."

"I'd like you to leave your eyes open and look at me during sex."

"I close my eyes so I can imagine someone else. I'm not trying to hurt you, but I've been with you so long that sometimes I don't get as turned on anymore."

If looking at each other during sex was out, so were the "open eye orgasms" I wanted to bring up next, so I crossed that off my list.

"I had a consultation with a sex therapist. I'd love if you could jump on the next call with him."

"I'm not going to talk to another man about how to have sex with my wife!"

I fought back tears. It seemed so hopeless. I remembered to use my sweet voice.

"I want us to be more affectionate during sex. I want to play romantic music or kiss or be more tender."

"Honey, sex is just physical," he explained, "and you know I don't like kissing."

"What do you mean, it's just physical?"

I did not believe him. He couldn't possibly mean that. Brad was one of the most loving men I knew. Didn't he feel our closeness and love in his heart when he was with me? I had seen images of men on the covers of romance novels and in soft porn, showing them in tender loving poses with women, and this proved to me that men could make love and be tender, and certainly they would show this side of themselves to a woman they loved, and Brad loved me, so what the fuck did he mean sex was just physical?

"Yes, sex is just physical," he repeated, "I show my love by doing things for you, not through sex."

Did that mean he would rather change the plumbing than fuck? He had never complained about his chore list.

Maybe if he were happier with me, he would not withhold in the bedroom, although I really wasn't sure if he was withholding at all. I ramped up my real estate sales work and applied for jobs at temp agencies.

Brad asked me on a weekend trip to Idyllwild. We stayed at a Bed and Breakfast and took some beautiful hikes.

A month later, in November, I went off the suboxone. I had been on it for six months. I was on no medication at all, and I didn't drink alcohol either. I had regained my weight and was back to 128 pounds and I looked healthy and toned. I wanted to make sure I stayed sober and off the pills, so I decided to attend 12 step meetings. The people in the meetings talked honestly about their feelings and lives in a way I liked. Admitting our weaknesses and flaws inspired me and made us closer. I got an NA sponsor, worked steps, and went to all the women's groups available. My heart opened wide and flowed in love in the women's' groups. I fell in love more with life. I hugged people instead of shaking their hand. I liked this new life without pills.

Periods, cramping, pregnancy concerns, young children, or pills no longer impeded my sexual desires. I wanted sex all the time. My sexual energy was a powerful force from deep inside my belly, hungry for expression. I was a beautiful woman in my sexual prime, ready to discover my humanity, femininity, and capacity for love. Yet it was all going to waste, because I was stuck with a man who kept ignoring and pushing it all down. I hated him and the entire concept of marriage, which held me hostage to the sexual desires of my partner.

"I hate your quickies," I said.

"That's just how it is, I can't last longer," he said.

I did not believe him. We had a whiteboard in our hallway for the kids to write on. I used the blue marker and wrote NO

MORE QUICKIES on the whiteboard. I didn't care if the kids figured out what that meant.

I watched porn to get the fucking I did not get at home. It just made me feel worse. I felt jealous of the lucky porn girls who at least could get a hard cock, and then I cried because my husband would not do that with me. Damn monogamy. I asked Brad again if he wanted to watch porn, and to my surprise, he did. He liked the hardcore fucking videos. They did nothing for me.

HOPE

That summer, I got a job for a company which consulted on facilities and finance for local school districts. I was bringing in money and no longer felt like a financial burden. My company liked me and offered me options for growing my career.

Brad and I talked about moving closer to his work. Our older kids had graduated from high school, and Oliver would be a freshman that fall. It was a good time to move. Brad liked south Oceanside, a coastal community in northern San Diego County.

We rented a cute older home a few blocks from the beach. The interior reminded me of a Restoration Hardware catalog. It was charming. My job was just a few minutes drive down the coast and we were happy, at least outside the bedroom. Brad finally had his beach home and a wife who worked. This should make him happy and improve the parts of our relationship running on hope: intimacy and sex.

"I love your laughter," he said often.

"I love how you open me up emotionally," he said.

"What can I do to be a better wife?" I often asked.

"Cook more," he said.

I wanted his answer to be about sex and not cooking, because I didn't like cooking that much, but I cooked more anyway. He never asked what he could do to be a better husband. Maybe he knew he would not like the answer.

I was still upset with his quickies. What was missing was his desire to please me, connect, and be tender and attentive in bed. Sometimes I felt sad and other times I was angry. We talked about it again, and Brad saw I had a point. He agreed to a one-hour sex date every week. This was moving in the right direction and gave me hope for marital satisfaction in our bed. He still gave me his quickies during the week, and I did not mind as much, because all week I looked forward to Saturday mornings.

I enjoyed the Saturday morning sex more. I liked the extra attention and closeness. He was going down on me, and he stayed for my orgasm. However, the quality was still severely lacking. On the oral sex, he had a 20-minute time limit, which he enforced. I was still afraid to sit on his face or rub my pussy on his legs because these things could repulse him. Also I didn't like that he made me wash up before he went down on me and that I had my orgasms from masturbating.

I could not recall the last time Brad had given me an orgasm. It was many years ago. Despite his hand jobs and oral sex with the time limit and all my instructions on how to lick me, his touch was not arousing. My orgasms always were better when I was alone, and I didn't like that. My orgasms should be better when I was with my lover.

Despite my sexual dissatisfaction and finding him unattractive, I was deeply in love with him. The only time in decades he was handsome was on the houseboat, because he was relaxed and his face softened. After the vacation, he reverted to his usual stressed state. His face showed the combination of lack of joy, repressed feelings, stress, premature ageing from sun damage, and the places he picked his face when under stress. He looked at least 10-15 years older due to the deeply creased wrinkles and age spots. His face was so wrinkled, that when we had sex in the missionary position, the skin on his face drooped down in many places. I felt old around him and decided to get a chemical peel as soon as I could afford it, so I could look as young as I felt, and to make up for his ageing. Yet I loved him and wanted him more than anyone. One night at dinner I realized, *I am looking past his ugly face into his heart because I love him from the inside out.*

I was getting concerned with my use of vibrators. I had used them more and more over the past two years, and the past few months I used them every time. They seemed like a crutch. I had stopped using the Hitachi after just a few tries, despite its popularity, because it was like a jackhammer on my clit. Within two minutes of use, my clit and entire vulva area was numb. If I did finally orgasm, I barely felt anything at all. Were the other vibrators numbing me too? Had they dulled my clit?

I longed to get more in touch with my body. I went cold turkey on the vibrators. I used my fingers to masturbate. I could not build up enough arousal to orgasm. I persisted in using only my fingers. For the next two weeks, I could not orgasm at all, regardless of how long I rubbed or how turned on I felt. And then, finally, I orgasmed. Were we all sold a bill of goods on the vibrators or did they actually enhance the orgasm for some women?

ADDICTION IS A CHOICE

I was still going to meetings and working the steps with my sponsor. I liked this personal development that I had put on hold my entire marriage, so I would not outgrow him. I liked my sobriety. I had no use for pills because they numbed my body. I loved sex too much to take pills again.

I started a women's NA meeting near my home. I had my 12 month sobricty day, and I took a tokcn at cach mccting I attended. Brad and the kids came when to one of the meetings when I got my 12-month token. My sponsor gave me my token at the women's NA meeting I had started. She gave moving speech about me, and gave me a heart shaped necklace.

"This is for you to realize all your dreams."

My heart felt warm and I teared up. I liked that word: Dreams. I had not even thought about dreams in years. What were my dreams anyway?

After one NA meeting in Oceanside, I was talking with some fellow 12 steppers. I wondered what they would think of me for liking sex with my husband, so I brought it up.

"I'm really enjoying sex with my husband more since I went off the pills," I said.

One of the old-timers smiled. "You know what I don't like about sex with a woman? I don't like if she has sex with me because she wants attention or approval or she wants to please me. I want a woman to have sex with me <u>because she loves sex!</u>"

He emphasized those last words and smiled, as if he remembered fucking a woman who loved to be fucked.

Wow. Really? I wasn't slutty or immoral for liking sex? A man actually preferred a man who enjoyed sex? An entire new world opened to me.

The next time Brad and I fucked, I remembered the old-timer's words. I allowed myself to like sex and not feel ashamed for it. I felt powerful, alive.

I was feeling less free at the 12 step meetings. We were living in the past, talking about a habit years after it ended. We had to label ourselves as addicts, although we were sober. We had to keep our attendance at meetings anonymous, in essence keeping our recovery anonymous as well. Keeping our 12-step attendance a secret may have empowered the organization, but it kept many addicts struggling alone. How I wished I would have known my neighbor and kids' teacher went to AA – they could have been sounding boards years earlier when I yearned I had someone to confide in.

Furthermore, I completely disagreed with many of the steps, particularly Step 1: We admitted we were powerless over "the substance". I wasn't powerless at all. I chose to take every pill. Why did they say "we are addicts" and speak on my behalf?

After 17 months of sobriety and working through 11 of the 12 steps, I stopped going to meetings. I drank a glass of red wine, and I did not "release my addiction all over again". Instead, I felt free and powerful for being able to do what others said could not be done. I drank a glass of red wine at every dinner from then onward, and sometimes I had a second glass. One night, I smoked pot, but I didn't like it.

I spent the next nine months deprogramming myself by reading everything I could find on addiction as choice, and took another good look at myself and why I had taken pills and for so many years. I concluded that addiction was a habit, not a disease. Habits were hard to break, whether the habit was watching TV, smoking cigarettes, or taking drugs. Something hard to change did not make it a disease. No research existed to show that taking drugs was a disease. All they had were brain scans of addicted people showing the brain changes. They never showed the brain scans of people after they quit.

The disease model made sense to take the stigma out of addiction. It made sense that people who had lost hope in life needed a helping hand. However, none of that meant they had a disease, were flawed, or were powerless. Wasn't it better to be honest and inspire people to reach for their dreams rather than make them feel weak and powerless? Wasn't all drug use really just a search for meaning and connection anyway?

It seemed the loss of a loved one was the main reason that people in "the rooms" talked about relapse. I was done with "the rooms". I remained grateful they had shown me the value of vulnerability and sharing ourselves honestly. Brad and the kids had attended meetings when I took my sobriety tokens, and they supported my decision to stop going.

I started having a glass of wine with dinner every night, and cookies with tea at bedtime. I gained a few pounds, partially because Brad liked me a little heavier but also because I used the wine and cookies for comfort. These things let me know everything was not alright in my relationship. I could masturbate to relieve the pressure in my pussy. I just didn't know how to relieve the pressure in my heart.

CHAPTER 7

MY OPEN MARRIAGE

One night when we made love it just happened. I felt so happy underneath him in the missionary position. My heart felt warm. I wanted to express my emotions. I knew he didn't like me saying "I love you," because he said it is something you show, not say. I figured he would let me say it in bed.

"I love you," I whispered to him as I clutched him tightly.

As soon as I said those words, I felt my heart open up and a deep intense pleasure deep in my vagina. I felt a definite connection between my heart and my body. I didn't need him to answer. I wanted to see what would happen when I said it again.

"I love you," I said again, softly.

"Why are you saying that?" he asked with anger, and briefly paused thrusting.

"I just wanted to say it."

I was emotionally stable enough to handle his rejection, so I returned to our shared passion, but I finally got it. For him, sex was only physical.

I hungered for a complete sexual experience in which the man adored my genitals, especially my clitoris, buried his head between my thighs, and from that position gave me an orgasm with his finger or tongue. I wasn't going to get that from Brad. I fantasized about other people licking my clit, usually women. I needed to get sexual satisfaction.

I turned to porn. I bought a subscription to vivid.com and watched some of the videos while Brad was at work. I liked the lesbian sex videos because they showed women being orally pleasured by someone who loved doing it to them (and men in porn never did it at all or only briefly), and educational videos about oral sex, pegging (a woman performing anal sex on a man with a dildo in a strap-on) and the lifestyle (formerly called "swinging").

SWINGING, OR THE LIFESTYLE

The lifestyle documentary featured a wife being fucked by the filmmaker while the husband watched. It was the hottest thing I had ever seen. My clit tingled when the husband told his wife to ride the filmmaker's hard cock a little faster. She smiled at her husband, and did as he asked. I wanted my husband to get turned on watching me have sex with another man, and watch him having sex with another woman. Perhaps being with other women would increase his sex drive and improve our sex life. I wasn't worried that he'd fall for another woman. I was sure he would never leave me.

The swingers were probably very good at sex and could give me vaginal orgasms, and other unknown delights.

I waited for a chance to suggest the swinger documentary. One night after dinner, when we were snuggled in bed, I brought it up.

"Do you want to watch a movie?" I asked.

"That sounds good. What do you want to watch?"

"Let's watch some porn. How about a documentary on swinging?"

"Sure!"

I started the movie. He seemed to like it, because he kept commenting on it.

"Do you want to have sex with other women?" I asked.

"Yeah, I want to have sex with other women. Why wouldn't I?" he said.

"Yeah, I want to watch you do that," I told him.

We spent the rest of the evening discussing swinging and what that might be like for us. Then we fell asleep in each other's arms. The next day we joined a swinger website. We learned to call it the lifestyle. Through the site we could access local events and meet other swingers online. We went to some meetups.

The lifestyle people we met at the clubs were not attractive like the people in the swinger documentary, and I couldn't picture myself having sex with any of them. Still, this new reality intrigued me. Instead of avoiding each other's spouses for the sake of propriety, we were supposed to desire them. The women flirted with my husband. It turned me on to think he might want to fuck them. I felt free, talking with their husbands and imagining myself having sex with them, knowing the women did not care.

Our main concern with having sex outside our monogamous marriage was getting a sexually transmitted disease (STD). We asked the couples a lot of questions about STDs. The couples told us they had never heard of anyone contracting any STDs. As we went to more swinger events and sex parties later on, we kept asking about STDs, and we always got the same answer: the couple had never had any STDs and had never heard of anyone getting an STD. I read up on STDs on the CDC website. We felt safe having sex with other people.

We went to our first lifestyle party. We paid the couple fee of $90. Single women could attend because they were desired for threesomes, but single men were not allowed. The party started at 7pm and went until the next morning. It took place at a large home and featured a DJ and delicious food. Guests could bring their own alcohol. I chose not to drink. Gina, a friend of the hostess, showed us around. A storage room held our purses and bags/change of clothes. There were many bedrooms, a large hot tub, a dance floor with a stripper pole, and a fucking swing. Women were allowed to walk around and watch others have sex, but men could watch only if accompanied by a woman, because they didn't want men masturbating while they watched others having sex. Apparently, masturbation was too taboo for even a lifestyle party.

The house was filled with couples. Some had been in the lifestyle for decades. Most were in their 30's to 50's and had children. The women were beautiful and well dressed. The men were mostly overweight and unattractive. I still couldn't see myself having sex with any of them.

An overweight man in the living room said he liked watching his wife be fucked by other men. His wife nodded her head and added that her husband had the final say on which man she could fuck. He smiled at her and said he wanted to see her be pleasured by the large penises she enjoyed. They had children in high school and had started swinging a few years earlier. He wasn't jealous she might leave him for a larger penis or stop enjoying him? They must have read my mind. They both said after the swinger party they always had sex again at home, and it was always the hottest sex.

I walked into the master bedroom with the intention to watch. The room was dimly lit, cozy. Several couples were having sex on the king size bed. A woman was giving an older unattractive man a blowjob. He looked around and our eyes met. He invited me to sit on the edge of the bed. I moved closer. He held my hand and asked me to join in. He repulsed me even more, so I walked away.

What I Did For Sex

A group of people were gathered around a large vibrator with a saddle-like seat and dildo attachments, the Sybian. Women took turns being stimulated to orgasm by the hostess who operated the device. Briana, a voluptuous 35-year old woman, with medium sized perky breasts, and long thick curly brown hair, put a condom on the attachment and sat on the device. I admired her beauty and bravery for sitting on that machine in front of us all. A man knelt behind her and played with her breasts and nipples while the hostess operated the controls. Briana's breathing picked up. She closed her eyes and breathed harder and moaned louder and then she orgasmed in front of us.

I wanted to orgasm so easily and in public, so I stayed and waited for my turn. I doubted I could. I had to be relaxed and feel safe to climax, which required a bedroom or other private place. A few ladies were gathered around, as I got ready for the Sybian. I was self-conscious, so I asked them to leave. I put a condom on the dildo attachment, and sat on it. The hostess worked the switches. I felt the movements inside my vagina and the vibration on my clitoris. It didn't feel that good and I was self-conscious, so I asked her to stop the machine. I was disappointed that I could not let myself orgasm in public. I definitely needed privacy to surrender into my arousal.

Brad and I liked the party enough that we attended several more. I was surprised how little sex was happening. It wasn't a free-for-all. Men had to court the women, and more people sat around talking than being naked. The sex I saw was just intercourse or women going down on men. Rarely did I see a man going down on a woman. I did not see anal sex, gay sex, BDSM, masturbation, couples watching each other, or anything novel. Maybe I wasn't going to the really fun sex parties.

At the next play party, held at a rooftop lounge at a hotel downtown, attractive couples were flirting with each other, while the less attractive couples were ignored. It didn't seem fair to leave them out, just because of their looks. One of the hot couples invited us to their room. When we got there, several couples and a sleeping woman were on the bed. A man stood next to the woman, and motioned to Brad to come over and told him something. Brad came over and whispered in my ear.

"See that woman sleeping on the bed, and the man standing next to her? That's her husband, and she's not really asleep. He wants me to fuck her and come inside while she pretends to sleep. It's their fantasy," he said.

"What? He's not worried about her getting STDs?" I asked.

"No, he wants the cum in her so he can lick it afterward."

"Don't do it." I didn't want him having sex without a condom.

"No, no way, I won't," he said.

The woman's husband talked to several men and then one man stepped up and fucked her while she slept.

I sat on the sofa and watched everyone. Briana was on the bed, being fucked by a young man. Brad thought she was hot and wanted a turn, so he removed his pants. His penis was limp.

"Schahrzad, come over and get me hard," he requested.

I stroked Brad's cock to get him hard, and sat back on the sofa. Briana's husband sat next to me. I was curious how Brad would penetrate her. Would he be tender with her, kiss her, and go down on her, all the things I wanted him to do to me? He proceeded to fuck her the way he fucked me, like an object. I was so embarrassed. The only saving grace was that his penis was so big, the woman was moaning louder than she had with the previous guy.

I didn't want Brad to embarrass me again with his pitiful sexual performance, so the next morning when we sat on the sofa drinking our coffee, I told him what I should have said decades earlier, "Your penis is not just for you to get off. Your penis is supposed to be a tool of pleasure for the woman."

Brad looked at me in surprise.

"Okay," he said.

At another play party, I met a young couple in their late 20's. It was their first event. I was in a mood to give a blowjob. I wanted to make sure she could handle it.

"Can I give your husband a blowjob?"

"Yes," she said.

She seemed nervous. He pulled down his pants and sat down again next to his wife. I kneeled on the floor and sucked on his penis. I kept looking at her to make sure she was comfortable with it. After a few minutes, he groaned and came in my mouth and I swallowed. Then I looked at her. She frowned, and got up and walked away. I understood her jealousy. I left it up to them to figure out what to do about it.

I liked giving blowjobs. While I did it, I imagined how good it must feel for a man to have his cock licked, kissed, and sucked. I didn't deep throat, yet all the men said they loved my blowjobs. They said it was because I really enjoyed it and I wasn't like the other women who gave blowjobs as an obligation. I didn't want to fuck at the sex parties. I wasn't attracted to any of the men, and besides, I already had a man. I was just at the play parties to get his sexual libido jump-started.

LOST IN HIS COCK

That fall, Chelli, my friend from high school, died of cancer. Her husband Eliot called me minutes after it happened. His voice was tender and he spoke slowly, deliberately. Chelli had died at their home in Denver. As he told me how she died, my heart was breaking. She had told me she was getting better all through her chemo treatments, and then just a month before she passed, she stopped taking my calls. I didn't want to push myself on a woman who was dying and didn't want to talk about her death. I just wanted to love her and be with her. I didn't get to do that. I could love her family instead.

As Eliot spoke, I wanted to hold him close in a loving embrace. He appeared vulnerable, perhaps in need of tenderness and love, and sex. I knew he and Chelli hardly had sex and she criticized him for everything. He definitely deserved a blowjob. I thought about her looking at us from wherever she was, and wanting me to give him love.

I told Brad about Chelli's death and my blowjob fantasy. Brad thought it was a bad idea to have sex with Eliot, because he had noticed Eliot's attraction to me over the years and he didn't want us to fall for each other. But since Brad was having sex with women at the sex parties, and I was not having sex with any of the men, I felt I had a right to tell Eliot about my fantasy. I emailed him after the funeral.

"I have thought of giving you a blow job," I wrote.

I nervously waited for his response. Would he be angry with me?

"The fantasy is mutual," he replied.

I was instantly aroused. Eliot said we needed Brad's approval. That night I asked Brad again about the blowjob. Brad was having sex with other women at sex parties and felt sad for Eliot's loss. He said he would think about it.

The next day, Brad called me at work to say I could go. Eliot immediately called and booked my flight to Denver. Over the ensuing days, our emails gained steam.

It was fun talking about sex with someone who actually enjoyed it. My arousal reached a level I had never felt. My vagina was tingly and so wet, my panties were damp all day long from the moisture. I went to the bathroom and looked at my vulva. My outer labia were swollen and huge and my entire vulva was engorged. I was horrified how ugly my pussy lips looked when they were swollen with desire. I wished the reason for the swelling was Brad. We told the kids I was visiting Sarina, who lived in Denver. They did not need to know about our open marriage.

"I'm curious if he can make you come," Brad said that night. Maybe he also wanted the sexual pressure off him.

On the flight to Denver, my pussy was still swollen, and my panties were damp. I washed up in the airplane bathroom before we landed. I hoped my vagina smelled clean, and Eliot wouldn't notice the swollen lips.

Eliot picked me up at the airport in his new Land Rover. He looked dashing in his suit. I felt sexy and important that a handsome successful man went to all that trouble to dress up for me. Eliot got out and gave me a warm hug and smile.

"It's a good thing I didn't come in to get you. I'm hard as a rock," he said.

He opened my car door and I fell into his leather seat. I couldn't recall the last time a man opened a car door for me. I felt like a woman being courted and desired. He got in, leaned over and kissed me. His determined hard tongue pressed with wanting against my own. I did not expect this at all. I thought Eliot would give husband kisses, whatever those were. I didn't know anyone who French kissed like that. Besides, the last time I was French kissed was in college. I was nervous with anticipation. He drove straight to the hotel, and asked if I wanted a bottle of wine he brought along. I did not. I wanted to do this sober.

We checked in. He had paid the airfare, so I paid for the room. I wanted to show him I was there because I wanted him, not because he paid for my trip, and I didn't want the burden of thinking I owed him anything. With Brad I had trouble asking for what I wanted in the bedroom, because he supported me financially and resented it. There with Eliot, I would support myself and there would be nothing in the way of me asking for what I wanted in the bedroom.

We took the elevator upstairs. We wore our wedding rings. I felt like a woman having an affair. Walking behind him, I admired his strong body. He was a few inches taller than Brad, about 6', and he cycled, skied, and did Crossfit. I couldn't wait to see him naked.

He opened the door to our room, let it fall close, grabbed me, and pulled me close. I let out a moan. He kissed my neck, breathed in my ear, while holding me tight. Pressed up against his tall strong body, I felt protected and a feeling of surrender came over me. I went weak in the knees and fell back into his arms. His strong hands gripped me tight. He walked me backwards to the sofa and I collapsed on the cushions. He reached forward and continued kissing me. My body ached for his touch. My moaning was louder. He lifted up my skirt and pulled my panties to the side.

I had shaved my pubic hair except for the landing strip. I was a little embarrassed about my enlarged swollen vulva lips. I hoped he wouldn't mind. He didn't say anything. He just moved his head down between my thighs.

His tongue touched my outer lips and I gasped. Nobody had been there in years. I loved that he didn't go right for the button part of my clitoris. He slid his tongue down and sucked and nibbled gently on my labia. I boldly pushed my hips toward his face. I would have never dared do that with Brad.

Eliot's tongue explored my inner lips and then my clitoris, as he circled and flicked it, moving on and off my clit, side to side, and softly just like I liked. Each time he made contact with my clit, a shot of pleasure shot through my entire body. He varied his technique, keeping me aroused and in suspense.

He was still in his suit, kneeled on the floor at my feet, and it was hotter than fuck, because he had the self control to keep his cock in his pants and make it all about me. He seemed to enjoy doing it. It didn't seem like he was just doing me a favor, but I had to know.

"Do you like doing that," I asked. "You're really good at it!"

He looked up at me. "I love it! You taste so good."

I couldn't believe my ears. I had wanted Brad to say that for years! I wondered if I would have tasted good if I hadn't washed up in the airplane bathroom. I let those thoughts go, and sank back into the pleasure of my body and Eliot's warm breath on my clit.

I allowed myself a few more minutes to enjoy the oral sex. It would take me at least 20 minutes to orgasm, and I felt guilty having him spend so much time on me when I hadn't done anything for him. I wanted to show him what I came for.

"Sit down," I invited.

Eliot got up and we hurriedly removed his shoes and pants. He wore Ralph Lauren plaid boxers. It was a welcome contrast to Brad's briefs. Brad always refused the boxers or sexy underwear I bought. The boxers were hot.

Eliot's penis was beautiful, hard as a rock, so erect it was almost touching his stomach. Surprisingly hard for a 52 year old man. I hadn't seen a penis that erect in years, not even at the play parties. I felt proud I turned him on so much and curious how fucking him would feel.

Eliot sat on the sofa. I sat at his feet and smiled at him. He was so handsome. Slowly I licked his balls, rimmed his asshole, and sucked his cock. He was moaning. Why did Brad never moan or make any noise during sex? Brad was quiet even when he climaxed. Eliot kept moaning and he pulled me up. My body hungered for him.

We went to the bed and did not use a condom, because both of us had been monogamous with our spouses for decades. Eliot got on top, held my body firmly, and slipped his hard cock inside me. He felt so much better than Brad, just because of his hardness. I had not felt so much pleasure in my pussy in years. I was really moaning. I asked to get on top and he let me. I rode him slowly, letting the tip of his penis head just come inside my opening, and then I experimented with different moves. I pressed my hips down on him as hard as I could, ground and slid on him. Eliot let me move as I liked. Having a man who enjoyed sex was really fun.

"Damn, you feel so good, I love how hard you are and that you stay hard so long and let me move how I like."

I buried my face in his neck and I rode him a little faster and pumped hard until I got out of breath. I sat up and looked at him.

"Ride me hard and put me away wet," I joked.

He laughed.

"I've got some ideas of my own," and we both laughed.

I liked that we could just be ourselves during sex. We could talk, fuck, and laugh. It didn't have to be so serious. Eliot pulled me close. He held my face in his hands, brushed aside my hair, and kissed me tenderly. Why didn't Brad ever want to kiss? Eliot thrusted again and my body went limp with pleasure. I buried my head in his neck and the pillow, and felt the pleasurable sensations as his cock pushed deep against the depths of my cunt, in a spot I had discovered only recently, a spot that Brad only teased because he lasted only seconds.

Eliot moved in me deliberately, with presence, instead of the quick rabbit thrusts I got at home.. Eliot used his penis as a tool of pleasure. The longer he fucked me, the more aroused and engorged I got, and the more I opened my body and heart in surrender to him. I was proud I could feel so much. I didn't have feelings for him. I was just responding to his loving masculine presence.

Why couldn't Brad make love to me like that? My heart filled with sadness, and my eyes filled with tears. *Don't cry, Schahrzad. It's so inappropriate to cry about my husband while I am sitting on this man's cock.* I quickly pushed all my sadness away. Eliot made a series of quick thrusting pulses, which paralyzed me with pleasure. My body opened up more, I got wetter, and I wanted his penis deeper inside me. Eliot grabbed my ass, which made me even wilder.

"Stick your finger in my ass," I begged.

His finger slid right in and the pressure of his finger in my ass amplified all my sensations. I did not know I could feel so much pleasure and respond with such lust. My moaning became a wail. I didn't care if the entire hotel heard me moan.

"I feel like a wild animal," I said.

He laughed with delight in his deep voice. That gave us a moment to catch our breath and I realized the patio door was wide open. I knew I was a loud moaner, so I asked Eliot to close the door. He got up and did it, and when he came back, instead of entering me again for his own need, he sucked gently on my clitoris. I didn't recall anyone ever sucking on my clit or going down on me after intercourse. My heart swelled and my eyes teared up for this man who tasted my feminine juices after being inside me. *Why couldn't Brad love my body and womanhood like that?*

I wanted Eliot to stay down there long enough for my tears to dry, because I did not want him to see. My tears and feelings didn't belong here, where he probably didn't want them, especially because they had nothing to do with him. I wished I could make love to a man who cared about my feelings so I didn't have to keep shoving them away. Eliot was good at oral, but I wasn't good at receiving it because I didn't think I deserved it. I had sworn years ago to be a women who could receive, but I sucked at it. I was convinced he was just doing me a favor and that he secretly resented every lick of his tongue. I had to make him stop.

"Come here," I beckoned.

He rose up to kiss me and I was surprised his cock was rock hard. I did not know a man could be turned on going down on a woman. I thought only women got turned on doing that. Eliot kissed me, but I didn't want his kisses. I wasn't into him as a man. I felt a little selfish, just wanting his cock. Eliot held me in a tight embrace and I felt so protected and pleasured all at once. He thrust faster as he kissed me.

"I'm going to come," he said.

Did he want my approval?

"Go for it, baby!" I whispered.

He pumped faster and faster, until he came with a loud long groan. I didn't know men made noises like that when they orgasmed. It scared me a little because I wasn't used to it. But I liked it.

Eliot looked relaxed, and sweaty. I gave him a kiss. I knew a man liked to retract after orgasm, so I was quiet for a little while. We held each other without talking. I imagined Chelli looking at us from heaven or wherever she was, and smiling at us. I was grateful Brad allowed me that experience and wished he wanted sex like this.

Eliot lay me on my back and then he went down on me and after a few minutes I didn't think he could make me come, so I told him I wanted to masturbate. Eliot lay next to me and kissed me as I pleasured myself. His kiss softened into a gentle tug on my lip. I felt warmth in my heart and that turned me on even more. I didn't kiss him back because I was focusing all my attention on my rubbing fingers and my clit. I briefly opened my eyes and noticed his eyes were open and he looked at me. His attentiveness and interest turned me on more. I got more and more tingly and then I came long and hard. He looked at me the entire time.

I wished that Brad would be excited when I masturbated and came. Was Eliot so turned on with me, because I was new to him? Maybe I expected too much of Brad.

As we lay in our afterglow, Eliot talked about his views and ideas on people, relationships, and life. I wished Brad liked people and thinking about his feelings. Eliot made it clear our weekend was just sex between friends. He left to go home and said he would be back in the morning.

Early next morning, I worked out, showered, and put on the tank top, booty shorts, and high heels that he had requested I bring along. I didn't feel slutty wearing that for him, because he treated me like a whole woman, not an object.

I heard a knock on my hotel door. It was Eliot. He looked so handsome, his blond curly hair a stark contrast to his black Patagonia sweater and jeans. I gave him a hug. His body felt strong and steady against mine.

"God, you look amazing," he said and eyed me in my sexy seductress outfit.

I felt sexy, alive, and desired in a way I could not recall.

"Thank you," I smiled up at him.

"Dance for me," he whispered.

"Come sit on the sofa," I said.

I played Stevie Ray Vaughan music. Blues were perfect for dancing and fucking. I felt his gaze on me as I walked around in my high-heel sandals and booty shorts. I could see how much he wanted me.

"God, you're so sexy!" he said.

I turned around and shook my ass, teasing him.

"Sway your hips for me just slightly, and then pull your shorts down just a little bit. Let me see you move like that."

I liked him telling me what turned him on and being his object of desire. Since I trusted him and I felt safe and respected, I wanted to be slutty and sexy. He sat on the sofa, leaned back, legs spread wide apart, ready for his performance. At first I felt a little shy, so I closed my eyes and felt myself as one with the music. If I had not been married to such a prude who refused to let me wear lingerie or dance for him, I would have had some practice. I wanted to cry. I pushed my sadness away.

Eliot was so handsome on the sofa. I looked him in the eyes as I moved my body to the sultry beat and gyrated my hips slowly. His eyes were fixated on my body. I pulled my shorts down over my hips ever so slightly and turned around and moved my ass the way he told me. I bent over like women at strip clubs and pulled down my shorts. I turned around, and laughed. He smiled at me.

I walked over to him and straddled his leg. He held me tight while I ground on him, and in less than a minute our clothes were off and we were in the bed again fucking.

Eliot drove me to the airport. On the flight home, I daydreamed about the sex scenes with Eliot., because I felt so alive. I would feel even more alive with Brad, because I loved and desired him. I was furious with Brad for not giving me the kind of sex that a man in his 50's clearly could deliver.

I wasn't my usual happy self when I walked into our home that evening. Brad didn't want to hear the details. He was washing the dishes.

It got worse over the next few weeks. I was sad almost all the time. I longed for having the same passionate sex with Brad, that I had with Eliot. Songs on the radio spilled over into my aching heart. I was lost in a gray, bland world of tears and sobs. I wasn't laughing anymore at Brad's jokes or anything at all. Everything I usually did to improve my mood, like changing my thoughts, saying affirmations, or a hard run, was not helping.

I dealt with my bottomless sadness by pushing it away and talking with my best friends Mindy and Mary over our weekly dinners. Mary was a 44-year-old divorced mother of two, and worked as a counselor. She was once my neighbor. Mindy was a 32-year old single mom I met at a 12-step meeting. They were the only people who knew what was happening behind closed doors at my house. I portrayed to the outside world that my life with Brad was happy, because I so much wanted it to be and also because I was embarrassed to admit what an utter failure my sex life was.

Brad saw me crying and walking around glum, and mistakenly thought I wanted Eliot romantically. He pulled out our book on open relationships and went straight to the chapter on jealousy. He became interested in being closer and improving our sex life. He put more effort into pleasing me. I felt happy once again.

That Friday evening, we lay on the bed and talked for hours, sipping chamomile tea and feeling the fullness of our togetherness. I found the courage to tell Brad something I had never told him in all of the years of our marriage.

"Honey, did you know I was a call girl in college?"

"I've known all along," he said while we were still in bed sipping on our tea. "It was in the newspaper when you were arrested."

What was a relief! I had been afraid our entire marriage of mentioning it, because I thought Brad would disrespect me if he knew.

Our improved sex life lasted only a few days. Brad's ED was getting worse and his interest in sex fizzled along with it. He didn't care about his declining desire. I wanted more hot sex, while he wanted less. Maybe I caused his ED by wanting so much sex. Maybe he hated me for not having worked all those years. He never said anything about it.

I had an idea to get the intimacy and romance that were ignored at home. I could have sex with another couple. I could watch them be tender together the way I wanted Brad to be with me, and lick the woman's clit the way I wished Brad licked mine. I asked Brad and he said I could do it. I contacted a few couples on craigslist, and nothing ever came of it. It seemed the woman's mood and the feelings in the relationship that day, determined how much they wanted a threesome. Looking for sex took a lot of time. I wished I could just have sex with my husband.

THREESOMES WITH OTHER COUPLES

One of the lifestyle women hosted a women-only party at her home. It was a chance to get acquainted. We brought appetizers and wine. Linda, a well-dressed large-breasted woman in her early 50's, asked me to sit next to her on the couch. She and her husband Roger were looking for a unicorn, a single woman in the lifestyle. She wanted to watch her husband fuck me, and since I was "fresh meat", she made sure to get first dibs on me. Maybe they could teach me about orgasms and I could witness their lovemaking.

When I got home, I asked Brad for permission to hook up with them. The lifestyle term was "hall pass", meaning I had permission to "play" alone. Brad said I could go.

"Maybe they can make you orgasm," he said.

The afternoon of our dinner date Linda sent me a text message. *"Be a good girl and wear something sexy for us"*. Their directions turned me on.

I met Linda and Roger at a restaurant in Encinitas. I wasn't attracted to either of them, but was hungry for new experiences. At dinner, Linda sat close, and flirted provocatively.

"It takes me a long time to come," I admitted.

"How long?" she asked.

"Probably 15-20 minutes, but it can be much faster or take even longer, depending on how turned on I am. How long does it take for you?"

"I didn't come fast until I met Roger. He gives me multiple orgasms, within minutes. He's so good in bed!"

She beamed at him. I wanted to find out if he could do that for me. He was attractive. Maybe I could fuck him.

"Take her shopping and buy her something sexy," Roger told his wife.

They invited me to their house the following weekend. I arrived at their home the following Saturday afternoon. Linda drove us to the sex boutique and I selected several outfits to try. Linda came in the dressing room with me and watched as I tried on the outfits. She bought two of the outfits for me. Back at their house, I changed into the bra/garter ensemble while she slipped into a short body stocking and then we presented ourselves to him. He no longer looked attractive.

They asked if I wanted to smoke pot with them. I didn't do drugs, so I declined and they went off to smoke alone. When they got back, Roger said he could fuck me for hours. It sounded horrible and I hoped he was kidding.

They took me upstairs to their sex room, a small cozy room with a queen size bed, red satin sheets, and dimmed lighting. I undressed, and he immediately fingered me quickly and hard, trying to make me squirt.

"That doesn't feel good. It feels sharp and like I have to pee," I told him.

"Just relax, it's supposed to feel that way," he said.

"No, I just don't like it," I told him.

They left to smoke more pot. When they came back, he said again he could fuck me for hours. I didn't want him fucking me at all, but my curiosity made me want to try. I went down on him to get him hard, but he stayed limp. He stroked his cock and he stayed limp. Since he could not have intercourse, he went down on me. He was really bad at oral.

"It doesn't feel good. I want Linda to go down on me."

Linda took his place between my legs and licked me in the most pleasurable way. I was sure if she kept that up for 10-15 minutes, I would come. After a couple minutes she stopped. I didn't know if he asked her to stop, or if she really didn't like licking my pussy. Wasn't she bisexual?

I was horny and wanted to come, so I stroked my clit. While I masturbated, he kept saying "pussy", which turned me off and made it impossible for me to come. The word "pussy" meant vagina, and anything put in my vagina didn't get me off. If he'd talked about my clit instead, he probably would have had more success. I didn't like him enough to tell him that.

They left again to smoke pot. When they came back, he wanted to fuck me again. He asked me to get him hard. Why wasn't he hard already? I sucked his cock but I couldn't get him hard enough for fucking. He stroked himself until he was partially erect, and then he fucked me doggy style while she watched and walked around us from various angles and took pictures. That's when I figured out that everything we had done, was for her husband Roger. I was just their toy, there for him to fuck, while she watched. After she had enough pictures, they left to smoke more pot. Why did they need to keep smoking pot when we were having sex?

After several hours and no orgasms for anyone, they suggested bringing out the sex toys. Linda brought out a basket of vibrators and dildos, and condoms. Roger said Linda and I ought to play together while he watched. She brought out a double-ended dildo and put a condom on each end. She inserted the larger end inside her pussy, and the smaller end into my pussy. She rocked rhythmically. It didn't feel good at all. She started moaning. Her moans sounded fake, as if she were moaning to try to turn me on, but I felt repulsed by it. I looked up and saw Roger standing at the doorway watching us. His gaze didn't turn me on either.

After four hours of sex with this swinger couple, we were all ready to call it a night. None of us had an orgasm. I left. I thought they might text me the next day to thank me for coming over, but I never heard from them again.

I still had curiosity to experience intimate lovemaking between a couple, and have a woman go down on me, so I looked for other swinger couples online. I needed to find a couple where I wanted to fuck the man and the woman, and the couple was also interested in me. This took a lot of looking. Finally, I found a couple in their mid 30's who had started dating just a few months earlier. We met for sushi.

"My boyfriend is so good in bed. He gives me multiple orgasms, and I never had experienced that before," she gushed over dinner.

After dinner, they walked me to my car.

"Kiss my girl," he said when we got to my car.

I kissed her and I didn't feel turned on. She didn't seem turned on either.

"Wow, that's so hot," he said.

We were kissing to turn him on. That was lame. I planed a date with them anyway to experience his expert sexual touch and have multiple orgasms too. And since she said she was bisexual, I was excited to go down on her.

I went to their house one afternoon while their kids were at school. They called right before to say she her vagina was sore from the hot tub and she would only be watching. It seemed like an excuse because he always made her watch while he fucked other girls and she went along with it because she was in love with him. I decided to go anyway because maybe she would go down on me.

She was dressed in a beautiful corset. I went to kiss her, and she did not seem turned on. She wasn't leaning in or moaning. Was she straight? Then she sat back and handed me over to him. He went down on me, but it didn't feel good,.

"I want her to go down on me," I said.

I Her tongue was exquisite, but after a few seconds she stopped. Did he tell her to stop? He put on a condom and we had intercourse while she watched. Soon it was clear he could not climax. He finally asked me to get into his favorite position, and then he came. Then I had to quickly leave before their kids came home from school. There were no orgasms for her or for me.

I was disappointed with the entire situation. I didn't get anything I wanted. I was done with women who pretended to be bisexual. Next time, I would start out with just the woman. If I was satisfied with her, then would I invite the man to join us.

I looked for more couples, but after dozens of hours online, I had no prospects. It was a hassle. Brad said I could keep my hall pass, so I looked for men on the swinger site, so I could discover my sexuality.

HE WATCHED ME MASTURBATE

Larry, a single man in his late 30's, had been in the lifestyle for many years. We met for coffee one evening. I was not attracted to him romantically or sexually. But he was a swinger, so he could probably teach me something and even give me an orgasm. I asked if I could come over. At his home, he spoke matter-of-factly.

"How would you like to have sex? What do you want to do, what positions or how to start?" he asked.

Yikes, this felt like a business transaction. I thought he would kiss me and just start doing something impressive and take charge in some way.

"Well, I like intercourse and I like oral sex," I said.

Larry nodded in agreement and walked closer and leaned over to kiss me. He stood far away from me and his lips were too soft and I didn't enjoy his kiss. I debated whether being there was even a good idea. Curiosity kept me there. Maybe he would do something really amazing.

We went upstairs, took off our clothes and lay on his bed. It didn't seem romantic or sexy at all. I had imagined I would be turned on enough that we'd tear our clothes off each other. He had shaved his pubic hair, and it reminded me of a goat. Why would a man shave his pubic hair? I later learned that the male body-shaving fad started sometime after I married.

Larry went down on me. His tongue was rough, and he used too much pressure. I thought of telling him to use a gentler touch, and I didn't because I was curious how the rougher touch would feel and if eventually it would feel better. I assumed other women liked it that way, so maybe I could like it also. I endured his oral sex for about ten minutes.

"Hey, why don't you get a condom?" I asked.

I had no idea if he was relieved he could stop, or whether he liked it. He put on the condom and we fucked, but he didn't feel as good inside me as Eliot or Brad.

"How do you usually come? I want you to come first," he said.

"I masturbate to come," I told him.

His eyes lit up. That made me excited, because I loved being watched. I was glad I stayed. I masturbated lying on my back with my head on the pillows, using my fingers to rub my clit, while he sat at the foot of the bed to get a good view. I liked that he was sitting with a clear view of my pussy. He looked turned on watching me. His eyes glanced across my entire body, from my face to my moving fingers on my clit. I thought he could be pretending to like it.

"Do you like watching women masturbate?" I asked.

"Yes. I love it! It's very sexy!" he exclaimed.

He sounded like he meant it. I believed him. I didn't know a man could be turned on watching me masturbate. Larry's interest in my masturbation was turning me on, and I came in only ten minutes, a fraction of the time it usually took with Brad. Would Larry still be turned on watching the same woman masturbate year after year, and was I expecting too much of Brad? And why didn't I know any of these things at my age?

After my orgasm, I was ready to go home. But first I had to make sure he had an orgasm too. He wanted a blowjob. I gave great blowjobs and I figured he'd come in a few minutes and then I could leave. I started out slow, and then sucked more vigorously on his penis while I stuck my finger in his ass. He spread his legs so I could put my finger inside. After ten minutes, he still hadn't come. He got out his phone and took some pictures of us in the mirror. My jaw was sore and I wished it could all be over. I doubled down, used my hand more than my mouth, and kept going until he finally came. Why did all the lifestyle men have trouble reaching orgasm?

"Wow, that was great, especially with you licking my ass and sticking your finger in it."

It wasn't great for me and I was relieved I could leave. At home, I wanted to tell Brad about my encounter with Larry, but he wasn't interested in the details. I did tell him was that Larry hadn't been able to make me come either. As the week wore on, I decided I didn't want to see Larry again, and I was done exploring men sexually for a while. My biggest sexual question at that time was whether anyone could give me an orgasm.

I didn't want sex with other men anymore. I was in love with my husband. He turned me on and I couldn't get enough of him. Yet I was sexually and emotionally deeply dissatisfied. I yearned for more closeness, romance, and sex that nourished my heart. I wanted to linger in bed in the morning with my lover and cuddle, make love to romantic music, walk together holding hands, and care about pleasing each other sexually and emotionally. I wanted all that without replacing my husband with another man.

I started to dream of a girlfriend with whom I could explore sensuality and sexuality. I imagined going places with her and holding hands in public. I looked for women on the lifestyle site. The few women who interested me did not want to meet for sex, either because they were not attracted to me, but usually because they only wanted sex that also involved their husbands. The lifestyle was mostly for couple swapping and threesomes.

LESBIANS

An Older Woman

I turned to online dating sites. Brad didn't mind at all. Maybe he was glad I met my sexual needs elsewhere and left him alone. I opened an account on OKCupid and within two hours I had a coffee date with a 61-year-old attractive lesbian. Finally I found a woman who liked girls for herself, not just as a fuck toy for her guy. S

Over coffee, she told me she and her past girlfriends had amazing sex. I couldn't wait to experience whatever amazing things she would do to me, as well as lick her clit. By the time we ended our coffee date it was close to 10pm, so we made hookup plans for another day.

Two days later, after work, we met at a nice hotel in Carlsbad. I wore my bikini and stripped for her, eager for the hot sex about to happen. She looked at me lustfully. She took off her clothes and lay in bed on her back while I went down on her. She was motionless and did not make a sound. Her long gray pubic hair kept getting in my mouth. I looked up periodically for eye contact. Her head was back on the pillow and obstructed by her round abdomen. This wasn't hot at all, but I was determined to make her climax and I did.

After her orgasm, I lay next to her and we held each other. She went down on me and she was terrible with oral sex, so I masturbated to come. She was a lesbian and experienced with women. She should know what to do.

Afterward, she said she knew this was just a one time encounter and we said our goodbyes.

Sex In My Minivan

I looked for more lesbians on OKCupid, and none caught my eye, so I opened an account on match.com with the handle "Megan".

I was smitten with the online photos of Emily, an attractive blond haired 43-year old lesbian. We sent each other long emails. She said meeting for a hookup was new for her. She asked many questions about my history with women, my relationship with my husband, if I had any children, how long I lived in San Diego, and what I was looking for. I thought those were a lot of questions for a hookup, however I wanted to answer them because wanted to talk to someone about my sexuality and desires for women.

I told her *I love to please a woman sexually.* She wrote back that I made her Wet, and that she loved men but mostly she wanted their sisters or wives. Fucking hot! She asked if my husband wanted to watch. He didn't and I was glad, because I didn't want to show him the lovemaking and tender side of me, and have him secretly think I was ridiculous. We exchanged phone numbers. She texted me a picture of her beautiful round plump breasts, her hand pushed down inside her pants.

This is what I'm doing now

I wanted my hand inside her pants.

I can help you with that

She wrote about the rhythm of our hearts, rubbing clits together, that it didn't matter how long it took for anyone to come, and how she could come just looking in my eyes. It sounded erotic and sensual and exactly what I wanted. We set up a coffee date.

Emily was seated on a leather sofa at the back of the café. Her blond curly hair fell just past her shoulders. She wore a white blouse, a deep red scarf draped across her shoulders, and tight jeans. She greeted me with a hug and beaming smile. I sat down next to her, and she faced me and just smiled. I really liked her. She kept touching my arms as we talked. I liked her touch. I felt sexy and excited to be in public with a beautiful lesbian. We drank our coffees and talked. She excused herself to go to the bathroom and when she returned, she wanted to leave.

"Let's go for a drive," she suggested.

We got in my minivan, and she leaned over to kiss me. She was so soft and smelled so good! I wanted her alone with her clothes off in a bed.

"Let's get a hotel," I suggested.

"Oh, let's just drive," she insisted.

She gave me directions to a nearby park. It was close to dusk and the park was already closed, so we parked in the dirt parking lot across the street. I pulled over to the edge of the lot and we started kissing again. I wished we were in a hotel.

"Let's get in the back seat!" Emily suggested.

"Sure!" I agreed.

I wasn't sure what she had in mind and why we weren't at a hotel. We jumped to the back seat of my minivan. Our kisses grew stronger and we pressed our bodies close. My panties were damp with excitement. I so much wanted to go down on her, smell and taste her pussy, and feel her clit under my tongue. I thought as the lesbian woman she would take my clothes off first, but I started it.

I unbuttoned her blouse. I pulled up her black lacy bra and saw her round full breasts with pink nipples. I sucked gently on her nipples, and I moaned because I was so turned on doing it. She moaned too. I licked her nipples more, and together we removed her blouse and I unbuttoned her pants.

"I'm on my period," she said.

"I don't care."

I was too turned on to care. We slid off her pants. I was very happy that she let me. I myself would have been reluctant to let anyone go down on me during my period, because I would be concerned about the iron-like smell of blood.

Emily spread her legs. Her pubic hair was shaved. I started slow. I kissed her pubic mound and outer lips, and pressed my lips against her vulva and my tongue on her clitoris. So smelled so sweet, she was so soft. I couldn't tell she was on her period. She had probably washed up in the café restroom.

She was moaning and aroused, so I gave her more direct stimulation. I licked her inner lips and clit and moved my tongue all around. She breathed hard and moved her hips up and down. Licking her clit made mine throb. I felt her clit swell under my tongue. And then it got hard…and harder…all the while I was getting aroused and wet and my own clit was hard too. I flicked my tongue sideways over the hard ridge of her clit. Her breathing got heavier. Her legs shook and trembled, she got wetter, and then her moans filled the car. I stayed right on that same spot through her orgasm until she pulled away.

After she came, I kissed her sweet vulva lips. She had a content happy smile. I sat next to her and we held each other, because it seemed that's what I should do. I didn't have romantic feelings for her, and I was sure she had no feelings for me either. I was horny, so I took off my pants and fell back comfortably on the back seat.

Emily knelt on the floor, and gave me oral sex. It started feeling good, but not spectacular. I closed my eyes and tried to get into it more. I looked down at Emily, with her thick mane of curly blond hair between my legs. It was dusk and soon it would be cold. I really just wanted to come. Although her technique wasn't that great, looking at a woman between my legs turned me on. I leaned back and let myself enjoy the pleasure. But my arousal was not building. *I probably should just masturbate to finish myself off.*

A flashlight shone into our rear window.

"You need to move your car, we are closing the park," a loud voice said.

We looked up and saw a park ranger. We looked at each other in part excitement, part worry. I hadn't been caught making out in a car since high school.

"Oh my gosh, are we going to get a ticket?" I cried out.

"Would the charge be indecent exposure in public?" Emily laughed.

"I can't believe he came over here!" I said.

We ducked so he wouldn't see us naked. I wondered if he was turned on seeing two women naked making out in the back of a minivan. Maybe that would prevent him from giving us a ticket.

"Let's get dressed!" Emily was looking around for her clothes.

"Where's my underwear?" I asked.

I rummaged in the dark through piles of clothes on the floor. I was still so horny and disappointed that my oral session was interrupted. I peered out the window. The ranger and flashlight had moved away from my car. His back was to us, and he was probably waiting for us to leave. It didn't look like he was writing up a ticket. We got dressed and drove off. The ranger just stood there until we were gone.

"I'm so horny. I just want to come!" I told her.

"I know," she said. "Just drive around and let's find another place to park."

We drove around and pulled into the far end of a parking lot at a community park. We got in the back seat. I pulled down my pants and leaned back against her and masturbated as she held me. I was aroused, yet my masturbation wasn't building into an orgasm. Maybe it was because I couldn't see her, kiss her, or touch her, and when I opened my eyes I was looking straight ahead at a parking lot. I closed my eyes and started fantasizing, but I was too aware of being in a parking lot and being exposed was a turn-off, not a turn-on. It took me a long time to come and it had felt like work. After my orgasm, I drove her back to her car.

Driving home, I wondered why this woman hadn't been able to make me come, why I could make her come, and why it took me so long to have an orgasm. Was it her technique? Was I really that difficult to get off? Maybe I wasn't turned on by women after all, or maybe only by some women?

When I got home, I was excited to tell Brad all about my crazy adventure and the park ranger. Brad thought it was funny and he encouraged me to get together with Emily again. I was really happy that Brad shared in my enthusiasm and that I had married a man who was secure in himself and supported whatever made me happy.

Emily e-mailed me the next day to say what she liked about our encounter. She said it was hot, that I was lusty and went for what I wanted, and that I was about to discover the rich world of lesbian sex and relationships. I didn't feel that way about women. However, I wanted more sexual experiences with women, and experience some of the tenderness and sensuality she described because I could never have that with Brad.

After some back-and-forth planning and some cancelled dates on her part, I met Emily at a hotel for a second date. I wasn't feeling as turned on by Emily anymore, because she had been so unreliable about when and where to meet, and she seemed preoccupied. My curiosity made me stay. I gave her an orgasm going down on her, and then she went down on me. It felt good but not amazing. After about 15 minutes she stopped.

"It's taking you too long to come," she said.

"Really? I have a thing about that, because my husband tells me I take too long."

"Well, that's your issue and that's on you," she said and lay down next to me.

I thought of women as giving and loving to give oral to another woman. I didn't expect her to have a time limit like my husband. I pushed my hurt away.

"Here, I'll just masturbate," I suggested.

I masturbated while she held me. There was nothing romantic or sexy about the way we did it. Then we got dressed and went to dinner, and afterward I dropped her back at the hotel. She didn't ask me to spend the night, and I didn't want to. The sex with lesbians so far was disappointing.

Her Skilled Tongue
I went back on match.com and was immediately attracted to Sarah, a fit attractive 51-year old professional woman. She looked a little masculine, and had thin lips, and both were a big turn on. We met for lunch. She was nervous, and her hands shook. Some of her tension was because she saw coworkers seated nearby, and didn't want to be seen on a date with a woman.

"I was married for 20 years to a woman," she told me. "I had artificial insemination and gave birth to two girls and a boy, and my wife adopted them."

I had never known a lesbian couple and loved getting a glimpse inside her life.

"Why did it end?" I asked.

"My wife lost interest in sex. We slept in separate rooms the last six years of our relationship. "

"Wow. My husband and I also slept in separate rooms for about that long too. Why did you stay so long?"

"For the children. But I have a high sex drive and I'm always horny, so I finally decided enough is enough and I left her two years ago."

"Wow, that's the same reason I left my marriage too! Good for you!"

"I haven't had sex since I left her," she told me. Her voice was still shaky.

All in all, she hadn't had any sex in eight years, and she was really turned on, so I could see why she was so nervous.

"What? Why not?" I was shocked.

"I didn't want to sleep around, and I was also self conscious about the weight I gained from the pregnancies. I've been working out and eating better, and now I'm fit and confident, and ready to get out there and date, and voila, you're my first date."

"Well, you look great!" I told her.

She invited me over, and we drove separately to the house she had purchased the year before. We went straight to her bedroom. As we kissed, I could feel myself very wet. Our breathing deepened.

"I want you to go down on me," I almost begged, and pressed my hips closer to her body.

"I can't wait to taste you," she said, looking in my eyes.

Her pupils were dilated. I wondered how wet she was and if she could make me come. We undressed. Her lips brushed my neck and then my nipples, as she slowly made her way down my body. By then my clit was throbbing.

I shuddered when her tongue brushed my thighs. I wanted her tongue on my clit, but she didn't go straight there. She licked and sucked on my outer and inner lips. Her tongue hit my clit and I gasped. She innately had the gentle touch that brought me to orgasm. She licked my clit so gently, just the way I liked. As her tongue circled my clit, I could feel the pleasure and intensity kept increasing, more and more, and my moans grew louder. The more I moaned, the more excited she got. She moaned and panted so hard, I looked up. She was so sweaty, her hair stuck to her forehead. When I saw how turned on she was, I relaxed mentally and that's when my orgasm started building from deep inside. My breathing got deeper and heavier, and then I felt my orgasm was imminent. Sarah flicked her tongue lightly on my clit, just teasing the orgasm out of me. It felt like my clit swelled up to reach her tongue, and then I exploded into a deep long intense orgasm that lasted for almost 30 seconds.

"Oh my God, thank you so much!! That's the first time anyone has made me come in about 20 years!"

She smiled.

"Wow, that was amazing, I can't believe you made me come going down on me."

The last time I climaxed from oral sex was decades earlier, on my vacation with Zoe. I didn't recall if Brad ever gave me an orgasm from oral sex. I remembered one boyfriend in college made me come from oral sex, but I didn't recall if any other man ever did. I was just thrilled somebody could make me come.

She lay on the bed. I went straight to her pussy and saw how wet she was. Soaking wet. She would enjoy this. I knew I was good at oral. I made every woman I was ever with come from it. Going down on her wasn't as much of a turn-on after I had already come, but I did it for the fairness and challenge.

I gently ran my tongue on her vulva, exploring her succulent region from the outside in. As Sarah's breathing deepened, I licked my tongue mostly on the ridge of her clit, and stayed in one spot. I knew she liked it because her breathing got heavier. She was so sexy as she got turned on. Her legs shook, and I knew she was close to coming. As she was closer, I licked the button part of her clitoris in steady rhythmic strokes. She moaned loud and pulled away from my mouth. I felt satisfied that I could please a woman. I lay on her and kissed her on the forehead.

"What we did was so beautiful! We each just gave each other an experience that got us all lit up. More women should have casual sex!" I told her.

Why could she make me come when other women could not? Could a man ever get me to orgasm? I was so thrilled about my oral sex orgasm, I scheduled a second date with her. She invited me for coffee at her house two weeks later.

"I met someone. I can't see you after today." She blushed and smiled. "She and I haven't progressed to kissing yet, but I'm horny, so I definitely want sex with you today."

That time we had sex in her living room, and it felt like it was just physical. I wasn't emotionally or mentally attracted to her, and the sex seemed boring because we just took turns going down on each other. We did not see each other again.

OUR COUPLE SWAP

On New Year's Eve, Brad and I went to a lifestyle party. A couple I had not seen before caught my attention. Tim, a handsome, dark-haired man in his early 40's, strode across the dance floor followed by Krista, a slender red-head in her early 30's, who wore a long dress and choker necklace. She exuded sexual energy in every step of her swaying hips and dreamy eyes. They walked up to the big bedroom. I waited a few minutes, and then followed them in to watch. Over a dozen naked bodies were fucking on the bed.

Tim held an attractive older woman, probably in her early 60's, on his lap. He bounced her up and down slowly on his penis, as they gazed in each other's eyes. I was surprised that a young man could connect so intensely with a woman so much older. Their eye contact during intercourse made me wet and aroused. Krista was in the middle of the bed, surrounded by naked bodies, and moaned loudly while riding a cock. She seemed like she was in the middle of an orgasm. Tim didn't seem to mind that she was having so much pleasure with another man's cock.

I returned to the main room and sat on the sofa, and watched people on the dance floor and stripper pole. A little later, Tim came downstairs and sat next to me.

"I really enjoyed watching you with that older woman. You made such an intense connection with her."

"Yes, she was quite erotic."

"Is your girlfriend bi?"

"Ask her."

Just then, Krista came downstairs and sat between us on the sofa.

"Are you bi?" I asked.

She looked me straight in the eyes. "Yes, I am."

She looked so beautiful. She told me they were on vacation from Virginia.

"We just went online to find out what to do for New Year's Eve, and we found this event, so here we are. We're only in town for three days," she told me.

I leaned forward to kiss her. Her lips felt soft, and kissing her made me wet. I pushed my body into hers and kissed her harder. She responded likewise. She breathed heavier and moaned softly, and she leaned forward into me. She was definitely bi. I looked up to see if Tim minded, or if he expected to be included. He was just watching the dancers. Brad sat on my other side.

"Can we go in a room?" I asked Krista.

"Sure," she said in a soft voice, as she looked me in the eyes.

She turned to her boyfriend. "Tim, we're going in a room. You guys can come later if you want."

Tim nodded in agreement. Krista took me by the hand and led me across the dance floor, through the kitchen, and down the hallway to an empty bedroom with a massage table. We kissed each other and took off our clothes. She was stunning, with her white skin, lean body, and small breasts. I liked her confidence and that she didn't need her man to be there with us.

She lay down on the massage table, and I kneeled on the floor, licking her pussy. She smelled sweet. Her vulva was beautiful, and her vaginal opening was barely noticeable. It was small and tight, just like those of other women who had not given birth. I found out later she gave birth by C-section. I was curious to someday see a pussy of a woman who gave vaginal birth and how her vagina and pussy looked, because I thought mine was ugly after giving birth. My vaginal opening was stretched open a little. No man had complained about it, but I thought it was unattractive

I had barely been licking her, when the men came in. I was still sure I wouldn't be removing my panties for Tim. I wasn't that attracted to him.

"I don't want to kiss you or have you fuck me, but I'll give you a blow job," I told Tim.

"Sure, that's fine," he said.

I liked that he was just going with the flow. Brad stopped kissing Krista and put on a condom.

"Stay standing," I told Tim.

I knelt on the ground and gave him a blowjob. A minute into it, he looked down at me and said, "Hey, let's watch them!"

"Yeah, I'd love to," I said.

Finally! These people that knew couple swapping was hotter if we could watch our partners give and receive pleasure. I watched Krista lay on her back on that massage table, writhing and moving, as Brad stood at the edge of the table and penetrated her deeply. She looked at him longingly with those faraway eyes, moaning, writhing, moaning louder, and apparently having many orgasms from it. I had never seen anyone look so beautiful or move so lustily during intercourse!

They noticed we were watching. I went back to sucking Tim's cock. I felt a warm rush of liquid in the back of my throat. I looked up at him as he finished coming. Krista was smiling at her boyfriend, so she and Brad took a break. I was curious about all the moaning she had done while Brad fucked her.

"Do you have orgasms from intercourse?" I asked.

"Yes!"

I was envious and at the same time hoped she could give me some tips on how I could do that. If I could have vaginal orgasms I could climax during intercourse, an activity that I could do with my man, and not have to rely on masturbation or oral sex, which seemed boring and tedious for a man to do or observe.

"How do you move like that during intercourse, how do you know how to move?"

"I just do what feels good. I just let go, and feel my body, and I move the way it feels good," she explained.

"Well, don't you have to move in a way the guy likes too? Brad doesn't like me on top, because it doesn't feel good, so I move the way he likes it," I told her.

"Oh don't do that. Don't worry about what the guy likes. Just move how you like. Be selfish."

Wow. I had never thought of that. I didn't have to move the way a man liked. I could do what I wanted. I couldn't wait to try that.

"How did you learn to look at people like that? Your eyes and your gaze are so sexy and seductive!" I told her.

"Oh, Tim taught me that," she said laughing. "He taught me the importance of eye contact and luring my lover in."

Krista turned to Brad, "Do you want a blowjob?"

"Yes!" He replied eagerly.

She took my husband's cock deep in her throat, all the way down. She sucked him and sucked him, and Brad's head was bent back in ecstasy. Finally he let out a loud roar as he came in her mouth.

"Oh my god, that was the best blowjob of my life!" he yelled out.

My heart dropped into my stomach. I was furious and extremely jealous! I couldn't believe he said it. Even if it were true, did he have to say it like that in front of me? I'd never be able to compete. I tried deep throating in my youth and gagged on the penises. I had written off deep throating as something I would never have to do because Brad loved my blowjobs. My reality shifted. To give him the best blowjobs, I would need to deep throat going forward. I didn't want to deep throat and that meant he would no longer like my blowjobs.

I fought back tears, because I didn't want to show my jealousy and ruin the fun everyone had. We had to walk through the large living room to get to the front door. I braced myself. All eyes were on the four of us, as the swingers gauged how good our encounter had been. I kept a straight face, because I couldn't force a fake smile.

In the car, I let Brad have it.

"How could you be so insensitive? I am sooo jealous!" I yelled.

"Oh honey, I'm so sorry, I'll make it up to you," he said. "Listen, when we get home, I'll go down on you until you come."

That was a nice offer and it settled me down. By the time we got home it was about 3 a.m. and Brad kept his word. He went down on me for 45 minutes. However, he couldn't make me come. In fact, I couldn't remember the last time he made me come.

Despite my jealousy over the blowjob, we had connected very well with Tim and Krista, and we all wanted to have more sex. Krista mesmerized Brad. Over the next three days, we met up again for couple swapping. Tim wanted to give Brad a blowjob but Brad refused to let a man touch him. Tim was an extremely skilled lover, with a hard cock, and one night after he warmed me up with several hours of foreplay and deep vaginal penetration, we had anal sex that left me begging for more. It was only the third time in my life I had anal sex. He said he was so good at it because he was bisexual and knew how to be gentle and make it feel good. He said the woman needed to be fully engorged and dripping wet before it should be attempted.

After they left town, Brad told me he was done swinging. He said he didn't like the person he had become. I understood what he meant. The constant search for new sexual encounters and the titillating pictures on the lifestyle site left us constantly horny and looking for something outside ourselves. We deleted our profile on the lifestyle site. But my desire and hunger for sexual and emotional experiences with were as big as ever.

"IF YOU WON'T FUCK ME, I'LL FIND SOMEONE WHO WILL"

A few days later, when Brad got up and left me in bed wet and horny, I ached for fulfilling deep long fucking. It wasn't the quantity of sex that was the problem: it was the quality and that was just getting worse.

"Honey, I really want to have sex with Eliot again and with other men," I told him later that morning.

"No. You could fall for one of them," he replied.

I didn't care if I could fall for anyone or if Brad wanted monogamy. I wanted satisfying sex, and if Brad kept refusing to give me that, I would get it elsewhere. I was a woman with sexual rights, not someone's property.

"I'm going to have sex with other men, and I don't care if you like it."

We argued about it. Eventually he said I could fuck whomever I wanted as long as he did not know about it. I wasn't concerned I would fall for someone else. I was in love with Brad. We still went for coffee after work and morning walks on the beach. We had our family dinners with Oliver. We talked about our investments and went to bed together and cuddled at night.

That week, Mary called to invite me to a polyamory potluck meetup. The event was held at Kamala Devi McClure's house in Pacific Beach. Kamala Devi was a nationally known polyamory spokesperson I had seen on a cable TV show about polyamory. The small living room was filled with about 30 people. She instructed us to do some group exercises involving eye gazing, which I found very uncomfortable. A man sat across from me, and we sat and looked each other in the eye. I wanted to smile or run away, but I did it. Kamala Devi's primary partner was the father of her young son.

"We have 11 lovers in our pod, and at our next meeting, we will discuss adding another person. Everyone practices poly differently, but one of our best practices is to only add lovers that are enhancing to the previously existing ones."

She and her lovers all practiced yoga, meditation, self-growth, and authentic communication, so their lifestyle had a much more alluring charm than just the random hookups I had seen with the swingers. Mary and I were totally intrigued by it.

I had questions for Kamala Devi. She lay on the sofa with a woman in a non-sexual embrace.

"Kamala Devi, can I ask you a question," I asked.

"Yes," she smiled at me.

"Brad thinks I will love him less when I have other lovers. Is that true?" I asked.

"That's a limiting belief," she said matter-of-factly.

"Wow, I love that. But he gets jealous. What can he do?" I asked her.

"Give attention to your existing partner in proportion to the attention you are giving your new partner," she advised.

"I have another question. I had sex with my high school friend's husband after she died."

She smiled. "That makes sense. And what a beautiful way to honor the memory of your friend!"

A few weeks later, I flew back to Denver for another tryst with Eliot. He was rock hard for a long time and made me feel like a real woman, even though he couldn't give me an orgasm and I masturbated to come. On the flight home all I could see was the big gap between the sex I had with Eliot and the sex I had with my husband. It wasn't okay anymore. I was no longer going to put up with the sex that Brad gave me. He needed to man up. I waited until after dinner and then I told him.

"I want with you what I had with Eliot. I want you to kiss me, to be hard for me, to look at me when we make love. I want to dance for you and wear sexy lingerie. I want you to stay hard long enough to go down on me and care about my orgasm."

He replied as he usually did. "Well, honey, sex is just not that important. I like what we have."

Damn it Brad, you better step it up or I swear this is over.

"You're not a good lover. I'm bored with you sexually."

Brad got up and went into Chandi's room, which doubled as the guest room while she was away at college, and slammed the door. I really didn't care what he did at that point. I loved him and I wanted him sexually more than anyone, but if all he had to offer was the kind of sex we had been having, I didn't want sex with him at all!

He didn't come out until the next morning. He didn't speak to me until that evening.

"I'll give you what you want, but I won't get testosterone treatments because those are bad for my body."

He looked mad and resigned. He didn't say anything about his resentments against me, and he didn't show any empathy for my longing or unhappiness.

In that moment, I lost all desire for him. His reckless disregard for my feelings turned me off. I no longer wanted the man who threw bits of married sex at me and then got up, leaving me in bed wet and horny. Even the porn women got better sex than that.

"I AM SO TIRED OF BEING TOLD NO"

I was crying over Brad more frequently. I was almost in despair. Why didn't he want me sexually? The passion I felt in sexual union with Eliot was so emotionally rich, it overpowered the pleasure I felt from San Diego sunshine, fluffy clouds, or conversations with colleagues at the office. I no longer derived pleasure from daily life, and I constantly longed for what I had a hotel room in Denver.

Fortunately, I had my monthly dinner with Mindy that week. I told her everything. I was completely out of my power and I didn't like it. I had tried everything I could think of and I was completely unhappy.

"Do people ever leave a marriage after 25 years?"

I couldn't believe those words came out of my mouth.

"Yes, they do," and she turned to look at me.

"Well, how would I support myself if I lived on my own?" I asked.

"Your life will be different, but you will still have a life," she answered. "Maybe you will live in an apartment instead of a house. Maybe you will live in a cheaper part of town."

That didn't sound appealing at all, and I didn't give it any further thought. A few days later, when I went out for coffee, I saw a colleague from my real estate days, seated outside. He had a faraway look in his eyes.

"Are you okay?" I asked.

"I'm so tired of being told *no*," Greg said as he shook his head side to side, his eyes downcast. "She keeps refusing to have sex with me!"

Why was he telling me that? I barely knew him.

"I'm so sorry," I said.

"And when we do have sex, she constantly asks if I'm done yet or says *hurry up, hurry up*. You know, that's what it must be like to get a hooker, " Greg looked up.

"Does she masturbate?" I asked.

"I don't know," he replied.

"What? You don't know if she masturbates?"

"No, I don't know. I don't see her do it," he replied.

"Well, does she like women? Is she gay?"

"No, I don't think so."

"Gosh, I'm so sorry Greg. Brad tells me *no* all the time and I'm tired of it too."

"She has no emotion during sex. She just lies there telling me to hurry up. Damn, she won't even let me go down on her. I just want to please her so much. And she doesn't go down on me at all, not ever."

"Is she Catholic?"

"No, she grew up in the conservative South though. And when we do have sex, she leaves her clothes on. I'm just tired of the constant rejection."

"Wow, I'm so sorry. Why do you put up with it?"

His mouth broke into a smile. "Have you seen my wife? She's gorgeous!"

Yes, she was. But still, how could be so in love with her, when she was so cold? Was he was a selfish lover? If so, why didn't she tell him?

"Have you guys gone to marriage counseling?"

"She won't go."

"Oh, that sucks. Brad tells me no all the time. I lay there in bed wanting him, and he tells me no. He won't kiss me, he won't go down on me, and he gets off quick and leaves me lying there. I cry over him a lot."

"I'm really sorry," he empathized.

From that day on, Greg's words kept ringing in my head: "I'm so tired of being told *no*. I'm so tired of being told *no*. I'm so tired of being told *no*. I'm so tired of being told *no*."

JENNA: SHE FINGER FUCKED ME LIKE A GUY

My match.com profile started with: *Ferociously bi and, please don't hold this against me you beautiful lesbian women, I am also married…*

That's where Jenna found me. I got a message when she marked me as a 'favorite'. I looked at her profile picture and she was hot! I felt a warm rush in my body and my heart skipped a beat. She was the type of lesbian who turned me on immensely, but was rare to find: beautiful, sporty, androgynous, slender, 5'10", with blond hair. She wore a baseball cap backwards. She was 49 years old and lived in Irvine, an hour away. I was immediately smitten and sent her a message.

Hi Jenna, you're so hot. I can't wait to meet you.

I'm just looking for something casual. I will be in San Diego in two weeks and stay at a hotel downtown. I will let you know.

It was cold and rainy the day she finally came to San Diego, She texted me after she was checked into her hotel, and suggested two restaurants for dinner. I liked that she took charge and knew of good places to eat.

I walked into the lobby of her hotel. A slim woman walked briskly toward me. She wore a heavy black leather jacket, jeans, and walking shoes. Her shiny hair fell just past her shoulders. She definitely looked lesbian. My heart raced. She took me by the arm, turned me around in the direction she was walking, and said, "Hi…let's go."

Damn, that was hot. I liked how she took charge. I walked next to her through the cold blustery evening, and tried to keep up. I liked her energy. I couldn't take my eyes off her. *God, she's so fucking beautiful and sexy!* She opened the hotel door for me, and guided me on our walk to the restaurant. She placed her hand on my back to move me past oncoming pedestrians. I liked her energetic gait and how she guided me.

At the restaurant, she walked up to the hostess and announced her name. This was new. When I went out with Brad, I put in our name, because he didn't like doing that. Having someone take charge like Jenna did made me feel protected and safe, like I was with someone who could handle the world.

The hostess led us to our table. Jenna walked behind me, teasing me about my online screen name.

"Megan, huh?"

I liked how she flirted with me. I got excited thinking that the people around us imagined what might be between us sexually. At the table, Jenna pulled out her smartphone and put on a pair of stylish reading glasses. She looked like a hot executive as she messaged someone on her phone and read the menu.

I ordered red wine. Jenna ordered scotch. *She's sexy as fuck, a woman who acts like a man!* I looked at her with the same wonder and admiration I had previously felt for handsome successful businessmen. I wondered how she would be in bed. Would she love going down on me? How would she kiss?

"My girlfriend left me," she said, and looked right at me.

Just like that. She just admitted it. They had been together for 14 years, and a few months earlier, the woman had just left. Jenna told me she was devastated by the breakup. I couldn't see it in her face..

"Wow, I'm sorry." I didn't know what to say.

"I did everything for her," she told me, and looked right at me. She must have sensed I was wondering if she'd do everything for me too, so she laid that to rest.

"I'll never do that again."

"How is it being single?" I asked.

"It was very difficult at first, and now I'm happy again. I'm very busy and I don't want a relationship."

I admired her for being so happy as a single woman. I loved being in my relationship with Brad. Would I be so happy if I were single?

"I love to watch porn of women masturbating. I'd love to sit across from you in a chair and have you watch me do that," I told her.

She took a drink of her scotch.

"I don't watch porn."

I took that as she didn't watch porn and she didn't want to watch me masturbate, and then I didn't want to tell her any more fantasies.

Over dinner, she told me about her math degree and her work in commercial real estate. She loved the San Diego Padres baseball team, had "pretty good seats" and went to most of the games. I imagined going to a baseball game with her. I had never been to a sports game because I really wasn't into sports. I would definitely go with her! The waitress came up and put the check in front of Jenna. How did the waitress know that Jenna was taking care of me, that she was like the man? It was so hot.

We walked back quickly through the cold, drizzling rain. Back in the room, I walked over the window to look out at the downtown lights. Jenna walked up behind me. I turned around. She came closer and leaned over for a kiss. Her kiss was ordinary. It didn't turn me on, but I was curious about what would happen next. We kept kissing and fumbled off our clothes and eventually we tumbled in that large soft bed that took up most of the small room.

She sat up, and took off all her Indian rudraksha beads and put them on her nightstand next to her incense. My heart beat a few harder beats, I felt hot, and my head felt light. I had never been with a lover who was interested in meditation. I imagined myself wearing Indian beads, burning incense, and meditating together. She placed all her beads on the nightstand, next to her Bhagavad Gita. We got under the sheets and lay next to each other, hungrily kissing.

"Do you like strap-ons?" she asked.

Her question took my by surprise. Why would we need a strap-on? If I wanted penetration, I'd be with a man! I hadn't thought about using a strap-on with a woman. Wouldn't women want clitoral stimulation? If they wanted vaginal penetration, wouldn't they get a man? I didn't know what a strap-on could do for me.

"No, I don't want a strap-on. Penises are overrated."

The words just came out of my mouth. Did I really not like penises? I liked men, but penises didn't give me orgasms and they didn't stay hard long enough and they moved too fast and they didn't always feel good and many penises were out for themselves and their own pleasure and let me down. I wanted a different kind of sex: sex that gave me orgasms. There was no need for any penises.

"I didn't expect that from you."

She seemed pleased. She motioned to her overnight bag in the closet. "I brought some strap-ons, but we won't use them."

Then she kissed me again. I kissed her deeply and took in all of her strength. I felt her hand pressing on my pubic mound, while she massaged my labia with her fingers. Her face was right up against mine, her eyes open, looking right at me, as if I were her little toy. I was a little uncomfortable kissing someone with eyes open. I looked at her beautiful face, with its smooth skin, her brown eyes, her blond hair thrown softly around her face. She didn't have any wrinkles, which was surprising for her age of 49. I wondered if she had a procedure done. Orange County women were known for that.

Her lips were tender and gentle, yet I could feel her power. My tongue merged with hers and I didn't want to stop kissing. I nibbled on her soft lips. She responded to my passion with fervor. I didn't know I liked kissing so much.

She rubbed her clit on my pubic bone while we kissed. She was getting more and more turned on, rubbing harder and harder until it hurt. She was so strong and used such force and pressure. I was a little scared for a few seconds. She was stronger than any man I had been with. I remembered she lifted weights and trained for marathons. Her grinding was making my pubic bone hurt a lot. I almost wanted to cry. I didn't want to ruin the moment and I was curious about what she would do. I decided we'd have a talk later about what we each liked, and for now I'd just endure it. She finally stopped the grinding and lay next to me.

She put two fingers in me, deep inside. Yesssssss, it felt so good. This was penetration done for my pleasure, not the pleasure of a man who just moved in me to ejaculate. She was doing what would feel good for me. She moved them in, out, slowly and sensuously, then a little deeper with each thrust. I was extremely wet. My whimper turned into a moan. I picked up a tempo of my own and pushed with my hips to get all of her inside me, as deeply as I could.

"Deeper, go deeper, deep, deep," I begged. "More, more more…."

I leaned forward and kissed her hard and pushed my tongue deep in her mouth with the same vigor she used to stick her fingers up my cunt. My moans were loud, like an animal. I wanted to be fucked deeply and have it never end.

Finger-fucking me turned her on also. She lifted me up and turned me on my stomach and fucked me doggy style. Then she moved me on my back and got on top, all the while kissing and finger fucking me. She fucked me like a guy, except she had her fingers in place of a penis. She tossed me around in bed, fucking me harder and deeper, her beautiful brown eyes intently on me.

She pulled out and sat up at my vulva. She spread her second and middle fingers apart, and slid them inside me. I wrapped my legs around her waist. She looked at me and wanted to bring me closer.

"I've got you," she said, and pulled me up.

"I don't know, I'm afraid to let go." My legs were still wrapped around her and I didn't think she could pull me up.

"I've got you," she repeated.

I trusted her and surrendered, and that turned me on more. She pulled me up, and I straddled her. I looked her right in the eyes and wrapped my arms around her. Her fingers penetrating me deeply were so pleasurable I didn't know why I ever needed a penis. I moved my hips up and down on her fingers. I felt like I was in a far away land, barely aware of anything but a pleasure spot deep inside my pussy.

My moaning was turning her on madly, so she said, "that does it", and she lifted me up, carried me over to the wet bar, sat me down, and finger-fucked me in earnest. My back must have bumped against the wine glasses, because I heard clanking. The noise took her out of her zone, because she slowed down a bit and carried me back to the bed.

I wanted to taste her and run my tongue all along and around her clitoris. I wanted to slide my tongue inside her and taste and inhale her deeply. I wanted to do all that while she sat on my face and smothered me with her strength and wetness.

"Can I go down on you?" I asked, too embarrassed to mention the face sitting.

"Yes."

She had long curly blond pubic hair, lots of it. It was sexy as hell. She tasted sweet. I licked her clit in many different ways, and at the end, I focused on the ridge, which was getting harder, and the knob, which was harder still, until she had an orgasm. Then I lay on her while we kissed.

"Will you go down on me?" I asked.

She hesitated, sighed, and said, "I don't know where you've been."

And then she did it anyway. I expected to be taken to new heights. She started to lick around my labia in places that didn't feel so good and she used too much pressure. She was horrible at oral sex! It didn't feel good at all, and after about two minutes she stopped and rolled on her back and looked at the ceiling.

"My neck hurts."

That sounded final. What kind of lesbian was she? I pushed the thought aside and reverted back to what I knew: masturbating. It was not all how I wanted to come. I lay next to her and masturbated while she held me close and watched me like her little toy. After about ten minutes it was clear I was having trouble building my orgasm. Kissing her and fantasizing did not help. Some women may have faked an orgasm at that point, but I had never done that and wasn't about to start. I was determined to come. I fantasized about a man watching me, and hoped she didn't sense my mind was far away. Finally I felt my orgasm building. I opened my eyes to look at her just as I was coming. She was looking at me too.

I liked her kissing, but the rest of the sex was horrible. Maybe we could talk about it and improve on the parts I didn't like. Maybe we could start dating, and possibly she could be my girlfriend on the side. I felt content and sleepy laying next to her. I looked at the clock. It was 2 a.m. I didn't want to leave.

"I'm supposed to go home to sleep, but I don't care what my husband thinks. I'm tired and I want to sleep with you."

"You can sleep here. You can use my toothbrush," she offered.

I was happy she wanted me to stay. I left in my contacts, and fell asleep in Jenna's warm embrace. Throughout the night and every time I woke up, I snuggled up next to Jenna and kissed her. She kissed me back. I didn't worry about waking her. She wasn't like Brad. She liked sex and I felt she would be happy to be awakened in the night if the reason for the waking was our kissing.

I dreaded the morning, thinking she would want to get up and do something that took us out of our cozy embrace, because that's what Brad would want to do. He would have skipped the sex and gone outside to explore. I drifted back to sleep. I woke at sunrise and saw her stretch her arms.

"Do you want to get up?" I asked.

"And do what?" she asked.

She kept lying there, all beautiful and relaxed. My heart felt warm and my mind raced with all the possibilities. I wanted to go lick her pussy again and started to move down on her body. I thought she would offer to wash up. She didn't. I was a little worried she might smell or taste badly and that I wouldn't like her anymore if she did. I licked my tongue all around her vulva. She tasted as sweet as she had the night before. Why did Brad ask me to wash up in the morning before going down on me? Jenna was proof that women's pussies were sweet and beautiful, and not some nasty thing that needed to be constantly scrubbed.

She came quickly. After she came, she fingered me for a short time and then she stopped probably because she wasn't turned on anymore and we both knew the fingering wouldn't make me come. She didn't offer to do anything.

"I'll masturbate," I said.

She didn't say anything. She lay next to me, and she watched me as she had done the night before. I was disappointed because it bored me. Afterward she kissed me, and I felt warm inside and happy. We drank coffee and talked.

"I like being in a relationship," I said.

"All women like being in a relationship."

"But you don't."

She didn't answer.

"I better go," I told Jenna.

She insisted on walking me to my car. When I got home, I was ready to defend my sleepover to Brad.

"It's okay you spent the night with her," he said.

I was relieved. Apparently, a woman didn't threaten him.

I texted Jenna when I got home. I told her I would love to see her again in two weeks. She texted back to say she had a nice evening with me, and was glad everything worked out. She didn't say anything about seeing each other again.

I was miserable that night, lying in bed with Brad. It was the first time in years I did not want him. What I wanted was kissing and connection, a kind he had never provided. I thought about Jenna. How could I ever be in love with him again, when he wouldn't even kiss me?

The next day, I replayed in my mind the most fulfilling moments with Jenna, particularly the kissing. Jenna was a flowing brook in my heart. I yearned to be with her again. I wanted to talk with her about spiritual things, go to a baseball game, have sex and experiment sexually, and I didn't want to wait two weeks. Although I was desperate, I could not show it. I used all my self-control and waited a few more days and then I texted her again. The minutes dragged on as I kept checking my phone for her reply.

Then, two days later, I saw a text from her on my phone. My heart raced. What did she say? I would have got in the car right then to drive to her house. Her text said: *Enjoyed your company, have a great week*. I wasn't a fucking real estate client, I was the girl who kissed her in bed and gave her orgasms.

My week wasn't going to be great at all. It was going to be freaking miserable. My chest felt heavy. Why didn't she ask to see me again? She said she had enjoyed herself. Was she holding back because she thought maybe I didn't feel the same? I could reassure her that I had a great time also (but I had already done that). Was she was afraid to be hurt again, and if so, then I could show her I was serious and she might trust me and let herself go. I battled the urge to text again or heaven forbid, call her. I didn't want to turn into some kind of stalker or desperate love-lorn woman. I knew I had to keep myself together. But I didn't *feel* together at all.

Maybe I could get her the same way a man got a woman: by persisting. I sent more texts, and I wrote her I *remembered how sweet it was to sleep with you and reach over and hold and kiss you.* Jenna didn't reply.

I kept going about my life as usual, working, meditating, grocery shopping, exercising, and dating. All of it felt bland. Brad was a gray rock, taking up space in the house without contributing anything to my broken heart. My heart longed for arms that held me tight, fingers that sought my pleasure, and lips that kissed me tenderly...arms and fingers and lips like Jenna's. My pussy longed for a hard cock that pleasured me deeply...a cock like Eliot's. I was done with a log in my bed. Jenna and Eliot showed me what was missing in my marriage.

I wasn't going to sit around and wait for Jenna or Eliot to want me, so I went back online looking for lesbians. I hoped to meet someone as enchanting as Jenna, who was equally interested in me. The problem was the small lesbian population in San Diego. In the age group of 40-50 years, in a heavily gay neighborhood, match.com showed 64 lesbians and 1900 straight women. Many of the women who responded online did not want to meet a married woman. I had some interesting conversations with Tina, who wanted to know if I was a top or a bottom, and who liked to top from the bottom. A Mexican Jewish girl sweetly declined, and wrote she was looking for a good Jewish girl. A woman with the email handle named after a flower wrote she didn't understand why I was still married if I obviously enjoyed sex with women. A woman named Mary seemed intrigued by both my bisexuality and my married status. *Might be kind of exciting,* she wrote. But the biggest problem was that most lesbians in that age range were unattractive and overweight.

I relaxed some of my criteria and arranged some coffee dates. On dates, I had a harder time relating to lesbians because our lifestyles were so different. Often they had not been married, and since there were no children they often had a series of shorter-term relationships. None of the women I met so far had children. I met a few of the women for dates. Mary was a beautiful 44-year-old lesbian, yet I felt no attraction for her. Over dinner, all I wanted to talk about were Brad and Jenna and my broken heart. It really wasn't fair to her. I was not dating material in the state I was in. I decided to stop meeting new women until I was not sad anymore.

Then, a text message came from Jenna. She said my persistence had paid off, and she could come see me the next weekend.

JENNA: "WHAT DO YOU LIKE ABOUT MEN?"

She stayed downtown at the same hotel. When I saw her, my heart melted. She was so strong and beautiful. Her shoulder-length blond curly hair rested on a stylish gray sweater. She stood at the door to her hotel room, and looked at me intently. She waited for me to come to her. It was such a confident move, and it turned me on.

"How was your day?" she asked.

"It was great. I had a really good run this morning. "

I put down my belongings. I had brought some overnight items that time. I sat in the chair. She lay on the bed, and propped her head on pillows.

"What sign are you?" she asked.

"Libra."

"I have to get up early tomorrow to meet my friends for brunch."

"I want to keep seeing you."

"But you're married," she said, and looked right at me to gauge my response.

"My husband doesn't mind if I keep seeing you."

I wanted him, and I wanted her. I wanted them both. I contemplated if I would leave my husband for her. No, I wouldn't leave one person for another. That's what emotional people did. I joined her on the bed and we kissed.

"Let's just get under the covers," I suggested.

We took off our clothes and snuggled under the warm down covers. We wrapped our arms around each other and kissed. I got lost in her again.

"What do you like about men?" she asked.

I liked her probing questions. What did I like about a man? Was it the penis? No, definitely not. Fingering felt just as good as a penis. Besides, on our first date, I told Jenna penises were overrated. My love of men had nothing to do with a penis. Then why did I like men? Hmmm...

"I like their strength."

Yes, that was it. I liked their physical strength, their mental strength, and their emotional strength. I liked that they were more logical and less emotional, I liked the security and protection they provided. I liked the stories they told. I liked that they liked to go out into the world and be outdoors, start businesses, take risks, provide. Then I realized, Jenna had all that. She had enough male energy to be all that and it made me want her even more. We went back to kissing and we rolled around in bed and it was enough.

"I just love kissing you. You're like a drug," she said, rolling me around in bed.

She had never done drugs. She just hungered for my sweetness. But besides kissing, the rest of the sex was mediocre. She got aroused finger fucking me and then came quickly from my cunnilingus.. I masturbated to come.

"I have to get up early," she announced, signaling it was time for me to leave.

"I brought my overnight things in case you wanted me to stay," I said, hopeful.

"No, I have to get up early tomorrow." She stared at me intently.

My chest felt heavy and my eyes teared up.

"Are you okay?" she asked.

I wasn't sure. I got dressed, grabbed my purse, and slowly walked to the door. She walked behind me. I turned around to face her.

"Yeah, I'm okay," I said through moist eyes.

"I'll walk you to your car," and she grabbed her jacket.

I fought back tears as we walked to my car. Why had she asked me to leave, when she had said kissing me was like a drug? At my car, she gave me a quick kiss and I watched her walk away.

"Don't forget about me," I yelled out.

She stopped and turned around. "How could I?"

I texted her a few days later and asked her how she felt about me. She said she didn't want a relationship. I was devastated. I hated how distraught I was. How could I cry and be so sad over a woman I met only twice? Had I transferred my longing for Brad onto her? Did I get attached to her because I loved her kisses, or wanted to be like her? I felt miserable and every song on the radio made me think of her and cry. My sadness felt like the cold winter that never ended.

I asked my friends for advice. I had not dated in so long, I really didn't know dating rules. Was there something wrong with me to be interested in someone who was not interested in me? Finally, I decided it did not matter whether she liked my emotions. What mattered was expressing my feelings.

"I'm going to send her flowers," I told Mary.

"Leave her alone," she said.

"But I want to express my longing and desire. I want to show feelings, not repress them. It's okay if she doesn't respond."

I sent flowers to her office. She didn't respond. A few weeks later, I called her. She didn't answer, so I left a voice mail message and told her I wanted to see her again. She didn't respond. I lay next to Brad in bed, night after night, longing to kiss. And since he didn't let me kiss him and she did, I longed for her instead.

THE GUESTROOM (MARCH)

A few days later, about two weeks after my second date with Jenna, I was snuggled up to Brad in bed. He had given me a foot massage and then turned to his Smithsonian. When I rubbed up against him, he told me no to sex. with such disdain.

I heard my friend's voice in my mind: "I am so tired of being told no. I am so tired of being told no".

Damn it, I was tired of being told no. I grabbed my pillow, stormed out of our bedroom, and lay in our daughter's soft comfortable queen size bed. I fell asleep right away.

I woke up early the next morning. Sunlight beamed through the beach curtains and filled my bedroom with light. I felt peaceful. I didn't miss him. I didn't want him. Brad had not come after me. Why had he let me go? What would the kids say?

I opened the windows and the ocean breeze blew the curtains around. I looked around the cheerful clean room, with the white bed, bright green desk, white nightstand, and oak wood floor. The walls were lined with pink bookshelves and memory boxes filled with colorful perfume bottles and glittering jewelry with large beads. It was an uplifting contrast to the bedroom I shared with Brad, with its brown carpet, brown bed, and brown rattan shades on the window, which blocked the light.

That morning I moved to my own rhythm. I did what I wanted and had stopped doing for Brad. I got up at 5:30 am, when I woke up, instead of laying in bed waiting for him to wake up and possibly make love to me. I played my Indian chanting music. I meditated.

When I came out of my room, I ran into Oliver. He looked puzzled.

"Mom, what are you doing?"

"I got mad at dad and I slept in Chandi's room."

"O-kayyyy." He looked at me for an explanation.

"I'm tired of crying over dad," was all I could come up with.

That night I was alone in my room. For the first time since that summer vacation three years earlier, I didn't want him. Yet I still wanted all the other parts of our life together: the financial security he provided, our cute beach house and its proximity to work, a home for our children, and a fulfilling forever marriage. I didn't want to move out. I just needed to find a new way to spend my evenings. Then I fell asleep.

The second morning, I woke up to sunlight streaming through my curtains. I meditated and went in the kitchen to make coffee. Brad had already left for work. I was glad he was gone. This wasn't just me being mad for one night. I didn't want him anymore. I had to tell the kids.

I called Chandi. "Honey, I'm staying in your room for now, so if you come home from college to visit we'll have to figure something out."

"That's fine, Mom."

"You're not surprised?"

"No, Mom, I knew you were unhappy. "

"So you don't mind?"

"No, I have my own life now."

Good, that was a relief. I didn't want her to be sad.

I called Matt, who had moved out a few months before. "Sweetheart, I'm sleeping in Chandi's room now. Dad and I broke up."

"Okay, Mom."

That's all he said, and then he was quiet like he usually was, so I didn't really know how he felt or what else to say.

What about Oliver? Maybe he would be sad. When he got up, I told him. "Oliver, we'll be sharing the bathroom now, so you can help me keep it clean."

"That's women's work," he joked, and we both burst out laughing.

What I Did For Sex

I hoped he didn't really believe it was women's work. He and his siblings started cleaning when I put child-sized brooms and mops into their hands as toddlers, and he cleaned my company's office on the weekends. Did he revert to joking as way to deal with what happened? Time would tell. I didn't want to tell anyone else, because I wasn't entirely sure what had really happened and what to say. I went for a run, got dressed, and left for work.

That evening, Brad and I tiptoed around each other making dinner. He didn't ask me to come back, and I didn't want to anyway. It seemed this could be permanent. I went into my room with a bottle of wine and watched The L Word on Netflix. It was a series about lesbian relationships with extremely hot sex scenes that made me wet and stirred my heart for intimate connection. I didn't feel good about all that wine and movie watching, but I thought it was okay temporarily, to take my mind off being all alone.

Being alone was nice. I could listen to my chanting music, get up when I wanted without disturbing anyone, and do my long meditations again. Chandi would need her bedroom when she came home to visit from college, but I would deal with that when it happened.

The next morning after Brad left for work, I moved my bathroom supplies, clothes, alarm clock, and personal belongings into my new room. I was surprised at how I went from being totally in love with my husband, to not wanting him at all. Was it over? Why would Brad just let me go and not try to get me back?

I did my aerobics, meditated, and got ready for work. I drove my beautiful route along the coast, under sunshine and a cloudless sky, and the blue waves crashing on the shore. I felt peaceful. At work, I told our secretary what happened.

That night, I lay in bed and looked at the beach curtains. Tears welled up and I let myself sob. Damn it Brad, why did you have to check out of "'til death do us part"?

That night, I was talking about it to Chandi. "Mom, maybe Dad will be happier with a new woman that he doesn't have all those resentments against," she suggested. She never said what resentments she had in mind and I did not ask.

I went online and researched passive aggressive behavior, resentments, divorce, and breakups. Maybe reading would give me some answers. I went to bed that night with my broken dream and cried myself to sleep.

Two weeks passed. I still did not want Brad. I started talking about it to my mom, siblings, colleagues, and friends, typically saying, "I moved into the guestroom because my husband keeps telling me no to sex."

"He tells you no to sex?" was the typical reply. People seemed surprised because I was beautiful, and it was assumed men wanted sex 24/7, and it was the women who said no and had headaches. I researched this and found out half the time it was the man saying "no" to the woman.

Brad still had not come after me, probably because he knew he could not give me what I wanted. He longer sang in the shower or made jokes, and he looked pale and had circles under his eyes. It was a little awkward living together in the same house, seeing his sadness and knowing I was the cause. I avoided talking to him. I didn't want to create false hope and I didn't want to talk to him at all. I wanted some space between us, so each of us could reflect alone on what had happened, and let it all sink in. I was processing a lot of emotions too. Although I felt right being in the guestroom and did not want him anymore, I felt sad about my imploded marriage, and often I cried for Jenna. I felt a deep sadness I could not cure. We were both sad.

Since Oliver and I had adjacent bedrooms and shared a bathroom, we saw each other more and became closer. In the morning, I kissed him on the cheek, and he did that awkward teenage move where he smiled because he liked it, yet also pulled away because he was separating from his mom. He was adorable. At night, I tucked him in and sang the German lullabies he loved as a child.

"Honey, I know my voice sucks but I love singing to you," I said, rubbing his back.

"Oh no Mom, I love your voice," he said.

I sang him the three lullabies and told him goodnight, and each time he said it was done too fast. I was proud of my 17-year-old son who liked affection and touch, cared about people, and still liked being tucked in at night.

"Mom, Dad wonders why you don't talk to him," he asked one morning.

I was frustrated Brad had no clue why I left him. I explained it to him in a long email. Brad emailed me back the next day and told me he loved me very much. He didn't like kissing me that much, and he thought he had just lost the sexual attraction to me over the years. He was willing to try testosterone and marriage counseling. It didn't change anything. I didn't want him anymore. Maybe if he did those things and I became attracted to him again, I would consider him.

I prayed for answers on what to do. *God, what is the right decision? Should I stay or should I go? I am willing to go either way God. Give me a sign.*

A month passed. I looked at the calendar to note the day I left our bedroom. I couldn't believe it. It was March 21, 2013, Persian New Year and the second day of spring. It seemed symbolic. Maybe leaving him was right. I was glad that Brad had made me go back to work. It made leaving him possible.

I was thinking clearly, but emotionally I was a wreck. I missed our affection, cuddling at night, hugs, dinners together, our talks, and how he made me laugh, and I missed having a man to please. My biggest problem was my sadness over Jenna. I cried a lot. Until a few years earlier, I thought people who cried over someone else were weak, needy, and immature. I was an adult and I had my life together, and I shouldn't be crying over people who didn't want me. I was embarrassed. I didn't like crying over all these people and losing control of my happiness, so I set about figuring out how to cheer myself up by working out, meditating, talking and being with family and friends, and choosing happy thoughts. I read a book on breakups. The book said one day the crying would end. I held on to that hope, while every minute dragged on in endless misery.

I met my friends and talked through my feelings. I took walks in nature, went to Crossfit, meditated., tried rock climbing, 3 kinds of yoga, and meetup groups. The kids were surprised and impressed with my new activities, especially rock climbing. Sultry music made me even sadder and upbeat music made me smile and dance. Sometimes I allowed myself to relive enchanting memories of my lovers, and other times I pushed them away and distracted myself. I thought of escape in a bottle or pills. No, I left Brad's bed to be more and feel more. Numbing myself would just be a setback to all I had endured and worked for.

Mama said I would find instant relief if I disassociated my feelings from my thoughts. "Just feel the feeling in your body, and let it pass. It's your thoughts causing the pain. Let the thoughts go and feel your feeling." I tried it and it almost worked and then I gave up and went back to what I knew: feeling sorry for myself and hating my feelings that were not joy.

I thought about having sex with men and dismissed the idea. Men and sex usually involved feelings, romance, and relationships. I didn't think it would be healthy to get involved with a man so soon. After a relationship ended, it was healthy to take time to oneself for a few months or years, before starting another relationship. I was sure a man wouldn't want to date me anyway, still married and living at home with my husband. I couldn't imagine bringing a man over for dinner. I was too sad anyway to go on dates. What would I talk about? My imploded marriage? Some day I would date men again, but not then. This was my time to explore lesbians. They would consider me, since I was not with men, and I may never get that opportunity again.

A PREVIOUSLY SCHEDULED VACATION (APRIL)

About three weeks after the separation, Brad and I took the boys on a previously scheduled one-week vacation to visit Chandi in Iowa, and our parents in Nebraska. I didn't want to be on the trip with Brad. I was mad at him for letting me down in our marriage. On the trip, he was sweet to me as he had always been. How could he be so nice to me, when I was the one who left?

Brad and I pretended in front of our families that everything was fine. I told my stepmom about my separation, because she was always supportive. I did not tell Baba, because I didn't know how to explain it in Farsi.

One night at dinner, Brad looked very handsome and I was horny, a dangerous combination. I wanted him that night, so we slept together for the first time since the separation. We fucked on the floor, so our parents couldn't hear the squeaking mattress. Our sex was hot and lusty. We spent the night together cuddled in bed, and he was tender and loving. I felt close to him and I thought we could possibly get back together. I still planned to go to counseling because a one-time hot hookup with my husband did not mean everything was going to be better.

When we got back home, he said he would never take testosterone and sex wasn't important to him, but he still wanted to go to counseling.

ANDREA: "DON'T MAKE ANY NOISE"

In my bedroom at night, I browsed lesbian profiles online and that's where I met Andrea. She was a 42-year-old lesbian who worked as a paralegal. We made a dinner date. She pulled up on her motorcycle. She wore a black leather jacket, jeans, and boots. She was dressed like a man. Fucking hot! She loved wine, so we ordered a bottle with dinner. Afterward, she invited me over.

We kissed on the sofa. She was a good kisser so she turned me on a lot, and my whimpers turned to moans. I wanted to play with her nipples, because that turned me on, so I boldly reached into her shirt.

"I don't like my nipples touched. I like my entire breast touched," and she showed me by rubbing her hand in circles on her breasts. She didn't seem so appealing anymore. Rubbing her breasts was complicated and felt like work. I considered leaving.

She finally took me into her bedroom. Her bed was comfortable and soft, the lighting cozy. We got naked under the covers. Her clit was large, and fun to lick. She got more turned on, but after about 20 minutes she had still not come. She didn't say anything at all. I considered she could be mentally stuck, as I often was. A friend had told me she had her best orgasm ever when a man who was going down on her grabbed her legs tight at the end, like he meant it. I decided to try this.

I leaned into her pussy and grabbed her legs tighter like I meant it. That turned me on more, and I started grinding on the bed and softly moaning. She responded. Her body felt warmer, her vulva and clit felt slightly more swollen, her breathing got a little heavier. I was thrilled with my discovery. I kept licking her, holding her tight. As she got more aroused, I went for the button part of her clit and licked it nonstop until she came. Then I gave her an obligatory kiss. I just wanted to orgasm and leave.

She put her mouth on my vulva and licked me all over. I wanted her to make me come, so I focused on the sensations in my body and gave her directions: softer, get into a rhythm and stay with it, softer, just stay in the same spot. I liked my courage to tell her what would feel good. But she kept moving and it didn't feel good and I was just wearing her out without moving the action forward. I was horny and wanted an orgasm without all the hassle.

"Here, come up here and play with my nipples and I'll masturbate," I offered.

She did. After my orgasm, I forced myself to cuddle and talk.

"Every time I have sex with a woman, we start a relationship," she said.

"You don't have to. You can just have sex for its own sake, for your pleasure," I told her.

She seemed to like that idea. She told me that next time, she would use her strap-on. I couldn't wait. So when she invited me back a few weeks later, I was excited.

"We really need to be quiet during sex," Andrea told me in bed.

She said that once, her neighbors said they heard her and her girlfriend having sex and she was embarrassed about that. Asking me not to moan was like asking me to not get wet. I felt repressed, but I stayed to experience the strap-on. We started kissing.

"Do you want to use a dildo?" she asked.

"Yeah, sure!"

"I'm not going to use my harness. We'll just use these dildos by hand," she said.

Bummer. I really wanted to experience the strap-on. She opened her nightstand and pulled out three small dildos of various sizes and a bottle of lube. I was surprised how small the dildos were. She picked out a very short narrow dildo to use on her. I put a little lube on it and penetrated her slowly. Her vagina was extremely tight. She moved her head back and moaned. I went in and out very slowly, gently. I kissed her and then I pulled out the dildo and went down on her. As her moaning increased, I put the dildo back in and moved it in and out while I licked her to an orgasm. She was very quiet when she came. She almost didn't make a sound.

"That was really good," she said after coming. I felt proud. Then she went down on me. It felt good and I started moaning.

"Shhh..the neighbors will hear," she whispered.

You suck, Andrea. What a turn-off. I love moaning. I wanted someone who encouraged me to make more noise, not less, someone who called on me to express myself more, not less. I didn't tell her, she had a right to want what she wanted. My arousal was not building from her oral, so I fantasized while I masturbated. After my orgasm, I wanted to leave. I understood why men left after sex. I just wanted sex and the sex was over.

She texted me a few months later and said she felt used. I gave her a good time and orgasms. How was that using her? I never saw her again.

SHANNON: "I FEEL YOU"

I had almost given up on women, when I saw a profile from Shannon, a beautiful 49-year-old attorney from Orange County. She had two toddlers and wanted a relationship. The kids were a turn-off for dating a woman, because I didn't want a lesbian as a life partner or even as a live-in girlfriend. Young kids needed time and attention and would be in the way of sex and going out. But she was so beautiful, I contacted her anyway. On our first phone call, she asked me about STDs. Shannon said she lost gay male friends to AIDS in the 80's, so she was super sensitive about catching an STD, especially AIDs. She asked me to get STD tested before we met up, even though I had just been tested three months prior and was negative for everything. I went to my HMO to get the full range of STD tests, and emailed her the results:

Attached are my test results. They are negative for Hep A/B, HIV, syphilis, gonorrhea, and chlamydia. I had my HPV test during my pap exam four months ago and it was negative also.

She thanked me for getting tested and told me that I was passionate and how much she appreciated my energy. She called me the next day.

"I spent all afternoon today driving around to find a nice restaurant for our brunch date, and I found a 5 star restaurant with an incredible menu."

It seemed needy, like she was trying to impress me because she didn't think she was enough. I did my first meetups for coffee, because it was easy to leave if we didn't click. Nonetheless, a nice brunch date sounded amazing.

I drove to meet Shannon for Sunday brunch at a beautiful restaurant near her home. I spotted her on the patio, a slender brunette in a fashionable low-cut shirt. She was sexy as hell.

"Hi. Are you Shannon?"

She beamed a smile and her beautiful eyes sparkled. She stood up to hug me.

"Yes. Schahrzad?"

"Wow, you're gorgeous. I love your top!"

She was drinking champagne and orange juice. We went to the buffet and I saw she was about my height, and from the waist down she was definitely butchy. She wore tight jeans and cowboy boots. While we ate, she sat close to me and leaned over to talk. Her hair was shiny and curly, and her full breasts and a black lacy bra peeked out underneath her brown low cut shirt. I felt like I was receiving a gift, being courted by this beautiful woman who made herself pretty for me.

As she spoke, she put her hand on mine. I was uncomfortable with her move. Handholding was something between two people who knew each other and wanted closeness. Was I resisting intimacy or was she taking liberties? I was new to dating so I didn't know. I left my hand under hers, to challenge myself and get the experience. The waitress put the bill in front of Shannon.

"Let's walk around," she suggested after she paid.

We walked through the hotel, and she took my hand again. I didn't like her doing that but I let her. We stopped in the restroom. I noticed an awkward moment as we both went into stalls and I was about to hear my date urinate. I figured I just had to get over it if I was going to date women.

Just as we walked out, she turned around and kissed me. Her lips were soft. She pressed forward and put her arms around me. Kissing her turned me on. She was getting turned on also, because she kissed me harder and grabbed me tighter.

"Come, let's take a walk," and she took me by the hand.

"Where to?" I asked.

She smiled. "Hmm…I don't know yet, let's just go.'

We walked around a park near the restaurant, and she took my hand. I let her do it again, even though I did not like it. Why did I want to fuck her, and not hold hands?

"Can we get a hotel?" I asked, hoping we could hook up.

"My babysitter leaves in three hours," she said.

Did that rule out fucking? Wasn't she horny too?

"Let's get my car," she said.

The valet brought her car, and we went for a drive. While she drove, she again put her hand on mine. I was uncomfortable with all the handholding. Why did she keep doing it, and why did I let her? I was gutless. I could leave my husband, but I couldn't tell this woman to stop holding my hand.

Shannon drove to an office parking lot and parked next to an apartment building. Sweet, she wanted to make out, but sex in a car was uncomfortable and reminded me of being in high school, with guys who did not value me enough to take me to a bed.

"Let's get a hotel," I suggested again.

"I need to be home in two hours because my babysitter is leaving."

She motioned to the back seat. I turned around and saw two car seats.

"Here, let's get in the back."

I wanted sex more than I wanted to avoid having sex in the car. So I got in the back and she followed behind. I took off my shoes and straddled out of my pants. I sat in the narrow space between the car seats and she lay on top of me, her chest pressed against mine, her breath in my ear, in broad daylight in a parking lot in Orange County. I laughed to myself at our lust and spontaneity.

And then, between two car seats, toddler books and animal cracker boxes, she finger-fucked me. She fucked me deep… well….long. She knew places inside me that I didn't know existed. I moaned louder and moved my hips to her rhythm.

"Feels so good," she whispered in my ear.

How did she know? I got lost in her, lost in her touch and her fingers, and the pleasure deep inside my body. I was wet and moaning loudly. She got so turned on by my wetness and moans, she took off her pants.

"Do you like strap-ons?" she asked.

"I've never had one used on me, but I'd like to try it."

"Yeah, you'd like that, next time I'll fuck you with that."

She laid on me and finger-fucked me slow and deep, and kissed me tenderly. Then she whispered softly into my ear.

"I feel you. When we're apart and I tell you that I feel you, this is what I mean."

She moved her fingers inside me. I made a mental note of how I felt, so I could remember it when I needed to.

Then she went down on me. My clit swelled in anticipation. I shuddered the second her warm tongue made contact. She hit me in the right spot. I struggled to spread my legs wide apart so she could really get closer, but the car seats were in the way. She flicked and circled her tongue around my clitoris until I was so close to coming, but she didn't have enough room in that backseat to really get between my legs the way we both wanted, so I masturbated to finish to orgasm.

I went down on her and she came within five minutes. Afterward, as she drove me back to my car, she put her hand on mine. That time, I pulled away.

CHAPTER 8
BROKEN DREAMS

MARRIAGE COUNSELING

The intake counselor, a friendly middle-aged licensed social worker, was tasked with evaluating us and devising a treatment plan.

"Why are you here?" she asked.

"I'm tired of being told 'no' to sex," I told her.

I was sure she would side with me. She looked at Brad.

"Sex just isn't that important to me," he said.

I was sure she would give him exercises to do, or tell him he ought to try to please me even when he wasn't in the mood, or to get him to be more in touch with his feelings. Instead, she looked at me.

"Sex isn't everything! You have a long marriage here and a man who loves you, and you would throw that all away for sex? Who will take care of you in your old age?"

I was furious! How did she dare she tell me what to do, when I came to her trying to figure it all out? Besides, I was married to an old man already. He had wrinkles, age spots, skin cancer, and erectile dysfunction, yet I loved him and yearned for more connection and closeness. I wasn't running from age, at least not consciously and at least not then. It seemed she was projecting her own beliefs onto me and not being a professional or even like any of the women I knew who all loved sex. I knew she had no ground to stand on.

"Is this your opinion or is this based on research?" I asked.

She looked at me and didn't say a word. Brad didn't say anything either. Maybe he was happy she sided with him.

"A relationship is more than just sex. Sex is just not that important in relation to all the other parts," she told me.

I knew she was giving her personal opinion and not being professional. I wasn't going to let her bully me like that.

"Is this your opinion or the official viewpoint of this California HMO?" I asked.

She changed the subject. We talked a few more minutes and then she wrapped up the session.

"Let me make sure I understand why you are here today. Let me repeat back what you both said."

She turned to me.

"So Schahrzad, sex is so important to you, that you left him because of it?"

I nodded in agreement. She turned to Brad.

"Brad, sex is just not that important to you. You were happy with how things were and you don't want to make a change to get her back?"

"Yes," he said.

"I recommend individual counseling," she said and jotted some notes on a paper. I thought marriage counseling existed to save marriages. She was sending us our separate ways, to our separate counselors. I had never heard of this kind of marriage counseling.

"You can book your session at the appointment center," and she got up, shook our hands, told us goodbye, and closed the door behind us.

Brad and I went to the front desk and made our appointments for individual counseling. My therapist was a woman in her 60's. She walked me back to her office and we sat on opposite sides of a low coffee table.

"What brings you here?"

"My husband keeps telling me no to sex, and if there's no sex, we're just friends, so I'm done."

I waited for her reaction.

"I understand that. A vital sex life makes a vital relationship."

Good. This woman was much better. I felt understood, so I told her about Jenna, my sadness, and my inability to express myself with Brad.

"I don't know whether to stay with him or leave. I really could go either way. I want to know what's the right thing to do."

She seemed impressed by how well I was handling everything and told me it was normal to be unsure of what to do, and to be sad about Brad and Jenna too. I felt better. She suggested that I schedule another appointment with her three weeks later.

At our next counseling appointment, she asked how my life was going. I told her I was still crying over Jenna, and filled her in on work and my new activities.

"What do your kids think about your separation?"

Her question surprised me. I didn't believe people should stay married for any reason other than it was the right thing for them. Kids needed love, but they didn't need both parents. Oliver and I were closer since I moved into his sister's bedroom. My older kids were at college so I didn't see them regularly. They seemed to understand. But the truth was that I wasn't sure how they felt. I could not see inside their hearts and minds.

"The kids are supportive."

"What do you want in a relationship?" she asked.

"I want my man to make love to me. I want him to want me. I don't care about jewelry, money, travel, or gifts. I want to feel sexually valued and loved, I want to be kissed and desired, I want to be playful and close and talk about our feelings and make love."

"Have you ever had that with him?"

The room went blank for a split second, and I teared up.

"No."

It was a profound realization. I wanted something from him that he had never given me, and maybe never would. In that moment, I gave myself permission to leave. I was no longer a woman giving up on a marriage. It was about what I wanted in a relationship.

With only half the session done, I looked for things to fix in my life. I wanted to take full advantage of the counseling and improve myself. I brought up something about my mom. She just smiled at me.

"Don't go looking for problems. You are doing amazingly well," she said. "We don't need more sessions, but if you ever want to talk, please call and make an appointment."

I left that appointment feeling free. I didn't have to keep trying to get something from him that he didn't want. I could let it all go and be free.

I called Eliot to tell him about the counselors and my sadness over Jenna. Eliot said maybe I had transferred my sadness over Brad on to her, and I was really grieving my divorce.

I lay in bed that night and thought about what to do. I needed to digest the idea of leaving my husband and my home. I still wasn't sure I could afford to leave him and I loved our little beach house. I could stay in the guestroom for another year while I paid off some debts, got more raises at work, and got used to the idea of leaving him.

The next day I was in Oliver's room and called one of my best friends in Phoenix to tell her my plan. Our kids had grown up together and our husbands knew each other.

"It's too hard for Brad to have you living there when he's still in love with you," she said. "You ought to move out. "

"Wow, you don't think I should stay with him?"

"No, not if you don't want to," she said.

"I don't think I can afford to move out. We have debts and I don't make enough money."

"Well, find a way to make it happen," she insisted.

Interesting. A few days later, I chatted with the cashier at our local organic grocery store. She was just 25, and into spiritual practices and yoga. I updated her on what had happened.

"You ought to move out. Don't worry about the money. After I moved into a place I couldn't really afford, my yoga studio needed me to teach more classes and I made the money I needed. Your money will appear too," she said.

I felt inspired. She called on me to be bigger and greater, and make something happen. I decided I could do it!

I thought about our children. They had handled the separation well, probably because Brad and I wanted to get along and we didn't argue. We didn't fight over money or who would take what, or talk negatively about each other to the kids. Both of us encouraged our children to stay in touch with the other parent.

Chandi was in Iowa and busy with her own life. She wasn't paying much attention to us, except when we talked on the phone. She had been in a 3-year relationship and understood the ups and downs of relationships, and she was supportive. She just wanted me to be happy.

Matthew had moved out a few months before, and I didn't see him much, because he went to school full-time and worked 25 hours a week. I had brought up the separation each time I saw him and asked him how he felt. He said he didn't care. I thought he cared a little bit, because he looked down when he said it. Maybe I read more into it.

Oliver blossomed during the separation. He had just received the highest score in his class on a chemistry test. He was setting personal bests at every track meet. Maybe he worked harder to be good to make up for what he thought was wrong at home, or maybe he just liked the extra attention I gave him. He seemed genuinely happy.

I asked our children what they thought about me moving into my own place. They said I should move out and move on. My friends were right. I had to move out. But first, I had to separate our money.

CAN I AFFORD TO LEAVE HIM?

I wasn't going to ask for alimony or child support. Brad had supported me our entire marriage and he didn't owe me anything financially and I still felt guilty I didn't work all those years and spent so much of his money. Also, I didn't want to be one of those women whose lifestyle was dependent on a man she no longer fucked. I was going to make my own way and build a career and make my way in the world.

I still wasn't talking to Brad, so I informed him I was filing for divorce and moving out via e-mail. He wrote back and asked when I was available to talk about the details. He said he was hurt and crying, couldn't sleep, and couldn't imagine dating. I felt a little sad for him, but I knew he would get over it within a few months.

MY OWN PLACE (MAY)

I found my dream apartment in just a few days. The apartment had been completely remodeled. The tan walls and light carpet set off the white doors and thick baseboards. A faux wood floor in the kitchen and bath areas gave an elegant cozy feel. The mature trees and stucco roofs were visible through my large windows. A preserve with running trails was just a few blocks away.

The apartment was available immediately. I signed a one-year lease. It had all happened so effortlessly, letting me know that leaving Brad was right.

I drove home, got the boxes from our last move out of the garage, and started packing. Then I emailed Jenna about my move. Maybe she would want to date me, because I was no longer married.

Brad saw the boxes stacked up in the living room and looked sad. He wasn't laughing anymore or making jokes. He had deep circles under his eyes. He said he wasn't sleeping well. How could he be so sad when I was so happy? He still did not ask me to stay.

I moved on a Friday, while Brad was at work.

Movers are almost here, I texted Chandi.

Mom, I'm so proud of you. You have so much courage, she texted right back.

CHAPTER 9
FREEDOM

I took just a few favorite pieces when I left him: my Persian rugs, baby grand piano, a few paintings, and Chandi's Pottery Barn bedroom set. She was still away at college and said I could have it. Everything else we had accumulated in 25 years of marriage, I left behind. I didn't want it. I wanted to be free.

My apartment was elegant and inviting for men. I planned to have a lot of men over and have a lot of sex, sex that was better than the married sex I had with Brad. I wanted sex with men and women. I definitely loved men, yet I wasn't sure a man could please me sexually. Brad had not given me an orgasm in years. Neither had any of the other men I had been with lately. I always masturbated to climax. Did something prevent me from getting sufficiently turned on by a man, or were the men I was with just bad lovers? I had been with women in my youth, and some of them gave me an orgasm going down on me. What if only women could give me an orgasm? What would that mean? I didn't want to be with a woman. I wanted to be with a man. Sometimes I wondered if something was wrong with me.

My new home was not a replica of what I had. The objects which had once represented success and security, like a china cabinet, outdoor furniture, a grandfather clock…even a silverware tray, interfered with visual beauty and simplicity. They had once denoted success and security, but now they were anchors and dead weight for future moving boxes. So were plants and pets, life forms that required feeding, watering, and caretaking, without giving anything useful in return.

I set my pictures on the floor, because this apartment was a temporary home. Eventually I would move in with a man who had a place, or we would get a place together. I didn't dream of buying my own place one day. I still didn't think I could ever afford it.

KEGELS

I unpacked my bathroom supplies and put the maxi pads in my cabinet. I took a second look. No. No, no way. The pads did not belong in my bachelorette pad. Maybe it was okay to wear maxi pads around my husband who was the reason for the pregnancies that caused my bladder to leak, but it was not hot or sexy for dating. I threw them out and promised to do Kegels to tighten my pelvic floor.

The next morning I went for a run. It was the first time in decades I ran without the maxi pads. I did the Kegels instead. I tightly squeezed my vaginal muscles and held the squeeze. I had a little leakage, especially when I ran downhill, and I squeezed tighter. The outdoor air felt freeing, refreshing. By the time I got home, I was dripping with sweat.

Shower, meditation, and a new outfit for my dates in Dana Point. Katie, 10 am, coffee at the harbor. Brenda, 11:30 am, lunch, at the Mexican restaurant next door. These women, who lived north of me, had chosen the adjacent restaurants, ninety minutes apart. It was so convenient and coincidental, giving me a feeling of being "in flow".

It was a warm sunny Saturday with a cloudless sky as I headed northbound on I-5 past the green hills of Camp Pendleton on my right and the ocean to my left. I opened my sunroof and inhaled the fresh spring air. "Feel This Moment" by Pitbull played on the radio. Yes, I was feeling this moment too. I had my dates and I wasn't impressed. Katie was boring, and Brenda had too many personal problems. On the way home, I picked up some Thai food, and that night, I went to sleep in my own apartment.

On Monday, I took my new route to the office, driving west through north Carlsbad.. The drive was scenic and relaxing. I opened the sunroof, blasted my music, and smiled.

"Good morning!" I greeted my colleagues at work, like usual, except my joy was brighter.

That weekend, Oliver and I bought his bedroom furniture, a loveseat for the living room, and a dining room table.

Every morning I exercised before work. I rode the spin bike in my apartment, did step aerobics in my living room, or ran outdoors on the trails. My bladder control did not return immediately. But it got better each time, and after one month, my pelvic floor muscles were so strong, I could drink coffee and do a 45-minute run, and no urine ever leaked out. I could sneeze while walking and do jumping jacks, and no urine ever leaked out.

In the first month in my apartment, I had sex with six lesbians. I didn't have feelings for any of them, as I had for Jenna, and the sex was boring. There was no hint of the raw energy I craved: hair pulling, throat grabbing, power play, being dominated, face sitting, ass licking, hot talk, or anything exciting. And although I gave every woman an orgasm from oral sex, few of them could ever do that to me. Shannon, the woman from brunch, was my only remaining prospect, but all she did was text or talk on the phone, without ever making another date. Sex with women was disappointing. I wanted hot sex. I needed a man.

MY TYPE OF MAN

I wanted a lusty tall strong man with a hard cock who could dominate me, fuck me with abandon, open me to new ideas and ways of having sex, and who got turned on by my moaning.

I also planned to keep seeing women, because I didn't know whether men or women would satisfy me more sexually. I still thought about Jenna, the woman who ignored me.

Fucking men meant I had to reconsider my views on STDs. I was no longer afraid of getting an STD from sex. Most of the sexually active people I knew never used a condom at all, including my friends and the swingers I had met. I had read up on STDs on the Internet and the CDC website. The articles recommended using condoms and oral dams, but there was still a risk of contracting herpes or genital warts through kissing and skin contact. I decided to go down on every man before I put his penis inside, and look for genital warts, and avoid bisexual men because they were likely to have unprotected sex with gay or bi men and have a higher risk of STDs, although maybe that was an unreasonable fear.

My type of man was professional, fit, at least 5'10" but preferably a bit over 6', confident and sensitive, who liked the outdoors, and didn't need alcohol. He was Caucasian, lean, and had a happy smile.

The man had to be professional and career driven. It wasn't about his money. It was about how he moved through the world. A man's physical movement, his energetic movement, and his purpose - that's what turned me on. I didn't want men who chose nursing or teaching or jobs that involved submission or following directions. I liked men who led others and created something: entrepreneurs, sales managers, and investors. I didn't want that man if he was winding things down and looking to retirement. I wanted a man filled with vitality and building his career.

I didn't want a man lonely after his children left, but rather a man who had dealt with all that and had a meaningful life post-children. Or the man could have younger children and I could be involved in raising them.

Many older men liked travel. I liked travel too, but the kind of travel that went inside myself. Geographic travel seemed like running from oneself. I eliminated men who sought a travel or activity partner, because that's not what I wanted, and men who were my age but never married and had no children. I judged them as having issues.

I liked a man who told interesting stories and made me laugh. He had to dress well: not expensively, but stylishly, so I could enjoy looking at him.

I looked for men within 25 miles of me. "What do you do for work and how tall are you?" were the first questions I asked, if it was not in the profile. If they wanted to meet for a drink, I deleted them. A proper man could enjoy the company of a woman without needing alcohol.

I used my match.com account with handle "Megan" that I had created for meeting women. I set up coffee dates with several interesting attractive men, ages 55-59, with careers in engineering and sales. Some of the men cancelled our coffee date before we ever met. For the dates I always wore my professional work attire.

"LET'S GET DRUNK"

I met Tom, a 49-year-old tall entrepreneur for coffee at 9am, on my way to work. We sat outside in the fresh spring air. I liked looking at him. He had a successful business and he had assembled some furniture for his daughter that morning. He leaned forward as he spoke, indicating his interest in me. His charm and flirtation turned me on. He was quite talkative. He told me about his business, including that he liked getting drunk at work. He didn't look like a drunk. Maybe we could date.

After coffee, we walked out together. I expected him to walk me out to my car, but he stopped in the parking lot. I hoped he would ask me out to dinner.

"Let's go out and get drunk sometime. It would be fun," he said.

"I don't get drunk, and I rarely drink."

"Alright then. Talk to you later." And he walked to his car.

Maybe he could get over the drinking thing. After I got to work, I texted him to reassure him I had a good time, because men were sensitive beings who needed reassurance, and if I didn't say anything at all, he could wonder all day if I liked him.

Shannon called me that night.

"I met a really hot guy for coffee this morning, but he just wanted to get drunk. What a loser."

"I'm glad you're exploring what you like," she said. But she did not sound glad. She sounded jealous, and that felt trapping.

The next morning, I had a text from Shannon. *You warm my heart and make my ovaries swell*

Her words brought tears to my eyes. I liked being exposed to this kind of poetic romance, but it seemed she was falling for me, and I didn't feel the same way.

Tom did not reply to my text. It seemed strange to ignore a correspondence from someone with whom a person had just shared a conversation and coffee. I went online to look for more men to date.

Brad called and said he would make dinner for Mother's Day. No, thank you. I didn't want to be friends with my ex. I was not attracted to him, and we had nothing in common.

That weekend, the kids came over. Chandi and I went to Crossfit and coffee. Then we picked up Oliver and had lunch and sat by the pool in my apartment.

"YOUR CANDOR IS REFRESHING"

I met more men in their early 50's for coffee. I wasn't attracted to any of them. I left our meeting before I finished my coffee.

Then came Rudy. According to his online profile, he liked cycling, live music, fine wine, and "Europe anytime". We set up a coffee date. Rudy was already seated and sipping his latte when I arrived. He looked as handsome as in his profile pictures. He stood up and shook my hand. I was glad he didn't grope me for a hug, like other men. Rudy was about 6' tall, lean and fit, with a flat stomach, which was very impressive for his age of 52 years. His hair was gray, and he had a nice tan and dimples.

Rudy started by telling me all about himself, mostly his success at work, his successful college age boys, and his many accomplishments. He then apologized for going on and on, and asked me about myself, specifically what I was looking for.

"I'm dating lesbians, however the sex so far is boring and I want a man to fuck on the side," I answered.

He leaned forward and looked me in the eyes, "I'm not used to women being so open." He leaned closer, "Your candor is refreshing."

"Thank you," I smiled. "I like to ask for what I want."

"I like a confident woman."

"Are you divorced?"

"No. Separated. My ex wife is a bitch and is dragging this out. She thinks I have more money than I do, and even her lawyer can't stand her," he explained.

Aside from talking poorly of his ex, Rudy seemed like a great potential sex partner. I had to see him in a relaxed environment so I could see his real self and decide if I wanted to have sex with him. We set a date for a trail run the next weekend. Then I left to meet Ed for coffee in Encinitas.

HIS VERY HIGH LIBIDO

"I have a very high libido," Ed told me over coffee.

He was a fit 54-year-old computer consultant, with wavy brown hair and a charming smile. I told him that nobody could make me come anymore, and I had my orgasms by masturbating. He assured me he was very good at oral sex. I liked hearing from a man that he enjoyed pleasing a woman. It turned me on. I wasn't sure if he was my type though. He had not been STD tested in almost a year, so he agreed to get tested before we had sex and email me his test results. We decided to make a date after he had his results.

A few days later, Ed texted to say his test results would be available in a couple days. He promised to go down on me, and, as he stated, "*looking forward to your evaluation of my oral skills vs. the women you have been with.*"

He invited me to his home for dinner on a Saturday evening. He served me the freshest juiciest salmon I had ever tasted.

"Oh my God, this salmon is the most delicious salmon I have ever tasted!"

"I bought this at the fish market this afternoon. It's fresh catch," he said.

"It's absolutely delicious. Wow. Thank you so much."

Over dinner, our conversation was about sex, particularly his massage table fantasy. It sounded hot and he was handsome, but I wasn't attracted to him. I had lost all interest in evaluating his oral skills vs. the women I had been with. I didn't want him to touch me at all.

"I don't feel like having sex with you or kissing you, but I'll watch you masturbate," I told him after dinner.

He got up from the table, quickly stripped out of his pants, and sat down in his kitchen chair. He began stroking his cock. I walked closer until I was about fifteen feet away. I watched as he stroked his cock, slowly at first, then faster and faster and faster, until his ejaculate shot all over the room.

"Did you see how far that shot?" he was beaming.

I really didn't care how far it shot, and it didn't turn me on at all, mostly because I had enough of men who were just into sex for their own pleasure, and also because I wasn't attracted to him.

"Yes, that was far." I didn't want him to feel bad. I just wanted to leave. "That was hot, I think I'll go now."

He got dressed and walked me to the door.

A few days later, we talked on the phone about his massage table fantasy. It intrigued me, because I wanted to try role-playing. Since it was just a massage, I wouldn't have to fuck or kiss him. I imagined him massaging me, then moving up between my thighs, and spreading warm oil between my labia, leading to an orgasm. Maybe he had a different scenario in mind, something with blindfolds or hot talk or watching me masturbate. I was really curious and turned on.

"Tell me more how this massage table fantasy goes," I asked.

"Well, you would come over and give me a massage, and then finish me off with a happy ending," he said.

What? He had to be deluded to think I would come over to give him a massage and hand job, with nothing in it for me.

"I don't want to do that."

He emailed me a few days later to ask about the massage one more time. He seemed annoyed and said I had led him on and I did not keep our agreements, which would make it hard to build trust. I wrote him back to say we were not a match and asked him not to contact me again. He didn't.

FILING FOR DIVORCE

May 28th was my 25th wedding anniversary. I had been in my apartment less than two weeks. It was a good day to file for divorce. I put on my grandmother's diamond necklace. When my mom gave it to me, she had said, "only wear this on special occasions." Filing for divorce was a special occasion because I took a stand for my freedom.

I filed the paperwork as if I were applying for a mortgage. I didn't feel sad. I paid to have Brad served. He would have 30 days to respond. If we moved through the process without any conflicts, our divorce would be final in six months.

"I'M HARD BECAUSE YOU MAKE ME SO HARD"

Rudy, the 52-year old man who found my candor refreshing, met me at the trailhead for our run. He was mostly a cyclist, in great shape, but not used to running. He kept up with me quite well for the entire hour. We talked while we cooled down afterward. He told me about his contributions to his clients, business partners, and children, and giving back to the world. He sounded like a great guy. I became more interested in him.

"You want to go for coffee?" I asked.

"Sure."

We relaxed over coffee and talked in detail about sex, and what each of us liked. He leaned in and was intensely interested in me, which, combined with my interest in him, made him more attractive.

"I love eating pussy," he said.

That got my interest. I was turned on by this man who appreciated and loved that part of a woman, that I felt had been neglected for so long. I wanted to spread my legs for him and have him lick my clit all over and see if he could make me come. We didn't hook up right then, because we were both sweaty from our run.

A CONDOM ON MY NIGHTSTAND

When I got home, I texted Rudy and invited him for an early morning sex session. My favorite time of day for fucking was early morning, and it had been years since I had that luxury of waking up to a hard cock. Fortunately, Rudy also liked morning sex.

At 7 a.m. the next morning, I was showered, in sexy lingerie. I heard a knock at my door. There was Rudy, with his gray hair, chiseled face, and manly cologne. He came in, and we immediately kissed and got out of our clothes. There was nothing romantic about it. I wanted his cock and he wanted my pussy. It was just physical between us, but not in a hot, I-need-you-right-now kind of way.

He took off his pants in my dining room, revealing tight red spandex briefs. He looked like a gigolo or someone about to do a strip tease. I had never seen a man wear such briefs. I pulled down his gigolo briefs, and his erect penis popped out. He was so hard, his cock almost touched his stomach. He was slightly larger than average, with a nice girth. It was such a relief to be with a man who actually got hard.

He followed me into the bedroom and I gave him a blowjob and teased him with my tongue to get myself more turned on. I kissed and gently sucked his balls and then I ran my tongue from his balls down to his ass and circled his asshole, rimming. I knew most women never did that, but I loved the smells, juices, sweat, moans, sounds, and playfulness of sex. I looked him in the eyes as I let my tongue circle the ridge of his head, and my mouth took in his entire head. He looked back at me in longing.

He was super hard and I just wanted to fuck him. I felt the wetness in my pussy. I thought menopause made women all dried out. Maybe I wasn't in menopause after all. I got a condom out of my nightstand, put it on him, and slid onto his erect penis. He slid right in because I was so wet. I shivered. Damn, he felt amazing! I moaned louder and louder. Rudy's cock fit me just right. I was getting wetter and wetter.

"God, you feel so good, you're so hard!" I told him.

"That's because you turn me on. You make me so hard."

I liked that. It was such a relief to be with a man who could get hard and stay hard. I kept riding him. He thrust his hips rapidly up and down in short quick strokes, a move which sent shivers up my spine. With each stroke, I felt pleasure deep inside me. My moans turned into a scream of sorts and I whimpered, "Oh my god, oh my god, oh my god, oh my god." I didn't want his deep thrusting to ever end.

"Do you have a vibrator you want to use?" he asked.

"While I'm riding you? Well, that's nice of you to ask, but I don't use vibrators because I have better orgasms with my fingers, and I can't masturbate to come when I'm on top."

"What position do you like for that?"

"I'm not really sure. I've only masturbated during penetration one time, and it was many years ago."

It was with Brad, before we had kids. I had been on my stomach, and we came at the same time. Brad thought it was great, but I didn't like it, because he missed out on my orgasm and I missed out on his. Masturbating during penetration with Rudy seemed too complicated, and I just wanted to enjoy myself and focus on feeling the sensations in my vagina.

"Do you want to try that now?" he asked.

"I can masturbate after you come, and you can watch me."

His eyes lit up. That indicated he would be turned on from my self-pleasuring, not bored like Brad. I rode him some more and he liked it a lot. I felt his cock get wider inside me and I could tell he was about to come. He let out a loud long moan and said, "I'm coming," which was hot. Brad had never told me when he came. I kissed him forcefully and deeply while his cock throbbed inside of me. Then his cock got soft and slipped out. He took off his condom and I put it on my nightstand.

He didn't offer to use his hands or tongue on me, so why did he say he loved eating pussy? I wasn't going to ask, because I only wanted it done if the man wanted to do it. I asked him if he would lie next to me while I masturbated, even though that was boring. I didn't know any other way to have it done.

Rudy held me and watched me eagerly while I masturbated, which was the opposite of what Brad had always done. I was getting more turned on by his enthusiasm, and I came much faster than I had with Brad. Rudy actually made it fun to masturbate. Afterward, we snuggled about two minutes.

"You can fuck all the women you want. I'm fucking other women too, and I'm not looking for a relationship," I said when he was washing up at the sink.

"I'm too busy with work to be fucking around."

Rudy had to leave for his meeting and I got dressed for work. It would be a while before Rudy and I could have sex again. His kids were visiting, and Oliver was coming over that evening to spend the week.

On the way to work, I called Shannon.

"Hey, I really want to see you again and try the strap-on sex," I said.

"We will. Soon."

"Well, let me know because I can come up there to see you anytime. How is everything going with your dating?"

"Well, I met a woman on match. She's from Sweden and seems just like my type."

"Oh wow, that's great."

"We talked on the phone for an hour last night, and we're meeting this weekend."

I was a little jealous about it, because I wanted to meet her too and this woman seemed to get priority because she was looking for a relationship.

"Hey, I had the best sex this morning. Oh my god, this guy's cock felt sooo good!"

"I'm glad you're exploring sexually," she said, but her voice did not sound convincing. She sounded jealous and that felt trapping.

That afternoon, Rudy texted me and said I was beautiful when I had my orgasm. I welled up with tears. Nobody had ever said I was beautiful when I came. I texted Rudy not to say things like that anymore because I didn't want to start liking him. I did not see him as boyfriend material, because he seemed closed off emotionally and wasn't funny.

I stopped at the grocery store on my way home to get cereal, apples, and chicken for Oliver. He was in his room, studying.

"Hi Oliver, I'm home."

"Hi Mom."

I went in and hugged him. Then I remembered the condom I had placed on my nightstand that morning. Had I flushed it? I went into my bedroom. Darn it, the used condom was still on my nightstand.

"Oliver, did you go in my room today?"

"Yes, mom."

"Did you see something on my nightstand?"

He grinned sheepishly, and we laughed. I didn't know if I should be embarrassed. This was real life, and it was good for Oliver to know his mom enjoyed sex. I went in my room and grabbed the condom and flushed it down the toilet.

HIS SISTER FETISH

Rudy came over a few days later, after Oliver left to go back to his dad's house. If he wasn't fucking other women, I could have sex without a condom. I wanted to feel the ridge and entire shape of the head of his penis, and his warmth. Also it would be more intimate. I asked about his sexual history.

"I was tested for STDs just a few months ago, and I hadn't had sex since then," he said.

"Great. Then we won't use a condom," I said.

We did not use a condom that time. Or the next. I liked Rudy's hard cock. He let me get on top, ride him just how I liked, and he stayed hard a long time. He would push his hard cock inside of me, and fuck me hard and slow, his strong hands grabbing my ass or hips. I clutched him and held on tight as he moved inside me. After about 20 minutes of penetration, when my pussy was swollen with arousal and completely wet, I asked him to ram his cock deeper inside. I usually ground my hand in circles on his back and scratched him. My moans became wails. I loved discovering my body and my pleasure. It felt so good, maybe I could orgasm from penetration one of these days.

I started liking Rudy the man. I googled his name to learn about him. I noticed whenever I was online on match.com looking for lesbians, he was always showing as "active". Why was he online looking for women when he had me?

"Are you a womanizer?" I asked him the next time I went down on him.

"No, not at all. I have been in a few relationships since my separation two years ago. Each relationship lasted about five months."

I sucked his cock a few more strokes and slipped him inside me. He felt so good. Maybe I liked him a little bit. Maybe I would be his next five-month relationship. We talked as he got dressed.

"Are you fucking other women?" I asked, just out of curiosity.

"No, I don't go sleeping around."

I felt a little guilty for having a much hotter sex life than he did. But at least he wasn't a player and I could keep fucking him without a condom.

"I'll stay the night sometime," he said.

After he left, I called my sister in Colorado and told her all about him. Sarina was also on match.com, so she asked for his handle and looked him up.

"He's hot!" she said.

The next time Rudy came over, I told him about Sarina. He asked about her match.com handle, and I gave it to him. After he left, I realized I was getting some feelings for him. I still could not see myself dating him, because he was too serious, had never made me come, and was not taking me out on dates. I wasn't sure what to do about it. Should I let myself develop feelings for him anyway, or just end it?

The next morning when I woke up, I had my decision. I would express myself and let him decide what to do about it. I texted Rudy and told him I was starting to get feelings for him, and asked him to come over. That day, I was out at a school opening, but I had my phone and kept checking for a text back from Rudy. Finally, a text message on my phone. But it was not from Rudy. It was from Sarina. *Rudy just sent me a match.com message saying I'm beautiful.*

I struggled to understand. Why was he texting her and ignoring me, when I had just told him I had feelings and invited him over, and I was in town and available and she lived far away?

Another text. *Rudy says I'm very sexy*

I called Sarina. "Rudy contacted you?"

"Yes, on match.com. He wants to meet me."

"That asshole! I just told him this morning I want to see him again and I'm starting to get feelings for him, and he never even replied." I paused. "Do you want to see him too?"

"Well, he's very attractive and successful, so I am interested."

I was mad at her for wanting him, and flirting with my guy but mostly I was mad at him for pursuing her behind my back. He could have just told me we were done, and he was interested in my sister, and I would have respected that. I didn't know family men who contributed to society and loved their children could be deceptive. How had I misread him like that?

And why did she want him ? She did not hookup and he lived far from her. Maybe fucking my guy would give her a feeling of adequacy. But I was insecure too. I did not want them to fuck, because I was afraid he would like her better in bed and that would prove I was sexually inadequate. I didn't tell her any of that because I was embarrassed, so I relied on the girl code instead.

"If you two have feelings for each other and want to date, I would be supportive, but you two just want to fuck. Go find your own fuck buddies. Come on, we don't fuck each other's guys."

"He's so sexy though," she continued.

"Well, I don't want you to see him. I like him," I argued.

"Okay, I won't see him then. But let's keep playing his game and see how far he will take it. I'll forward all his texts to you."

That seemed like a fun game. It served him right to be strung along like that.

I was mad at myself for having sex with him without a condom. He seemed to go after women so readily, and he wasn't honest. He could be fucking a lot of other women. I called my doctor and made an appointment for STD testing.

That evening, Shannon called. I told her about Rudy's pursuit of my sister.

"What a weasel!" she said.

We talked about our dating and meditation and sex. After we got off the phone, I sent her some sexy pictures, knowing I turned her on.

Momma she texted back.

I can feel my hair brushing the inside of your thigh
Baby

Nobody had ever talked to me like that. I welled up with tears and I felt warm in my vagina and heart. I remembered how my body opened up when I told Brad I loved him during sex. What else would my body do when I felt loved? Someday I would find out….with a man.

A few days later, my STD tests came back: negative for everything.

And then a text from Sarina: *He wants to come to Denver to see me*

I was furious with Rudy for doing all this behind my back. A real man would just man up and be honest about his intentions. Since he was not answering his phone or returning my calls, I confronted him via text: *Hey, my sister says you want to hook up with her*

His text message came a minute later: *Consider she contacted me first*

It was a lie, and it seemed like he sought to pacify me. Why didn't he just say he was done with me and wanted her instead? Maybe my sister understood people better than I did, so I asked her.

"Why is Rudy lying about contacting you first?"

"Some people lie and it's how they go through life. They start with a lie, and they get away with it, and eventually everything becomes a lie. You can ask a guy like that where he's going and he'll tell you to the bank when he's really going to the gym."

I didn't want any people like that in my life, but it intrigued me. What was the point of lying about everything? Although I was turned off about the lying, I still lusted after his hard cock, and as much as I didn't like to admit it, I held out hope there was just a big misunderstanding of some sort and he didn't want my sister after all. Why did we both still want to fuck him, even though he lied to us?

The next afternoon, Rudy called and invited me to a concert. It was a sold-out show. I was impressed he could get tickets. Maybe he had changed his mind about my sister and wanted me instead.

"Oh wow, I love that band. Sure!"

"Ok, I'll call you in a day to confirm. Do you like sushi?"

"I'm not into it ….But sure, I'll try it."

"Great, we can have dinner before the show."

Rudy called the next day and confirmed our date for the concert. It was my first live band concert since high school. He probably was no longer interested in Sarina, since he had asked me out. I never asked him though, because I wanted to be a good fuck buddy who had no relationship expectations. Besides, he would just lie anyway.

At dinner, he talked about his misguided neurotic selfish money hungry wife, and their divorce proceedings that were years in the making. She was probably a nice woman. If I hadn't been so horny, I would have just ended the date right then.

The live music was exhilarating. Rudy stood behind me, his hard cock pressed against my ass, as we watched the band and moved to the music. I ground up against Rudy, and he put his hands on my shoulders and hips. Nobody had done that in years. Sometimes I turned around and looked up at him. His head was turned to the side every time, as he looked out over the audience. He was probably looking at other women, but I didn't care. His cock was hard, and I knew it was for me. After the concert, he came over to my place. He was good in bed, like always, except he still had never made me come.

The next day, a text from Sarina: *Rudy is coming to see me in Denver.*

Somehow, that time, it struck me as hilarious. He didn't mean to be bad, he just couldn't help himself.

I texted him: *You have a sister fetish?*

He didn't reply.

That weekend, Mary and I met for dinner in Carlsbad. I told her all about Rudy. She asked his last name and I told her.

"Oh my god, I know his wife. She volunteers in our church nursery. She is the most amazing beautiful woman. The kids just love her."

"Really? Rudy said she is neurotic and selfish and just after his money."

"That's hilarious. He sounds like a jerk."

I kept replaying the pleasurable intercourse with Rudy in my mind. He was a weasel, a jerk, and a liar, but his cock sent me into ecstasy. Was I bad for lusting after a man just for his cock and getting attached in the process?

I texted Rudy: *I want to meet you to talk. I am starting to get feelings for you*

He didn't reply so that evening I left a voicemail, "Can you please call me to talk because I am starting to have feelings for you?"

He didn't reply, so the next morning I gave him an ultimatum. If he didn't care how I felt, I was done.

Please let me know if you can meet me tonight, else I can't see you anymore.

His reply came two minutes later: *Take your combat tactics elsewhere.*

I no longer wanted him. I was done.

CHAPTER 10

LESBIAN HOOKUPS

HER LEATHER STRAP-ON (JULY)

Shannon and I finally set a date for strap-on sex. We arranged a meeting at a hotel in LA near her home, to minimize her time away from her children.

I drove to LA, full of anticipation. I imagined having sex, lunch, maybe some shopping, and drinks afterward. She had already checked in when I arrived, so I went straight to her room. She was beautiful, as always.

"Hi Shannon. You look great!"

"Hi, it's great to see you. I only have two hours, because my babysitter needs to leave."

I swallowed my disappointment. I didn't want to tell her anything about my expectations, because she had a right to do what she wanted. But why did she only plan for two hours when she pursued me for months, and was a highly paid professional woman who could easily afford a babysitter.

"Come here, look what I brought," she said and led me to the bed.

On the bed lay a red velvet pouch with a drawstring.

"Hmmm…let's see which size you might like," she said, and pulled out three dildos of various sizes, materials, and colors: a 6" tall (1.75" wide) blue dildo, a 6" tall (1.5" wide) pink dildo, and a 4" tall (.75" wide) neutral toned dildo. I didn't know dildos came in so many sizes and colors, and I thought they were all very narrow and small. Still, I was impressed with the assortment she carried.

"Wow!" It was all I could say.

I had no idea how to put all that into action. She took a leather harness out of a different bag, put it on, and adjusted the straps. Fuck! She looked so sexy. I wasn't thinking about being fucked by her anymore, because I wanted to do the fucking. I wanted to wear that harness. I hoped she would let me have a turn.

She placed the 4" neutral colored dildo into her harness. It looked small, but I didn't tell her that. I was open to the experience she wanted to provide.

"I don't have sensation in the dildo, so I move by how it feels to you, not how it feels to me," she explained.

I lay on the bed and she climbed on top of me and we kissed. I wasn't feeling that into her anymore, especially because she reduced our big date to only two hours, and the dildo seemed very small. She put the tip of the dildo inside of me, and pushed gently, until it slid in, and then she used my wetness to push in deeper with each thrust. Once she was all in, she moved in and out. It didn't feel as good as being fucked by a finger or a penis. I tried to get into it. I held her tight and kissed her and focused on the sensations in my pussy. I still didn't enjoy the sensations. She could tell I didn't like it, so after about five minutes she stopped.

"I'd like to try doing that to you," I said.

I didn't ask to use the strap-on, since it could be considered a personal item like a hairbrush or vibrator. She didn't reply, so I took that to mean she didn't want to share it, or maybe she didn't like penetration with dildos.

"Lay down, let me go down on you," I suggested.

She laid her head on the pillow and looked at me. I climbed on top of her, kissed her breasts and stomach, and moved down to between her legs. Her pussy tasted and smelled sweet, she was engorged and wet, and I licked her clit until she was close to coming, and then finished off by licking her with steady rhythmic strokes on the little button part of her clitoris until she came.

She went down on me and I came very close to coming but couldn't. I hated when it was hard to come. I masturbated and fantasized alternately about Shannon going down on me and then about a man watching my clit and pussy, until I came.

After we both had an orgasm, I wanted to leave. There was nothing holding my interest in her after the sex was over. Our two hours were up anyway.

Shannon put away all her dildos. "I love this Aslan Jaguar leather harness. I'll send you the information on where you can buy it."

That evening, she called and gave me the name of the Canadian company where I could buy the same leather harness she had used on me.

"Leather gives and takes well as you move. Get a cock that fits the harness and is long enough so you can move and have fun with it."

"Ok, well, I have a dildo at home already. It's 8" long and thick."

"I didn't know you're a size queen. Was I too small?"

I didn't know what to say. The dildo was small, but dildos never felt as good as a penis or finger.

The harness came in the mail a few days later. I put it on and adjusted the straps. I slipped the dildo into the opening and looked at myself in the mirror. Fuck, I was so sexy....a real stud!

I called Shannon and told her I would ride my Girl the next time we were together. Since she was a "top", I knew it was unlikely she would let me. The "top" was the masculine energy and got turned on doing the penetrating, while the "bottom" was the feminine energy and was turned on being submissive.

I poured a glass of wine, so I got a little looser in the conversation.

"Have you ever had phone sex?" I asked.

"Yes, many times," she replied.

"I never have. I want to try it."

"Yeah baby, let's do it," she whispered.

I took the phone into my bedroom. I slipped out of my panties, leaned against the wall, and faced my closet mirror. I pulled up my dress and watched myself masturbate in the mirror.

"I'm rubbing my clit," I said.

She talked to me while I masturbated, and then we both masturbated. She told me all the things she was going to do to me and I got more and more turned on listening to her voice in my ear, until I came. Then she said she had to go.

I liked her sexual openness, and how free I felt sharing my fantasies. I called her the next day and asked when we could get together again. She had an excuse that time, and every time.

"I'm so busy with work."

"You can get STDs from men, and it's not safe. I have children to raise. I'm just not comfortable having sex with you while you are having sex with men."

Other times, she would call and talk for an hour. She also sent me regular text messages and made comments about 'our engagement', which was odd because I could never see myself marrying a woman and we were not dating.

"It seems you are avoiding me. I want to get together again," I told her.

"I love you. I'm there for you. I have to reconcile my own issues before I can make myself vulnerable to you. I have opened up again and realized what love is, and started yielding to you, until you texted me an equivocation and then all my warmth turned sour and my ego took control. I know I failed you."

I had no idea what she was talking about and I couldn't believe such a successful businesswoman was all over the place in her emotional life.

EMPTY NEST

I was too excited about my freedom to notice it at first. It was my loneliness. My family of five, a dog, and two cats were replaced with the void of an empty apartment. Gone were the dinner conversations, piles of laundry, Oliver's clothes strewn all over the house, and pets running through the kitchen. I missed the companionship of a man, watching him shave in the morning, sing in the shower, and speak in his deep voice. Nights were hard, because I missed snuggling up to a man. I stayed up until I was exhausted, somewhere around 1am. Maybe I needed a roommate, but I couldn't imagine living with anyone but a man or my children..

It was better when the kids came over. Oliver and I ate dinner together and talked about our day. He sometimes invited his friends for sleepovers. Chandi moved back from college that summer, and we spent time together almost daily, going to Crossfit or coffee. She talked for hours about her feelings, and her depth was too much and often I had to end our conversations because I felt suffocated in them. Is that how Brad felt around my feelings too, or was she being needy?

"You have no empathy, Mom," she often said.

I put empathy on my bucket list.

I saw Matthew only once a month, so that wasn't really helping me feel connected. The only downside to having my kids over was that I couldn't have sex. If I had been still married or had a boyfriend, I could have merged motherhood and sex.

How could I be sexually active as a single mom, when my kids were too old to be handed off to a babysitter or sent to school? I often wished they would leave for a couple hours so I could have a guy over. Once I was so horny, I just came out and said it.

"Kids, can you leave for a few hours? I want to invite someone over."

"I don't like coming over here, when you just ask me to leave," Oliver said.

"Yeah, I feel the same way," Chandi said.

"I know, I get that. I don't know what to do."

"Mom, how can you prefer some random over us?" Chandi asked.

"It's not that I like him more. I don't even know him. It's just that I have needs you cannot fill."

Being a single parent sucked sometimes. Maybe the empty nest was good, because I could have sex. I just had to make friends with my loneliness.

TELLING MY DAD ABOUT MY DIVORCE

I had not talked to Baba since our trip to Omaha that spring. We only talked a few times a year, so there was nothing unusual about it. Father's Day was a good day to tell him I left Brad and filed for divorce. I called his cell phone and he answered.

"Hi Baba. I left Gene. I am divorcing." I said, in Farsi of course.

"I know. Jackie told me," he said, in Farsi of course.

Jackie was one of his friends, who was my friend on Facebook. She had read it on Facebook and told him. What a gossip.

"I didn't know that you knew."

"Yes. I knew. Why did you leave a 'nice guy' like Brad?" he asked, disapproving.

"I wasn't happy."

"Be grateful for what you have! You saw your mom and me get divorced, you know that divorce is hard on kids. Brad gave you a stable life. What you have is due to him. Brad is a good man. "

I was angry he did not see my strength or abilities. Our kids were grown, so how could it be hard on them? He didn't even know how they felt because he never called them. What about me, and how I felt, and what I needed in a relationship?

"I had a purposeful independent life before I met Brad," I reminded him.

"No. You'll never find someone as good as Brad again!"

I would have liked a little more support. He really didn't know me very well. I was glad to get off the phone. There was no point in arguing with someone who communicated by lecturing, and it wasn't fun to talk to him because he was always right and made me speak in Farsi. I knew he loved me, so I told him I would call more often.

Sarina called and informed me of her upcoming date with Rudy.

"We're meeting in Denver," she said.

I was furious. Why was she boasting about it anyway?

'I don't want to talk to you anymore. I don't like that you're seeing him when I asked you not to."

The next time she called, I did not return her call. She kept calling, and I did not return her calls.

NOELLE

I had a great job, but I was not focused. I liked sex more than work. I spent hours online each week, while I was at work, looking for men and women for sex. I didn't bill for those hours, but my distraction lowered my productivity.

When I saw an attractive man online, my body felt hot. I sent messages to those men, and rarely received a reply. I didn't like being titillated with a palette of men I could not have. Maybe I wasn't hot enough for them. I lowered my requirements to men who were an 8 out of 10 and then succeeded in setting up several coffee dates. Many men cancelled at the last minute. I thought match.com was for people looking for a relationship, but Rudy was right when he had said "the purpose of match.com is to keep people on match.com." They accomplished this by continuously presenting attractive profiles. I had a few coffee dates, but the men bored me and I left before I finished my coffee.

I was immediately smitten with Noelle when I saw her profile on match.com. She was a 47-year old professional woman with radiant brown eyes that signaled confidence, passion, and strength. She had the long thick hair that I had always wanted. Her write-up indicated she was smart, witty, and educated. I sent her a message, and was thrilled when she replied. We messaged back and forth a few times, and she asked for my number. She called me right away, and our conversation quickly turned to sex. She told me she was a top and 'always in charge'.

"I'm very confident sexually. Taking charge sexually is what I do."

"Wow, that sounds amazing! I like to be submissive, and I love strong beautiful lesbians."

"Thanks. You're really hot yourself."

"Thanks," I giggled. She fascinated me. What would she do to me as a "top", and how was she "in charge"?

"What are you looking for exactly?" I asked.

"I'm looking for fun. I don't want to be exclusive. I'm going to date several women, and once it's not fun anymore, I move on."

"Wow! I love your openness and sexual appetite."

"I love sex!" and she laughed.

"I do too. I like men also and I'm having sex with men. Are you okay with that because if you're not you don't have to meet me."

"Actually, I am concerned about getting an STD. I'll have to think about this and use protection like a dental dam and gloves."

"Hardly anyone can make me come, and the lesbians I have been with were boring in bed, " I said, hoping I wasn't offending her.

"I can get a woman off better than any guy. Best sex you'll ever have!"

"Oh wow, that's hot.

"I am amazed by my beautiful feminine body, yet sexually I often feel like a man and completely relate to straight men in that way."

She went on to tell me that one night she spent two hours at a bar telling all her 'secrets' to a straight man on how to please a woman sexually. The man was so grateful, he almost kissed her feet. My head was spinning. She seemed so confident, a force of her own making. What would she do to get me off? Did she give good oral sex? Would she turn me on more than a man, and how would she do that? Could I take charge of women and be a "top", like Noelle and the women in The L Word?

I made a brunch reservation for Noelle and me for the coming Saturday at a restaurant with an ocean view. Then I texted her about the plans.

I like strong femmes. So HOT that u made a restaurant reservation with a view so I can see the ocean, but in reality I am always in charge.

That Saturday morning, I drove to the restaurant full of anticipation. Noelle was sitting in the lobby of the hotel. She was beautiful, just like her picture.

"Hi. Noelle?"

She smiled. A smile that lit up a room.

"Yes. Schahrzad?"

She got up and we hugged. She was about 5'10", with a strong toned body. I liked how she felt in the hug. We got a table with an ocean view and ordered brunch. Over coffee, she told me about some of her prior lovers, her work, and what she was looking for. After brunch we went across the street and walked on the beach. I felt proud to be seen in public with such a beautiful woman.

Then we took a drive drove up the coast. Noelle kept putting her hand on my legs and saying we had chemistry. I didn't feel the chemistry yet. Noelle said she was concerned about STDs, especially HIV. She asked about my sexual partners. I told her everything.

"I brought latex gloves that I will use when we have sex," she told me.

I felt a little hurt and disappointed about the gloves, but I heard her say she had brought gloves for "when we have sex", so it sounded like I was going to get laid that afternoon. Maybe the gloves would not detract from sex, or maybe they could be a turn-on. I also wanted to honor her need to keep herself sexually healthy and safe.

"Do you want to come over?" I invited her.

"Yes, of course!"

Fisting Felt So Good

We drove back to the restaurant, so she could get her car, and then we both drove back to my apartment. She brought her overnight bag in with her. I offered her some tea, and while the water boiled, she walked over to me, grabbed me, and leaned down for a kiss. Her kiss was delicious, strong and tender. She was strong like a man, yet soft like a woman. I felt safe and trusted her, which turned me on even more. I moaned softly in response to my arousal. As our kisses grew more demanding, my moans turned to almost a whimper. I just wanted to rip off our clothes and go on my bed, where I thought sex was the most comfortable. We went in my bedroom, and she tenderly took off my clothes.

I lay on my bed, naked. She kissed me and then she moved down to my hips, sat between my legs, and put on the latex gloves. I didn't mind the gloves. I liked that she was sitting by my vulva, looking at it, really present to giving me pleasure. My pussy felt so wet! She rubbed my labia for a while then slowly inserted one, then two fingers into my very wet pussy. Her touch was very gentle, not at all like the rough touch I'd had with some of the men. It felt good and my moaning increased. Her fingers started moving in and out, gently, slowly, and I really liked how it felt. It felt so good, I forgot where I was. I was moaning quite loudly. I lost sense of space and time. I went into some kind of zone and lost track of everything but the feeling of pleasure deep in my vagina. I realized I lost myself and I had to catch my breath. I came to enough, to raise my head.

"Feels so good. What are you doing?"

"I'm fisting you," she smiled.

I was alarmed. I had seen fisting in porn. It seemed gross and violent and painful. But here I was having it done, and it felt good. I couldn't decide whether I should be scared and ask her to stop, or let her continue because it felt so good.

"It feels really good, so just keep doing it," I said, and I sank back into the pillow.

Noelle kept pleasuring me with her fist, then she took out her hand, slipped off her glove, and licked my clit in circles and back and forth strokes until I came. Then she came up to my face and kissed me and we held each other a little while. I wanted to go down on her too, so she lay on her back and I sat down between her legs.

Her vulva was beautiful. Her dark curly pubic hair framed her thick outer lips. Her inner lips were purplish, her clit large and engorged. She smelled sweet. I started licking her for a while, sometimes looking up at her face. She lay there so beautiful. Her head was turned to the side; her long curly thick hair fell next to her on the bed. She looked relaxed. She started moaning more as she came closer to orgasm, and then she grimaced and smiled and moaned loudly in an orgasm that seemed to last for a full minute. She was gorgeous when she came. I wondered if I looked that good when I came. I was sure I did not.

"Include Me In Your Fantasy When You're With Me"
It was late. I turned off the light. I lay on top of her and kissed her. I started rubbing my body against hers, and getting all turned on again. I was too tired to have sex again, but I was turned on. I wanted to masturbate while she held me. I buried myself in her arms and rubbed my clit. I pushed her out of my mind and started fantasizing about a man watching me.

"I want to continue this with you, what we're doing, but I can't when you remove yourself and don't stay connected," she whispered to me gently.

What? It had never occurred to me that going into my own head and fantasy was pulling away, and much less that someone could sense that. It was pitch black in our room, and I was physically as close as I could get.

"Oh, you could tell? What do you mean? How can I fantasize?"

"Fantasize, yes. When you're with me, include me in your fantasy, make me a part of it," she explained.

That made sense! If it were daylight, I could open my eyes and look at her. Or if I fantasized, I could have her and the man watching me. I could have her watching me. In that instant, I came up with many scenarios that included her. I closed my eyes and masturbated with her in my fantasy also. I was so tired though that I kept drifting off to sleep, then waking up and masturbating, then drifting off to sleep.

"You're moving away again," she reminded me gently.

"Yes, I'm just so tired. Let's just go to sleep," I said.

"I'll get familiar with your body while you sleep."

She turned on the light on my nightstand. I snuggled up against her and was asleep within seconds.

The next morning, I awoke to that beautiful woman in my bed. Noelle said she had noticed the dimple in my elbow, my smooth skin, and the mole on my back, my fingers. Nobody had ever wanted to know my body in that way. I wasn't sure if I liked having this much attention given to me by someone I had just met the day before. I tried to be open-minded to being more loving and in the moment. But I didn't want to explore her body like that. Maybe I was just too selfish.

We had more hot sex that morning. I thought we could keep having sex that entire day. We didn't have penises that had to get hard and recharge. Lesbian friends told me about spending days in bed having sex when they first started relationships.

Noelle and I got out of bed, because she had plans for later that day. I checked my phone. Shannon had sent me about 30 text messages, because she was upset she couldn't reach me. Her neediness was a turn-off and I wanted to figure out how to get rid of her. I didn't even want to reply. I just liked being with Noelle. I felt free and easy around her.

I made us a delicious breakfast and we talked as we ate eggs and fruit and drank hot strong coffee. We talked about Brad.

"You've been deeply hurt," she said.

"I don't feel hurt. I'm happy." I said.

But her words were unnerving. Noelle sounded so sure of herself. Perhaps there was something I had withheld, something hidden so deep it had not come to the surface before. I wanted to look and examine all of myself, so I could keep growing mentally and emotionally. I decided I would make another appointment with the counselor.

After breakfast, Noelle told me I was smoking hot and she wanted more of the hot sex we had, and then she left. She texted me later that afternoon to say my scent was still on her and brought up memories of being so deep inside me. She liked the sound of my moans, the feel of my tongue on her lips, and the expression on my face when I came. Men never talked like that.

MY MALE ENERGY AND MENS' CLOTHES

Noelle's male energy and how she got turned on penetrating women intrigued me. I wanted to dress like a man, take a woman sexually like she took me, and be strong and powerful like she was. I already had a harness and dildo. I pictured myself in men's' clothes, my strap-on tucked neatly inside my pants. I longed to take and pleasure a woman the way a man took and pleasured me. I would make love to her and finger fuck her slowly and deeply. I'd watch her arch her back and moan from the touch of my hand. She would submit to me in utter sexual pleasure, and get lost in me.

However, my greatest reason for wanting men's clothes was my intense craving for the masculine energy. I missed a man in my home, watching him shave in the morning, and belts, ties, and pleated pants. In my man's shirt, I could be a man and take the edge off my craving. I pictured myself in public, the petite girl in heels and a tie, teasing men to be more alpha than I was. Secretly I wished they would pin me down, pull my hair, and throw me up against the wall.

I went to the men's department at Nordstrom's. Bright racks of shirts and carousels of colorful ties beckoned. I felt aroused walking through the department and selecting shirts to try on. I walked up to a salesman.

"I'm looking for a man's shirt for myself."

I waited for his reaction. He was matter-of-fact.

"Let's look for a narrow size 14. I have a wonderful new shirt that will fit you well."

He returned with a lightweight blue and white-checkered Hugo Boss shirt.

"This is a wonderful shirt. Notice the spread collar."

He showed me into the dressing room.

"Put it on, and I'll call alterations when you're ready. Just come out."

I went into the dressing room. The buttons were on the right side of the shirt, opposite of a woman's shirt, and it was huge on me. A seamstress from the women's department came to measure me for the alterations. I asked her to include darts. She pinned the shirt to fit my petite body.

A week later, my shirt was ready. I would wear it to work. The next morning, I put it on. I looked cute, but what if my co-workers thought I looked like a man? I couldn't let fear stop me. I wore it with a fitted brown pencil skirt, pink sapphire necklace, and high heels, to be sure I wouldn't look like a man. The pants, tie, strap-on, and flat shoes would be for another day. I felt immensely sexy. On my way to work I stopped at the dry cleaner and Starbucks. It seemed like more men noticed me, and they looked at me longer. Could they sense my sexual allure or know I wore a man's shirt? Perhaps the spread collar gave me a powerful look.

"I love your shirt!" the barista at Starbucks told me.

"Oh thanks, it's a man's shirt," I boasted.

I was nervous walking into the office. Thankfully, one of my co-workers complimented me on my shirt. In a morning meeting in our conference room, I felt more powerful. It seemed men treated me with more respect. Out at lunch, I started to feel confident in my shirt. Nobody was teasing me. Maybe I was cute. Women who waited on me at stores smiled flirtatiously at me, and moved their bodies while they talked. My shirt brought out a polarity between us. Their words and movements filled my being with refreshing delight. No wonder men found us women so enchanting. That afternoon, I sent a selfie to Noelle.

She texted, *Your lesbo look is adorable and sexy and makes a girl like me hard! I can't decide whether to scoop you up in my arms and kiss you, or throw you down on the bed and fuck you*

Fuck! I finally found a hot lesbian girlfriend! I wanted to be like her. I wanted to feel all my male energy and wear my man's shirt but next time with pants and a dildo inside, and throw women on the bed and fuck them. She definitely didn't fit that mythical lesbian joke of "What does a lesbian bring on her second date? ….A U-Haul." Noelle was way too powerful to be so easily uprooted from her own life and into someone else's. I felt free around her, and it boosted my confidence that a sexually experienced, smart, and capable woman found me sexy.

I didn't have that same feeling of freedom around Shannon. I had one more date with her and then I used all my courage to tell her we weren't a good match.

I had my appointment with the same counselor I saw about my divorce. I liked her.

"I'm here to make sure I have no hidden pain from my divorce," I explained.

She asked me about my kids, work, Brad, and my dating. I told her everything.

"You're doing amazingly well," she said.

"Thank you, " I beamed. "Well, since I am here, maybe we can talk about my mother. Everyone has mother issues, right?"

"Don't invent problems," she smiled.

We ended the session 15 minutes early. I learned to not doubt myself so much.

NOELLE: "LET ME SEE HOW WET YOU ARE"

Noelle and I took our trip to Las Vegas the end of July. Maybe she was a man inside, but she packed like a woman. She had a huge suitcase with several changes of clothes and a half dozen stylish sunglasses. That night she wore her Armani suit, and she looked like a man, and she was hotter than fuck. I felt proud to be seen walking around with her.

One afternoon, when we had returned to our room, I started changing so we could go to the pool. Noelle sat on the bed and watched me undress. She smiled at me sweetly.

"Go sit on that chair," she said.

I walked over to the armchair facing her bed, and sat down.

"Spread your legs. Let me see how wet you are."

A rush of electricity shot through my clit and my body felt hot. My pussy was wet immediately. I lifted my dress and spread my legs for her as she watched. She looked at my pussy. I was turned on. I hoped I was wet enough for her. I trusted her. I was certain the wetness was not visible to her, but maybe she knew how aroused I was.

"Come here," she instructed.

I walked over to the bed, full of anticipation of what she would do. She grabbed me and kissed me.

"You're such a good girl to be so wet for me," she whispered in my ear. I felt weak in my knees and leaned forward into her.

"You're so beautiful, so sexy. I brought something special for you," she said.

"Oh, really? What is it?" I was touched she brought me a gift.

"I brought a dildo that I picked out for you."

Wow. I felt love and appreciation in my heart. She reached into her bag and took out a harness and the most beautiful thick, blue, and translucent dildo I had ever seen. I undressed while I watched her put on the harness, and place the dildo inside. She came toward me with her cock. She kissed me to get me more aroused, and then she penetrated me slowly in the missionary position. I wasn't sure I liked it. I moved my hips and held on tight. I couldn't tell what she was getting out of it.

"You're really turned on by this, but you're not being stimulated," I said.

"I'm feeling pressure against my clit, and fucking you turns me on," she replied.

I finally understood. The "top" was turned on by penetrating and giving, not by genital stimulation and receiving. She moaned to the rhythm as she fucked me slowly, gently, deeply, and then harder. I opened my body and tried to get into it, but the dildo did not feel as good as a finger or penis. I grabbed her tight and moved my hips up to get more of her cock inside me, hoping I would start to enjoy it. I wished she would finger fuck me instead, or I could try using that dildo and harness on her. Noelle could tell I wasn't enjoying it.

She put away her harness and went down on me. When my breathing quickened and she felt me closer to coming, she put her fingers inside me. I felt my pussy get tighter and clamp down on her finger. My face pulled into a grimace as I came with a long loud moan. I hoped she saw it. I looked at her and smiled. She took her finger and put it up to my lips. I licked it. I tasted so sweet.

I was happy to go down on her next. Noelle had a beautiful vulva with a sweet taste. I loved how she turned her head to the side as her pleasure grew, how she smiled when she came, and that her orgasms lasted almost an entire minute. Afterward, I asked if I could use that dildo on her sometime. She said she only received penetration in a relationship.

The next morning over breakfast, I told Noelle about my public masturbation fantasy. Her eyes lit up. She wasn't like Brad, who hushed my sexual fantasies. Back in our room, I slipped out of my clothes. Noelle sat on the bed, watching. My skin tingled with anticipation. Slowly, I walked to our large hotel window overlooking the back parking lot. I reached down and touched my clit. It felt good. What if someone saw me? I turned around to look at Noelle for reassurance. She leaned forward, staring at my body. She looked turned on. I better be a grown woman and finish what I started. I looked out the window and rubbed my clit. At first, it was hard to let go because I didn't want anyone to actually see me. It was just hot when it was a fantasy. I finally decided nobody could see through the tinted windows. That's when I relaxed and my arousal built and I had my orgasm while she sat on the bed and watched me.

"I need to tell you something," she told me after our trip. "You remember the woman I told you about. I like her a lot and I'm going to be monogamous with her."

I was happy for Noelle, and sad for myself. I wanted to meet more women who were hot and sexy and free spirited like her. I went back online. It was hard to find women for sex. Most were unattractive. Others wouldn't hook up with me, because they wanted a relationship. The hot ones lived far away. Mostly, it was very time consuming to keep checking profiles and correspond with so many women. Most women started with a "wink" or marked me as a "favorite", instead of sending me a message. I finally gave up and started looking for women in real life.

A 23 YEAR OLD MARINE

My girlfriends had often invited me to join them for dancing in downtown San Diego. It had been decades since I went out dancing, because when I was married, I wanted to be home with my family. I put on some jeans, a James Perse beaded tank, and flats. Then I headed downtown.

It was a gorgeous August evening. Mary, Ellen, and I walked to several clubs. The nightlife and music felt exhilarating. I danced alone, encouraging myself to move without concern about how I looked. I drank water instead of alcohol, so I could be sober and take it all in. I noticed a few women on the dance floor. I asked several of them if they were bisexual. All of them said they were not. After several hours, I was sweaty from dancing.

"Oh my god, I'm having so much fun!" I told Mary.

"Yeah, me too!" she said, and motioned to a group of men in their early 20's standing a few feet away. They were all at least 6' tall, fit, with very short hair, tight jeans, and plaid shirts.

"Wow, check them out," she said. "They're probably Marines."

They were so young. What could she possibly want from them, or they from us? Besides, I wasn't interested in meeting anyone that night. One of the men left the group and walked over to us with a confident gait. As he came closer, I saw he was 6'4", Caucasian, and lean. He came right up to me.

"Do you want to dance?" he asked in a tender voice.

"No," I said, surprised.

I had no idea a man that age would find me attractive. He looked like one of my kids' friends, clean cut and nice. It seemed inappropriate to take him up on his offer. The young man walked a few feet away and talked with his friends. I glanced over at him. Hmmm..he was kind of hot. His young chiseled face, brown eyes, and dimples reminded me of the men I saw on the covers of romance novels, the kind of men I could never get because I was too old, and my time with hot studs was over. Or was it?

I walked over to him and smiled up at him. I was surprised I remembered how to flirt.

"How old are you?" I asked.

"23, Ma'am."

Wow, he was so young! I loved that he called me Ma'am. He smelled like alcohol, but barely, so I continued the conversation.

"I have kids your age. They are 17, 21, and 22. How old do you think I am?"

"38, Ma'am."

"I'm 51," I laughed. "What's your name?"

"Nate."

"I love your name! I'm Schahrzad," I smiled at him, acting shy in a way I thought men liked.

He repeated my name and it sounded hot. I stroked his arm. He was so strong. I was instantly turned on.

"I'll dance with you!"

He grinned, took me by the hand, and twirled me out on the dance floor. A slow song was next. I wanted him so badly. *Please, don't leave. I need this so much.*

"Dance with me," I whispered with great longing.

Nate smiled and wrapped his arms around me and we moved slowly to the music. I was only 5'3", about one foot shorter. I loved his height. I looked up at his handsome young face in the soft glow of the club lights. I wrapped my arms around his neck and nestled into his strong chest, being careful not to rub against Nate's groin, because I was a prim and proper girl. My panties felt damp, and it wasn't from sweat.

I longed for Nate to grab me tighter, kiss me, and shove his hard cock deep inside me. Would he come home with me? How would he make love to me? How often would he be available for sex? He was a young man, so he was probably horny all the time, and we could have sex daily, or as often as he could come over. I couldn't wait to run the friends-with-benefits idea by him, and find out what his plans were for after the club.

"Let's go outside to talk," I suggested after the dance.

Nate nodded and led the way outside, to the side of the building, where it was quiet. He grabbed me by my hips, and lifted me up in the air. I playfully wrapped my legs around his waist and then we kissed and laughed some more.

"I want to ask you something. I just lost my fuck buddy, and I need a replacement," I explained.

"I can help you with that, Ma'am," and he smiled and kissed me.

"What do you do for work?"

"I'm a jet engine mechanic for the Marine Corps."

Jet engine mechanic. Not white collar or officer, but it sounded hot. I invited him over and he eagerly agreed. We said goodbye to our friends and walked the few blocks to my car. That gave me a chance to finally ask him some questions.

"Why do you like older women? Younger women have younger bodies, no wrinkles, and more in common with you."

"Having sex with a young woman is like having sex with a plastic doll. I prefer sex with older women."

Did that mean younger women just lay there and did nothing? Did I just lie there when I was younger? It seemed he was exaggerating. Still, I was definitely more sensual, confident, and passionate than I had been at his age, so maybe there was some truth to what he said.

"Is this a common thing, for men your age to want sex with older women?"

"Yeah, almost all my friends want to have sex with older women, but not all have the confidence to go after it."

If many younger men liked fucking older women, why had I never heard about it happening outside of porn and occasional tabloid stories involving rich actresses? I had heard the term *MILF*, or Moms I Love to Fuck. Was that what he meant with older women? The term MILF implied bored housewives with breast implants and bleached blond hair that would fuck anyone, including young men. I never wanted to be so indiscriminate in my fucking. I didn't ever want to be a MILF. I had also heard *cougar*, which implied an inequality in power, hunting prey, and taking advantage of someone. I wasn't going to take advantage of him. I didn't want to be a cougar. I had also heard of rich older women who had *boy toys*, meaning the man was only there because she paid his way. I didn't want to have a man because I paid for him.

By the time we got to my apartment, it was 2 a.m. I went into the kitchen to cut a cantaloupe. Nate leaned down, his lips barely touching mine. He tenderly held my lower lip between his. A soft moan escaped my lips and I fell forward into his strong body. I felt my vagina relax from deep inside, and a release of lubrication. *Yes, I am a real woman, so responsive to a man's touch.*

Nate kneeled on my kitchen floor, pulled down my jeans and panties, and ran his tongue all around my labia and clit. I hoped I smelled fresh and clean. I looked down at his handsome young face between my legs. I felt courted, in a way I had once been pursued in college. He took a piece of cantaloupe off the cutting board, rubbed it all over my vulva, and stuck the sweet fruit in his mouth. Why had my husband never done that? Nate slapped my ass lightly.

"I don't really like that."

Most girls must have liked that, because he reached his hand back to do it again.

"I really don't like that."

"I'm sorry."

"Did you bring a condom?"

"No, Ma'am."

So he just went around fucking without condoms?

Nate unbuckled his leather belt and unzipped his jeans, revealing plaid boxers. He unbuttoned his shirt and I gasped. His chest was lean and toned, and he had six pack abs. I stood back and stared at him. He didn't have age spots or wrinkles, and his body was young, strong, and toned. I touched his chest.

"Wow…oh my god! You're so strong!"

"I've gained a few pounds. I've been drinking a lot lately, but I'm going to quit and start working out again."

"You're gorgeous!" I said, and pulled down his jeans and boxers. His cock was stiff, pointed to the ceiling.

"Wow, you're so hard."

"You like my dick, baby?" he asked softly.

"Yes," I whispered back. "Do you like calling it *dick* instead of *cock*?"

"Yes, baby, I do," and he smiled at me.

He took off my shirt and bra, and when he saw my firm small breasts, he leaned down to lick my nipples, sending shivers of pleasure straight to my clitoris. I whimpered and moaned. I loved my moaning. Nate kicked off his pants and boxers, picked me up, and carried me into the bedroom. I felt too heavy to be carried, 128 pounds.

"I'm not too heavy for you?"

"No, not at all," he laughed.

He gently laid me on top of my down comforter with the paisley bedspread. I scooted up on the bed and turned on the lamp on my nightstand. I lay back on the pillow. Nate went down on me, and I spread my legs. Nate's tongue moved all over my clit, first in circles, then in up and down strokes, then in more circles. He was so young, yet so skilled. I was glad I had shaved my pussy morning, even though I wasn't expecting sex. I had a sexy landing strip. Did that turn him on?

I felt completely comfortable with my naked body, which was toned and muscular, yet still had enough curves to be feminine. I didn't feel the same way about my pussy, aside from the landing strip. Would he like my scent, long labia, and the ugly enlarged opening from childbirth? Brad didn't like going down on me and always made me wash up first. Did I smell and taste good? Did Nate enjoy himself or was he just doing me a favor?

Nate gently slid two fingers deep inside me and because of my wetness, he slid right in. Waves of pleasure spread out from deep inside my body.

"Wow, that feels amazing," I moaned.

Nate licked my clit while his fingers stayed deep inside me. His face was buried between my legs, his hands on my thighs. I knew I needed to let go completely, to orgasm. I still wasn't sure I deserved to be pleasured, but I was determined to try, so I lay back down, closed my eyes, and put all my attention on Nate's warm tongue on my clitoris. I failed utterly at letting go.

"Do you like doing that?" I asked, because I had to be sure.

"Yeah!" and he nodded his head while he kept licking me.

"Come here, I want to taste you," I said, because I did not believe him, and also I was eager to get to the penetration.

Nate looked up. His chin was wet from my juices. Very hot! He wiped himself dry with the back of his hand and lay down. I climbed on top and he wrapped his arms around me, stroked my back and held me tight, while we kissed. Then I went down on him. I kissed his balls and ran my tongue lightly all over them. He gasped and moaned. Nate's sounds turned me on.

"You smell so good," I whispered, as I inhaled the musky scent of his balls.

I carefully put one ball in my mouth and sucked gently. I licked my way down further, to his perineum and beyond. He let out a louder moan. I licked all around his asshole for about a minute, which turned me on a lot and I was wet. I loved how I made him moan and how hard he was. I licked his dick from the bottom to the top. I looked him in the eyes while I slowly flicked my tongue under his fleshy ridge. Nick looked at me. He didn't keep his eyes closed like Brad.

"That feels good, baby," he whispered, still looking me in the eyes.

"You like it?"

"Yeah, I love seeing my dick in your mouth, baby," he said softly.

The way he talked to me turned me on even more. I wanted him inside me. I took a condom out of my nightstand, unrolled it down his shaft, and straddled him.

I gasped as he slid inside. I tilted my hips to get him deeper. Nate held me tight into his warm strong chest, as I rode him slow and deep. I nestled my face in his neck. A wave of pleasure spread deep inside my vagina. Nate grabbed my neck with one hand, my ass with the other, and pulled me close while he slowly pushed his dick to my depths. He gave a series of forceful slow deep thrusts. I lay on him, almost paralyzed with pleasure. I moaned louder, and then my moaning turned to a whimper and finally a wail. Nate grabbed my buttocks with each hand, which made me instantly wetter. He pushed me up and down on his cock by with his hands on my ass. I became more demanding. I wanted his strength.

"Deep, deep, deep. Hard…Stay deep inside, give me that deep pressure," I begged. He thrusted faster.

"Yes! Yes! Yes!" I was almost screaming. I knew I wouldn't orgasm from it, yet it felt really good.

"I want to come inside you," he whispered in my ear.

"Do it, baby," I whispered back.

I liked a man to come inside me. It seemed so loving and intimate. Nate held me tight. I felt his dick get wider and harder, and right when he started feeling even better than I thought he could, he moaned and throbbed inside of me. He immediately pulled out, removed the condom, and went in my bathroom.

I heard the toilet flush. He came back to bed. He looked tired. If he had a car, he probably would have left.

My hot encounter with Nate didn't seem so hot anymore. His ending reminded me of boring married sex where the man comes from intercourse and the woman is left to fend for herself. I hoped Nate would spring back to life and finger my clit, or do something I had never heard of before to give me an orgasm. If I had to give myself an orgasm, why did I need him?

He didn't offer anything, so I asked him to finger me and play with my nipples while I masturbated to climax.

We fell asleep and in the morning we had sex again. Then I made us some eggs and coffee. Over breakfast, he said he had been married once. He had cheated on her, and that ruined everything, but he just couldn't help himself for liking variety. I drove him back to the base at Miramar, and dropped him off at the shopping center across from the base.

"Can I have your business card?" he asked as he got out of my car.

I handed him my card. I wasn't sure if I'd ever see him again and that was fine, because I didn't have any feelings for him.

A few weeks later, when I was horny, I wanted to fuck him again. Nate had impressed me sexually. He stayed hard a long time because he used his penis as a tool to pleasure me, instead of using my vagina to get off. Maybe it was because he was married once and knew how to be with a woman. I wished I had his number so I could invite him over. Then I remembered him telling me many young men liked sex with older women. I didn't need Nate. San Diego was full of young men.

SOCIAL NORMS AROUND WOMEN AND CASUAL SEX
I felt at the top of my game, going after what I wanted. There was no reason to keep my exciting sex life to myself. I spoke about sex everywhere I went: to colleagues at work, on Facebook, my kids, retail clerks, manicurist, people at meetup groups.

"I have a date with a lesbian tomorrow."

"I have a beautiful woman in my bed."

"I had amazing sex last night with a 23 year old man."

The reaction was always wonder and amazement, so I kept sharing. One man said my sexual openness reduced his shame around sex, " I always have felt 'dirty' for wanting a woman's body because women seemed to get mad about it."

It made sense that men also had shame around sex. They were raised to believe they shouldn't want just sex from women, yet their testosterone and attraction to the feminine radiance made them desire women constantly. Maybe we would all be better off if we acknowledged that humans are sexual beings who often feel horny and enjoy physical touch.

"When it comes to sex, I feel playful, like a butterfly in a meadow," I often said, referring to having many sex partners. "I want to land on that flower, and that flower, and that flower. They are all so beautiful. I don't want to stay on just one flower."

Almost all women said they could never hookup like I did. They thought meeting men online was dangerous, even if the meeting was in a public place like a Starbucks. Others said they could only get naked if they knew a man, could not orgasm anyway unless they were in a relationship, and did not want sex outside a relationship. It seemed women who hooked up were doing it at bars, after they were drunk. Others had a hookup buddy. I didn't know anyone who fucked from curiosity.

Some of my friends didn't like it. Valerie, a friend from years earlier, sent me a FB message, *You're an amazing and sweet person. But I had to block you because I don't want to read about all of your broadcasted sexual activity. It's annoying. My friends are asking who you are and I don't have the energy for that. Sex is something private between two people. I really wish you all the best.* I was hurt, and yet I also understood. A few days later, a friend I had known since high school unfriended me because his aunt inquired about me, and he didn't want to explain it. Couldn't adults choose their friends without having to provide an explanation?

Was my friend Valerie right to say sex was something to private between the people having it? No, they were all just too timid. Everyone loved sex, and it was natural, not some dirty thing to be tucked away and brought out only in dimmed light for our lovers or in giggled conversations with girlfriends. Maybe the other people liked me because they also wanted to be free.

KRIS: SHE EXCELLED AT ORAL SEX

I kept meeting lesbians for coffee, but I wasn't interested in hooking up with most of the women I met, because they were not attractive enough. Kris was an exception. She was in her late 40's and overweight, but she had something I wanted: years of BDSM experience in a long-term lesbian relationship. We met for lunch. I imagined myself kissing her, but was repulsed at the thought. I debated whether I could have sex with her anyway.

"Do you want to come over and have sex? I just don't want to kiss."

"Sure, that's fine," she agreed.

Kris was amazing at oral sex. Her tongue moved and slid on my clit in all the right places. I moaned louder and I knew she could make me come. She was so turned on, she moaned and got really sweaty, and that helped me relax. My orgasm built and I came, and came hard. It confirmed that giving me an orgasm was about a person's technique, not my feelings. I just needed to know the person enjoyed it so I could relax. I returned the favor for Kris, and then I couldn't wait for her to leave.

The tryst with Kris seemed like a low point. I wanted to halt the meaningless hookups until I figured out what I wanted.

ABSTINENCE

I went abstinent. It was easy the first few days. But after one week, I missed physical affection and sex. Maybe humans really did thrive on touch and connection. I reminisced about good times with Brad. Maybe I would have been better off if my marriage had lasted. It seemed such a shame to throw it all away.

The truth was, I just didn't want him anymore and it wasn't just sexual. I did not even want to be friends. Aside from our children and years together, there was nothing between us.

"Mom, you changed and he didn't," my daughter said.

The kids told me he hadn't been sleeping well. They said his bedroom lights were on all night, and he had big circles under his eyes. I called Brad and asked how he was doing. He said he was trying to find meaning in life and move on.

SNUGGLE PARTY

Mary asked me to go to a snuggle party. Kamala Devi and Michael McClure, the couple featured on the Showtime series Polyamory: Married and Dating, hosted the parties. According to www.Kamala Devi.com/events:

> *A Sacred Snuggle Party is a sweet sensual event where we gather to flirt, touch, massage, run tantric energy, play, laugh, cry, share intimacy, vulnerability or whatever else spontaneously arises. It's a drug and alcohol-free party where we can relax and connect with like-minded people. More specifically it is a social laboratory to practice expressing what feels good and what doesn't, asking to get your needs met, setting boundaries, and perhaps even overcoming rejection!*

The full list of rules can be found at: http://www.cuddleparty.com/rules/. The biggest difference was that cuddle parties were non-sexual events, whereas nudity and sensual play was welcome at sacred snuggle parties.

About 30 people sat in a circle on pillows in Kamala Devi's living room. After introductions and icebreakers, Kamala Devi and Michael gave us instructions for our sensual play interactions. Throughout the evening's play, the rules were the person who was asked to be touched could say yes or no as follows:

If you're a yes, say *'yes'*.
If you're a no, say *'no'*.
If you're a maybe, say *'no'*.
When you are told *'no'*, say, "*Thank you for taking care of yourself*" to honor that the other person was just doing what was right for them.

You can change your mind at any time.

It was okay to change my mind? These people really understood me. I changed my mind often on things, even on such basics as whether I wanted a relationship or just sex, or whether I would get dessert after dinner. It didn't mean I was weak and unsure of myself. I liked this honesty.

Kamala Devi and Michael stood next to each other and demonstrated, "If you want to touch someone, you ask for permission. Let's say I want to touch Michael's arm. I will ask him. If he wants his arm touched, he will say yes. If he doesn't, he will say no, and if he is a maybe he will say no," and she turned to her husband.

"Can I touch your arm, Michael?"

"Yes, you can touch my arm."

Kamala Devi put her hand on his arm. I was struck by how respectful that was. I didn't like how men I met for coffee just grabbed me for a hug, without even knowing if that's what I wanted. Kamala Devi said we had to ask for each experience we wanted with that person, unless we already had a relationship or an agreement in place.

"Michael, can I hug you?"

"No," he replied.

Kamala Devi looked at Michael and said, "Thank you for taking care of yourself."

She turned to the group, "Notice when he said no, I was left free to go find someone who wanted a hug. I'd rather hug someone who really wants it, than someone who said yes just to please me."

That made a lot of sense. It seemed sometimes people said 'yes' to avoid disappointing the other person, and thus got into inauthentic situations and avoided reality. I wanted reality. I didn't want avoidance, withdrawal, or pretend.

Michael joined in, "This is how we deal with rejection. When I said 'no', Kamala Devi thanked me for taking care of myself. When you thank the other person for saying 'no' to you, you acknowledge that 'no' was only to take care of themselves. The 'no' has nothing to do with you. There could be many reasons I don't want a hug. Maybe I have an injured back, maybe I was worried I smelled bad and didn't want anyone too close, or maybe I just don't like hugs. It's so important to say 'no' if you are a 'no'. If you never tell me 'no', how do I know your 'yes' is real?"

He had a point! Kamala Devi nodded her head. Michael spoke again.

"Kamala Devi, I changed my mind. I want a hug," he said and turned playfully to his wife. The couple laughed and hugged each other.

After the instructions, each of us stood up in turn to share one experience we wanted that evening, and one experience we did not want. I liked this clear way of talking, and of thinking about what we wanted and sharing that. After the demonstration, we broke into groups of three and started sensual play. Within minutes, the room was alive with people taking ownership of their experiences.

I noticed several men sitting alone on the perimeter of the room. There were more men than women at the party, and unattractive or less social men did not find partners. It wasn't right that just because they were physically unattractive, they were excluded. I asked one very large man if I could hug him, and he said yes. I sat behind him, wrapped my arms around him, and closed my eyes. His body felt warm, strong. My heart warmed and I felt happy. I forgot he was large and unattractive.

"I like this," I said.

"I haven't been hugged in years," he told me.

He told me he lived alone and broke up with a girlfriend about three years earlier, and had not hugged or had any intimate touch since then. I was surprised that anyone went that long without touch. I was sure he wasn't the only one. I felt close to him and I wanted his touch.

"Will you hug me?" I asked.

"Yes."

I sat in front of him on the pillows and he put his arms around me. I leaned back and relaxed into his strong arms. I felt comforted. This was nice. Why did I choose people based on their looks, when the hugs had nothing to do with looks? If I were blind, maybe I would date unattractive people.

The next day, Nate texted and asked how I was doing. Abstinent, I replied. He texted me a few more lines, because he wasn't a man who treated women like objects. He was hot, but I really was more interested in my abstinence.

The only problem was missing human touch. I would go without sex, but I would not go without touch. I went to another sacred snuggle party. The hugs filled me emotionally. I always went home alone because I wasn't attracted to any of the people.

At one of the sacred snuggle party events, I was introduced to the Zegg Forum, an intimate container designed for personal growth and understanding. We sat in a circle. One person could step into the middle of the circle and share something deep and meaningful. A trained facilitator guided the process.

Aiden, a fit lean man in his late 20's, got up slowly eyes downcast. He said he got drunk and almost shot himself in the head a week earlier, because he was so depressed about not having had sex in years. My heart felt warm and tears welled up in my eyes at the thought of his loneliness and lack of touch.

"I haven't eaten pussy in years," he lamented, looking sad.

A man actually was depressed about not having a pussy to lick? This man craved giving what I craved receiving. I had an idea. My heart raced. I imagined lying under his tongue, my spread legs apart. As soon as he was seated, I jumped up into the circle to grab my turn. I needed unburden my shame. I walked around slowly, and looked down as I spoke.

"My husband never went down on me the first 22 years of our marriage, and when he finally did, he always asked me to wash up first."

I talked more as I walked the circle, and then when I passed Aiden, I turned to him, laughing, and said, "Where have you been all my life?"

Everyone laughed. Aiden laughed too. I wanted to find a man like Aiden, a man who really wanted to go down on me, so I could relax and enjoy it and see if a man could make me come that way. I looked at Aiden throughout the evening. Every time I saw him, he had a huge smile on his face. Sharing his pain had given him relief.

It had been three months since my last STD test, so I called my doctor's office and requested a full STD panel. My test results came back negative for everything.

ASHLEY: "ARE YOU SURE YOUR KIDS DON'T MIND?"
I met Ashley for a sushi dinner date in mid-September. She was a 34-year-old horse trainer, blond, with radiant eyes, a warm smile, flawless skin, and a body toned from working with horses all day. Our conversation was easy and comfortable. I liked her confidence. Ashley was lesbian, yet she had no issues with me also seeing men.

Despite her vivaciousness and beauty, I wasn't attracted to her at all. Maybe I would get turned on once we made out. We took a walk after dinner, and when we stopped and I stood close to her, I still felt no urge to kiss her. She must have felt the same way, because neither of us made a move. She walked me to my car, and then we finally kissed, and I didn't feel turned on.

I liked Ashley, so when she called me a few days later about cooking together, I invited her over. I checked with the kids, and they wanted to meet her. I suggested she come on a night they were here. The kids didn't like me having men over, but they had liked meeting my lesbian dates Noelle and Shannon. It really made no sense, but it was probably based on the meanings they gave my relationships with women versus men.

Ashley looked stunning. Her blond hair was in a ponytail and she wore a cute tank top and jeans. She brought all the ingredients and cooked most of the dinner. We ate with the kids. The kids liked her. During dinner, I debated why I wasn't attracted to her, and if I wanted to have sex with her anyway. After dinner, the kids went into Oliver's bedroom, while Ashley and I cleaned the kitchen. I was still debating whether to have sex with her. Would going down on a woman end my abstinence? Could I do it even though I wasn't attracted to her? Was it appropriate to have sex with her while my kids were in the next room?

I would have never considered taking a man into my bedroom with my children at home, but I had a different way of viewing sex with women. My mom often said women were more refined than men, and that men just wanted sex. She didn't get mad when she found out I had sex with a lesbian in high school. I figured sex with women wasn't something to be hidden away like sex with men. I had heard of emotional damage to children exposed to their mom's revolving door of men, but had never heard that in regard to women.

We put away the dishes.

"Do you want to go into my bedroom?"

"Maybe," she glanced over at me. "Are you sure your kids are okay with this?"

"Yes, they're fine, come on."

Ashley wasn't convinced. She disagreed with me and we went back and forth. I went into Oliver's room, and told the kids Ashley and I were going into my bedroom. They looked at me quizzically, but didn't object.

"Yeah, the kids don't mind," I said.

We went in the bedroom and closed the door. I still wasn't attracted to her, but I couldn't wait to go down on her.

"Can I go down on you?"

"No," she said.

I learned at the sacred snuggle party to respect and even encourage others when they were a "no", so I didn't try to talk her into it. She wanted to go down on me and I let her, but she wasn't good at it and I didn't come.

"Do you want to watch me masturbate?" I asked, expecting an enthusiastic response.

"No, I'm tired. I need to go," she said. "Send me a picture of you masturbating."

After she left, I finished myself off masturbating, and texted her some pictures of myself naked on the floor, in front of my closet mirror, with my fingers on my clit.

The next morning, I was in the kitchen washing dishes. The kids came in.

"Mom, we didn't like you having sex in your bedroom while we were home. That made us really uncomfortable, " Chandi said. Oliver nodded his head in agreement.

"Ok, I'm sorry, I thought you wouldn't mind since she was my friend. Thanks for letting me know."

Should I pat myself on the back for being such a good mom? The kids told me their feelings and I modeled that sex wasn't a bad thing to hide away. Or had I totally blown it, because a good mom would put her sexual desires aside when her children were home. She would wait hours, days, weeks, or years, however long it took, until her kids were out of the house, and only then would she have sex. She would be so devoted to her children, she wouldn't miss the touch of a man, a cock deep inside her, or cuddling at night. Maybe she would never date at all, like my mom.

Then I felt angry. My kids were no longer impressionable children who needed lots of attention and could be emotionally harmed by a revolving set of lovers. They were all grown up. I should be able to fuck whomever I wanted in my own home.

A few things were for sure. Whatever I did with Ashley was definitely sex and ended my six weeks of abstinence. Also, I was done having sex with women.

CHAPTER 11
YOUNGER MEN

I no longer wanted sex with women. I was done with soft lips and taking turns at oral. I was finally over Jenna. It had been weeks since I even thought of her. I was glad she blew me off, because I did not want to be in a relationship with a woman. I wanted the strength of a man, especially a tall handsome young man with a hard body and hard cock. I hoped it was common for young men to like women my age, so I texted Nate to ask what he liked about older women. He texted me back:

> *I love older women because they know how to appreciate my young hot sexy body- I'm 6'4" and I'm muscular. They know how to enjoy a nice glass of wine and they know how to actually have passionate intimate good sex. I don't mind that you're 51 - that's hot. I love the way u look.*

Damn, that was hot! If he felt that way, surely more young men did too. I just needed to find attractive men for sex. Bars were not the place, because I wanted sober sex. I rarely encountered the type of man I liked when I was out socially or at work functions, and on the rare occasions I did see a man who was attractive enough, he was with a woman or didn't return my glances. So I went online.

My bold profile asked for what I wanted, like I learned at the cuddle parties. I wrote "I like oral sex, intercourse, and eye contact", and posted pictures showing off my body in a bikini. I set the age range from 22 – 55 years old, and I looked for fit, tall, professionals whose pictures showed a love of the outdoors and a healthy lifestyle rather than bar flies. I had a huge wakeup call as I browsed the profiles of men over 50. In general, men my age had bellies and looked like they were tired out from life, and drank too much. I never wanted to end up that way.

I focused on the younger men. Their strong hard bodies and handsome faces turned me on, but I didn't need to see their bodies. An man with an attractive face, or outdoors, or in a suit at work were the biggest turn-ons. His lean face and posture indicated his energy, vitality, and fitness. My body felt warm and even sweaty just looking at their pictures. I hoped at least some of them liked older women.

JUSTIN, 20: "I LOVE OLDER WOMEN"

My plan was to meet for coffee, as I had done with the women. I sent messages to every man who turned me on. I rarely received a reply. Almost all incoming messages were from men I found unappealing. Finally, one incoming message caught my attention.

"I hope you're still on this site in two years when I'm 22. I'm Justin."

I clicked on his profile and liked what I saw. Justin was 20 years old, 6'3", and slender. He had a cute sweet face. I was touched by his honest desire to just meet me. Apparently Nate wasn't the only young man who liked older women. How old did these young men want their older women to be? 60, 70 years old? Could I really go down in age to a 20 year old? I felt aroused thinking about having sex with a man my kids' age, mostly for the novelty and perhaps also for the taboo.

What are you looking for? I messaged.

I love older women and I'm looking for a hookup.

I loved his honesty. We set a coffee date for after work later that week.

September 25. Justin, 20, student.

I arrived at the Starbucks before Justin, so I took my latte and sat in an armchair by the door and scrolled through my Facebook posts. I felt sexy in my skirt, silk blouse, and pumps. I kept looking up to check the door. A few minutes later, a tall young man with thick brown hair and a gorgeous long wool coat typically worn by men in colder climates, walked in. I felt aroused by his purposeful energetic walk and his classy coat. It was a warm evening, so he probably wore it to look sophisticated. He saw me, nodded, and came right up to me.

"Hi, I'm Justin," and he reached out his hand.

Impressive. His handshake was classy. And he was cute!

"Hi, it's so nice to meet you!"

He sat down, turned toward me, and looked me in the eyes, "How was your day?"

Wow. Nice opening.

"It was really great. Oh my god, you are soooo handsome!"

I loved saying what I thought and giving compliments and being forward like that. I asked him what he did, and he said he was a full time marketing student at a local community college. He also worked 30 hours a week at a retailer, and had to study after our date for a test the next morning. His discipline and work ethic raised my interest.

"I'm going to get a coffee," he said. "Go ahead and grab a table outside and I'll meet you out there."

It turned me on that he took charge. I sat at a table outside. It was the last week in September, and the nights were cooling off and I was chilly. Justin came out with his coffee. As we talked, all I could think about were my wrinkles. Did he regret meeting me because I looked too old?

"So you like older women?"

His eyes lit up and he smiled, "Yes! I do."

That was just hot. I was turned on knowing the age difference aroused him. I was probably part of some fantasy that excited him.

"What do you like about them?"

"They know what they want sexually. They are interesting," he paused. "What do you like about younger men?"

I imagined his naked body against mine, and his eager hard cock inside me. "I like their strong hard bodies," and I smiled at him.

"Oh yeah?" he smiled.

It occurred to me that a man liked to be wanted just for his body. Women seemed to resent only being liked for their bodies, but maybe men liked it.

"You want to come over?" I invited, because there was no sense in continuing to talk and I was getting cold.

"Yes," he replied immediately and looked me straight in the eyes.

I texted him my address in case we got separated. I met him in the parking lot at my apartment complex. As he walked up behind me to my second floor apartment, I wondered if he was watching my ass. He stayed right behind me as I unlocked the door.

"I like your apartment!"

"Oh, thank you!"

Justin followed me into the kitchen.

" Do you want some tea?"

"No."

"What music do you like?"

"Play what you want," he said.

I plugged my phone into the speakers on my kitchen counter and played the Passenger station on Pandora. It was slow and romantic. He walked over and leaned down to kiss me. His lips were soft and I melted into a warm soothing feeling that started in my heart and washed over my body. I felt open and receptive and yearned to be taken.

His strong hands gripped my waist and he pulled me close. He tugged tenderly on my lips, and then his tongue met mine, and I kissed him back slowly. I moaned softly. He didn't grope me, or push himself on me, or try for a quickie like Brad. I felt dampness in my panties, my body felt hot, and I wanted to take off my sweater. This was much better than being with women. I hungered for his strength and presence. I opened my mouth more and forcefully pushed my tongue deep in his mouth. I didn't care if he was too young or inexperienced to handle me. But he did. He hungrily kissed me back and gripped me tighter, his rock hard penis pressed against me. I was surprised a young man could be so aroused by a 51-year-old woman.

I felt weak in my knees so I asked Justin to sit on the sofa. He sat down and watched me come to him. I pulled up my skirt and straddled him, wrapped my arms around his neck, and looked at his young face. His beard wasn't even fully in. Much of it was still soft hair. I snuggled closer into him, and pressed my chest tightly into his hard body and we kissed. I didn't know kissing could make me so wet. I didn't recall if I liked kissing so much before I got married. It was so long ago.

My panties felt so wet, I wondered if it was soaked through to the other side and got on his pants, and whether he minded. I would never have dared do that with Brad. Would it be okay for me to grind my crotch on his leg, or would he find me rude? Maybe he would like it and be turned on by it, since he enjoyed sex and wanted me to enjoy it too. Worst-case scenario he would tell me to stop. I decided to go for it. I rubbed on him and moaned and got myself more and more aroused. He didn't ask me to stop like Brad would have done. Instead, he picked me up and carried me into the bedroom and set me down on my bed. I turned on my nightstand light so I could see him. He slowly unbuttoned my blouse, unhooked my bra, and slid off my skirt.

"You're so sexy!" he said.

I felt sexy and desired. He slid off my lacy thong, and I helped him take off his clothes. I looked at his penis. It was curved, hard and erect, and pointed straight to the ceiling. I was surprised that he was so turned on by someone as old as I was. Didn't men love younger women, and that's why older men got those younger trophy wives? I lay back on the bed, submissive, waiting for his next move. Justin went straight for my pussy, licking, flicking, and sucking. He was really good!

But my beliefs got in the way. I thought men provided oral sex as a favor, and did not like it because it strained their tongues. It made no sense because I could go down on a woman for an hour and not get tired. I wasn't that confident in how my pussy looked and smelled. I was worried about how long it took me to come, and whether a man would get bored or consider if unfair, since he would need only a fraction of that time.

I had a concern about his abilities. My orgasms seemed elusive at times and often required me to fantasize or focus, so I would get frustrated when someone brought me just to the brink, then made a slight change in technique and the entire buildup was gone. I would rather masturbate than be frustrated in that way.

I would only offer my pussy if a man really wanted it, and I wasn't sure Justin was that man. I had to stop the entire thing. I invited him to lie down so I could go down on him. He didn't say he wanted to keep licking my pussy, so that proved he was glad to stop. Maybe he only licked to orgasm with women he dated, and with the others it wasn't worth the effort.

What I Did For Sex

He switched places with me and then I gave him the same blowjob I gave every man, starting with the balls, down to his ass, and then long strokes on his shaft. I looked up as I licked him. His head was raised off the pillow and he was watching me. I looked him in the eyes as I used my mouth on him, which turned me on a lot.

"I want you inside me. Did you bring a condom?"

He took a condom out of his pants pocket. Very hot - a man who came to coffee knowing he would get the girl. I helped him put it on. I got on top and we both moaned when he pushed inside me. He grabbed my ass with both hands and moved me up and down, and I immediately got wetter. Brad never fucked me liked that.

Justin slid in and out easily because I was so wet. I rode him how I wanted, without regard to whether he liked it. This was still new for me, because I used to fuck men the way I thought they liked it. The longer I rode him, the more engorged and wet I got. His cock was hard and pushed on a pleasure spot deep in my vagina, a spot I had discovered only in the last years. I got so wet, I could barely feel him.

"I don't like being so wet. I'm not getting enough friction."

"I love how wet you are. You feel so good."

Justin thrusted from the bottom in a set of little pulses, which was extremely pleasurable, so I lay there on top of him like a dead weight. Maybe I was one of those girls who lay there like a plastic doll. But it felt too good to move. I wanted to scratch his back, but maybe that would hurt and he would be mad. I would do that later with a boyfriend, when I could talk with him about these things first.

"Deeper, go deeper, deep, deep, deep," I moaned in his ear.

He pressed harder to the end of my vagina, barely moving. It was the most pleasure I could fathom, and I wondered if it could grow into a vaginal orgasm. Then the pleasure subsided, darn it.

I sat up so he could see my whole beautiful body. Justin smiled. Then he flipped me over on my back and his penis stayed inside me, and his skill in doing that excited me.

Justin had excellent erectile function, so I could try masturbating while we fucked, something I had never been able to do with Brad and his premature ejaculation. I reached down to stroke my clitoris but his hips kept hitting my hand as he thrusted, and I didn't have enough room. I eventually gave up. Justin's breathing got heavier and faster, and his cock felt bigger and harder, and then he panted hard. After his orgasm, he remained on top of me, and kissed me and held me tight. I was a nice hostess and took his condom and offered him a warm washcloth. I patted his soft penis and balls gently with the warm washcloth, and he thanked me. He was so sweet.

"Do you swallow?" he asked.

"I like a man to come in my mouth and I always swallow," I told him, and threw the washcloth in the sink.

"I have a fantasy of coming on a girl's face," he said.

"Oh, I would never do that. That's so degrading."

"You think men do that to disrespect women?" and he laughed sweetly.

From his gentle voice, I immediately got it was not disrespectful at all for a man to come on a girl's face. I realized it was a huge turn-on and an act of love and connection, because a man associated his cum with his orgasm. Men were proud of their cum, including how much there was and how far it shot.

"Next time, you can come on my face," I told him, because it seemed fun to try.

I masturbated, while he stroked my nipples. The way he touched my nipples turned me on even more. It went straight to my clit from the inside, while my rubbing was on my clit from the outside. I was getting double stimulation, and the extra physical sensation overpowered all those thoughts in my head about whether he was bored. I was too turned on to care. It took just a few minutes, and then I came also. When I opened my eyes I saw he was hard again.

"Can you spend the night? I have a parking pass we can put on your car."

"I still have to go home and study for my test tomorrow."

I walked him to the door.

" I like you. I'd love to see you again," I told him. I loved my authenticity.

"I'll spend the night next time," and he gave me a kiss and left.

The next day at work, my report on a facilities project seemed bland compared to my passion of the previous night. I sent Justin a text, inviting him over. He didn't reply. I was disappointed, because I liked him and also because I was horny and had no other prospects. I didn't know it would be so difficult to get sex. My vagina was warm with arousal. Is that how men felt and was that why they wanted sex all the time?

That afternoon, when I was alone at the office, I closed my door and masturbated. I just needed to relieve the pressure. Then I got back to my report. I stayed at work until 11pm, when I was satisfied it was good.

Over the next few days, as I replayed the sex scenes in my mind, I got attached to Justin and started fantasizing about him, which led to missing him, and crying. I was mad at myself for crying over a man I barely knew, and not knowing how to let go of my pain. I decided crying was good for me, because at least I was feeling.

MY EX CAME FOR DINNER (OCTOBER)

It was October. I was grateful to live in San Diego, where it was still in the 60's even at its coldest. It had been a week since I had seen the kids, so I stopped by at Brad's house after work. I still had a key to Brad's house, so I just walked in. Brad was home and asked if I had a nice birthday. I didn't want to see him or talk to him. I told him about my interest in young men and he shook his head disapprovingly. Yes, I always talked about sex and he didn't like that and that's why I had left him, so no loss. I said hi to the kids and left.

I wanted to get over my resentments with Brad and get along. I invited him, my brother, and the kids to dinner. I had lived in my own place for five months, and he had not even seen it. He had always hated apartments anyway. I cooked a meal and set the table and then there was a knock on my door and they were all there: Brad, my brother, and our three children.

Brad noticed my bare wall and three pictures slanted up against the wall.

"These pictures should be hung. Why are they on the ground?" He glanced around, " Do you want me to hang them up?"

His excitement over hanging my pictures reminded me how he was excited about doing home improvement projects and completely out of touch with my feelings. Why would he would rather hang pictures than ask me how I was.

"How dare you come in here and fucking tell me how to decorate my apartment? I put those pictures on the ground on purpose," I yelled, my heart racing.

My kids and brother looked at me in amazement. I didn't care.

"I didn't ask for your help!" I continued.

I didn't tell Brad how I really felt. I didn't tell him I wanted to get along and talk about what was happening with each of us emotionally in our lives, and why I had those pictures on the floor. The pictures leaned against the wall reminded me that I would never be one of those single women who spent the rest of her life in an apartment because that's all she could afford. Some day, I would buy my own place, or move in with a man.

"You know, I'm just going to leave now," and he took his jacket and they all left.

I was a total bitch. I needed to get a handle on that but I didn't know exactly how. Maybe with the passage of time all my resentments would go away. I texted him the next day to apologize. But I hadn't changed my view of him so the apology didn't change me and I still had that to work out.

POLYAMORY RETREAT

I yearned for affection so I went to a snuggle party. I liked their teaching about authentic communication and marveled at their open relationships built on agreements and personal expansion. The hosts talked about a polyamory retreat and I immediately wanted to go. PolyPalooza 2013 was a clothing-optional takeover of a hotel in Desert Hot Springs, CA.

On my drive to the desert, I thought about Justin, the 21-year-old man with the long wool coat. I would rather have been home with him, but he had ignored my texts. I was also extremely horny. My panties were damp for days leading up to the retreat, but I was busy at work and put off making sex dates, figuring I would get plenty at the retreat.

I arrived at the hotel, which was booked with about 100 people of all ages, couples as well as singles. The retreat featured morning yoga, sex parties, bondage demonstrations, an elaborate rope tying demonstration, snuggle parties, BDSM and flogging demos, a costume party, STD and communication classes, Zegg Forum, and fresh vegan food three times a day. The Red Room, named for its red sheets and décor, was a public room available 24 hours a day for sex. It was for those who liked to watch, and be watched.

I propositioned the only two men I found attractive for sex. Both men told me *no.*. I envied the couples that seemed so in love. I wanted to be part of a couple. I checked my phone for a text from Justin. Nothing. No man propositioned me for sex. How did these participants get so many relationships, and I did not have even one? I envied them for getting all the sex they wanted, sex that presumably was good or better than the sex I was having.

The first evening, we gathered in a large room for a sexy costume party. It was the scene for a play party, or orgy. I wore my sexy schoolgirl outfit with my leather harness and dildo. I hoped someone would touch my dick. I was standing up talking with some friends, when I heard a man's voice.

"Can I suck your cock?"

I turned around and saw a large man in his 60's.

"What?"

"I'm Edward. We met at the last group exercise. I want to suck your cock. You're so beautiful, and I've always wondered what it was like to suck on a cock."

I wasn't sure whether to laugh at his playfulness, or be turned on getting a blowjob. I admired him for his courage to ask me and try something so new at that age.

"Absolutely! Here, let me lie down," I said.

Edward kneeled between my legs and he sucked on my cock with vigor. He put my entire cock in his mouth and sucked up and down. I'd never had someone suck my cock. I let myself feel like a man getting a blowjob from a man, and I pushed my hips up and down in rhythm.

"Do you like sucking on my cock?" I asked.

He looked up, "Yes, I do."

He kept sucking on my cock and I wished I had more sexual courage and could have pretended to come all over his face or in his mouth.

One of men who had refused to have sex with me asked me for anal play. Ah, my turn to be the dominant partner and deliver pleasure. He took off his clothes and got on all fours. I got some oil, put it on my finger, and slid it barely into his ass. He started moaning. Since he liked it, I gave him more. I slid my finger in deeper, slowly. He moaned louder, so loud I was almost embarrassed. No, I was proud I could deliver so much pleasure. I moved my finger in circles and went in deeper, then in and out. His moaning got louder, and he stuck his ass higher in the air. I realized he had saved our sex play for the group party. Did he like being watched?

"All the people are watching you be fucked in the ass," I told him, and his moaning became a wail. I liked the power of turning him on like that and everyone seeing how hot I made him get. I finger fucked him, in and out, in and out, and then since he was just on all fours and not even touching me, I got bored with it and told him I was done.

I sat in a chair and observed the large room of people engaged in sex acts. It looked like an orgy. However, it wasn't a free for all. People had sex only within the confines of their relationship agreements, and with others to whom they felt attracted. Aiden, the man who was sad over not eating pussy for years, was having sex with a beautiful woman, and I felt happy. I had no desire to get naked in front of all those people. They did not deserve to see me naked, and I needed privacy to let go and relax. I just needed to find a guy to fuck that I could take back to my room. I lowered my looks requirements and found a man who was reasonably attractive and invited him back to my room, since my roommates were out. We had boring vaginal sex in my bed, but least it took the edge off.

The next day, Edward told me he realized he was bisexual. After he sucked on my dick, he gave his first blowjob to a man at the sex party and he very much enjoyed it. I admired him greatly for making such bold sexual leaps at his age.

At the afternoon meeting, I noticed an attractive couple in their late 40's. Erin was one of the most beautiful women I had ever seen. I felt nothing for her boyfriend, Bryce. Erin was so in love with Bryce, that I was sure he was an excellent lover. Here was a chance to have the couple's experience I had wanted years earlier. After the meeting I went to the pool and ran into Aiden. He was glowing, presumably from the sex last night. I told him about my couples fantasy with Erin and Bryce, and he encouraged me to just go for it. I went into the dining hall for dinner and the first people I ran into were Erin and Bryce. It seemed preordained! I blurted out, "Do you guys want to have a threesome?"

"Yes," they said in unison. "Sit with us at dinner."

Over dinner, Bryce shared his fantasy. He wanted a threesome where Erin and I did all the work, and we would take turns fucking him. I couldn't wait. How would he make love to us? What was that magic between them?

Bryce emphasized repeatedly, "I want you to do all the work. Spoil me. I don't want to do any of the work."

"Yes, honey, that sounds great," Erin agreed.

"Totally. We'll do all the work," I said.

"I want to be in the Red Room," he added.

The Red Room was empty when we walked in after dinner. We took off our clothes. Bryce lay on the bed. He kissed me grossly so I didn't want to kiss him anymore. I put on a condom and slid Bryce's cock inside me. His eyes were closed. I rode him, but without the eye contact, there was no connection, and he didn't feel that good. He asked to fuck his girl. She was his favorite, he said. I couldn't wait to see how he made love to her. He must have changed his mind about being passive, because he asked her to get doggy style, and then he fucked her like a rabbit, in short quick thrusts with his eyes closed. My heart sank in disappointment. Is that how he did her, that beautiful woman? She deserved so much more!

The scene was a replay of sex in my marriage…my husband fucked me just like that….so unconnected, lacking feelings. Did she sense it too? I looked at her. She moaned and was smiling. Did she really love it, or was she just so in love with him, that she didn't even realize what was missing? Isn't that how I was with Brad? So in love, that I overlooked the bad sex? Yes, that's how it was. I didn't ever want to fall in love with a man and be fucked badly and deal with it just because of my feelings for him. No, I would not end up like that again. I would continue having sex on the first date, to make sure the man was passionate in bed.

I watched him fuck her like an object, and then said he wanted to come on our faces. I agreed, only because I had done that with Justin, a man I actually liked. Bryce pulled out of his girlfriend, and we lay on the bed near his hard cock, as he gave himself a few finishing strokes and his ejaculate shot out onto our waiting faces. We rubbed it in. Another couple came into the Red Room right after that. Too bad they had missed our play. Bryce jumped into the shower and I gave Erin a hug goodbye.

On the way back to my room to shower, I ran into Aiden. He smiled when he saw me. I blurted it out, "Aiden, I just had the threesome with Erin and Bryce, and I have cum all over my face!"

His eyes lit up and he leaned closer, "Wow, that's so hot! Can I do that too?"

I felt loved that this man wanted me, even though I had just fucked another man and had his cum all over my face. This was also my chance to get the oral I had wanted for so long. Nobody had given me an orgasm in years! I did not recall if any man had ever given me an orgasm from oral sex. If any man could make me come, it was Aiden.

"Yes, and will you go down on me?"

"Yes!! Of course," and his eyes lit up.

My heart skipped a beat and my clit felt tingly. He was going to give me an orgasm! My big day had come.

"Ok, let me just take a shower and I'll come right back," I told him.

"No, come dance first," he insisted and took me into the party room and twirled me around.

There we danced to the DJ playing music, with Bryce's ejaculate dried on my face. Aiden led me confidently, and twirled me around.

I went in my room and washed the cum off my face in the shower. My face was smooth and silky from the ejaculate. I came back to Aiden. He took me by the hand and led me to an empty room just off the party room.

He lifted me on a table and gave me oral sex that would not stop. His tongue and hands were determined. My clit was hard and engorged, and I felt the hard ridge of my clit under his tongue. I was so turned on, at the brink of on orgasm for 30 minutes, yet I couldn't come. Aiden's tongue kept the same intensity and pace. I felt frustrated and guilty for taking up his time and wearing out his tongue.

"Is your tongue tired?" I asked.

"I love it," he said and he didn't even lift his face off my pussy to answer.

I could tell he meant it. I sank back into the table. I told him I had to stretch out and tense my legs. I repositioned myself and put my legs together and tensed them. Aiden just put his face right on my clit and spread my labia apart. I played with my nipples. And then it started. My orgasm grew from deep inside, and I knew it was inevitable. I could feel my orgasm building, and it grew and grew, and because he had been licking me so long and I was so aroused, it was massive. My orgasm was so strong and powerful, I erupted in a screaming roar that lasted for half a minute. Aiden kept stimulating me with his tongue, but not right where I was sensitive, so he could draw out my climax.

"Who's making all that noise?" I heard several people ask.

I looked up. Several people had streamed into our hideaway. I was proud. Damn right, that was me making all that noise. It was me claiming my orgasm, my womanly power, my right to pleasure, and letting everyone know it. The people left the room.

"Thank you, Aiden. Oh my god, thank you. Thank you!!"

I felt elated. Relieved. Ecstatic. There was nothing wrong with me! I didn't have a secret block against men. A man could make me come. If he could make me come, other men would too. It was just a matter of their technique.

Aiden stood up. I knelt at his feet and kissed his balls and penis, and then I licked him while I looked up at him in gratitude and smiled. When he was moaning harder and close to coming, I took his penis out of my mouth and let him ejaculate all over my face. He looked at me with tender sweetness, and rubbed in his liquid. We held each other in an embrace lasting at least one minute and went back to our separate rooms. This wasn't a hookup where we would exchange phone numbers or start dating. This was love with no strings attached.

The next morning, I ran into Aiden. He was glowing. It was time for the morning meeting. I got up in the room of 100 people and gave my tribute to a man whose act had transformed us both.

"Everyone here knows that I haven't been able to have an orgasm from oral sex by a man in over 30 years, and I didn't know if something was wrong with me. Last night, Aiden made me come from oral sex."

The entire room cheered and clapped. Aiden got up next. His presence felt strong, and the entire room was silent. Aiden held his hands together as in prayer. He started with the man closest to him. He looked the man in the eye, closed his eyes and bowed, and then moved to the next person. A reverence filled the room as he walked around like that. He never said a word. And when he had thanked everyone, he sat down and smiled.

Sex was a powerful healer. How could anyone say sex was bad or dirty? My whole life I repressed my sexual power, because I believed good girls did not show their sexuality. The men at the retreat freed me. I would take this feeling out into the world.

CUNNILINGUS: CAN HE MAKE ME COME?

After the retreat, cunnilingus was at the top of my mind. Could other men make me come? If I let more men go down on me, could I get more comfortable with my pussy, and love it like I loved the rest of my body? It turned me on to look at it, but I was sure men did not like it. My pussy had all those shades of pink, and various folds and long inner labia lips, and didn't look like the ones I saw in pictures. Sometimes I felt repulsed by my lubrication and discharge and maybe it was gross and dirty. I wanted to get over that and like my pussy, just like men liked their penises.

I changed my online dating profile to ask for what I wanted. Other women might want a man who joined them on travels or helped them host dinner parties, but I wanted oral sex and an orgasm. I updated my online dating profile to include "Looking for men who enjoy giving oral sex."

I always asked men their height and what they did for work, because I could only fuck them if I respected their jobs. Most of the men who messaged me online were gentlemen, meaning they were respectful, used proper grammar, and did not talk about sex. If a man sent dick pics, asked to come right over instead of meeting for coffee, or inquired about my favorite position, I blocked him.

"I Love How Open You Are About Sex"
October 26. Scott, 28, salesman.

"Do you like older women?" I asked him over coffee, because I was still insecure about my age.

He looked right at me and smiled, "Yes."

I felt warm and my clit throbbed. I forced myself to go over my STD status, like I learned at the polyamory retreat. Here was the script: "I want to review our STD testing results. I was last tested for STDs two months ago. All my results were negative. I was tested for HIV, hepatitis B and C, chlamydia, gonorrhea, and syphilis. I was last tested for HPV in the spring of 2013 during my pap exam." Then I asked the man, "And you?"

Scott said he was tested 3 months ago, was negative for everything, and always used a condom. I liked that he was responsible.

Scott invited me to dinner, which meant he wasn't embarrassed to be seen with an old woman. Sitting in the restaurant booth across from him, I felt self-conscious. Why did he look me in the eye, when my wrinkles were so ugly?

The waitress brought our food. I told him about my hookups. Scott didn't act jealous or leave because I liked sex and talked to him about other men. I shared my frustrations.

"It's really hard to find men for sex. I wish I could meet men in person, not just online. And I don't want to go to bars, because I like sex sober."

"You can totally do that. Go up to a man at Starbucks, and just talk to him."

"What? I could never do that. He could tell me to get lost."

He laughed. "No, that won't happen. He'll be taken aback and flattered. He'll ask you to sit down."

"Well, maybe I could try that one day," I said.

"I love how open you are about sex," he said.

I invited Scott over to my apartment. His cock was extremely hard. *Thank you, God.* After years of a soft cock, I was still grateful when a man was hard. We had over an hour of amazing sex that included lots of kissing. How common was it for men to enjoy kissing? Maybe my friends were right – Brad didn't kiss me because he was gay.

Scott stayed in my bed for almost two hours afterward. He said he was almost ready to settle down and start a family. His presence in my home ignited my craving for male energy and affection. I put on my man's shirt that night and went to bed.

The next day, I emailed Brad and asked him if maybe he was gay. He sent back a funny email and said he definitely was not gay, and had been on a few dates with women.

"I Don't Go Down On Girls"
October 28. Mark, 20, biology major.

I met Mark for coffee after work.

""How's your experience on OKCupid?"' he asked, when we were seated.

"Great. I've met a lot of awesome men and had a lot of great sex."

I waited for his reaction. Would he leave because I was too slutty?

"That's hot," he said.

"You don't think I'm a slut?"

"No. I wish more girls were as open as you."

Mark told me he broke up with his girlfriend because she wanted too much of his time, and that interfered with his studying. He had his own place. I followed him over.

I liked his kisses and I went down on him. He had a hard curved cock. I had never seen a curved penis and was curious how it would feel.

He was very hard. I still couldn't believe a young man could be so turned on by an old woman. After a few minutes, I lay down, waiting for him to do that to me.

"I don't go down on girls."

"Not at all? Not even for a taste?"

"No, never. I've never done it."

"Well, you don't have to do that with me, but what about a girl you're dating?"

"No, I don't do that."

What a loser. I debated leaving, but I wanted to feel his curved cock. I got on top and just a few seconds into it, I was in ecstasy. I had never felt a penis that good in my whole life. He came in the condom and then he got up and said he had to prepare for a test tomorrow. I wanted an orgasm too just out of fairness, but I wasn't going to push myself on him because it seemed he was done with me.

There was no way I would ever go back to a man who refused to reciprocate on the oral and didn't care about my orgasm, so when he contacted me again a year later, I told him to get lost.

After the encounter with Mark, I started asking men if they liked oral sex before agreeing to meet them for coffee.

"I Love Going Down On A Girl"

October 29. Martin, 22-year-old communications major.

Martin lived with his parents, again due to the high cost of housing in San Diego. I knew from our messaging that he loved performing oral sex. We set our coffee date for a day that Oliver was not at my place.

Over coffee, he asked how my online dating was going, and I told him about all the men. He smiled and said he wished more girls were that honest.

He looked me straight in the eye over coffee, "I love going down on a girl."

That was all I needed to know. I invited him over.

Once we were in bed, he went straight for my pussy. I couldn't tell exactly what he was doing, but it felt really good. His tongue moved in all the right places and my arousal built and I thought I might orgasm. I had to make sure he could keep going and not leave me hanging as I got close.

"Is your tongue tired?"

Martin didn't answer. Instead, he grabbed my legs tighter and kept licking. Mentally, I let go. Within two minutes, my orgasm built from deep inside, and then it was inevitable and it happened. I climaxed with a long loud roar.

"Oh my god, thank you. Oh my god. This is only the second time a man made me come in years!"

Martin was beaming. He wiped my pussy juices off his face. I liked that he could give me an orgasm, and that he wanted me to come first. Unfortunately, the rest of our sex was not that exciting, so the next few times he asked to come over, I told him I wasn't interested.

TOMMY, 21: THE CONNECTION BETWEEN MY HEART AND MY PUSSY AND HIS OPEN EYE ORGASM

October 30. Tommy, 21, skateboarder, surfer, retail clerk.

The next day at work, I so was horny, I didn't want to work on my reports, and I didn't care about the cunnilingus. I wanted to go home and fuck. But there was a problem: motherhood. Oliver was scheduled to come over. I hoped I could sneak in a hookup before he got home from school.

What time are u coming home? I texted Oliver.

Going to a game. Around 10.

Good. I had time for sex. I went online and met Tommy. He was not that good looking, but I was horny and could overlook such things. We set a coffee date for that afternoon.

Tommy looked much better than his online dating profile pictures. I was glad I overlooked his poor photos. He was 5'11", lean and strong, with curly brown hair and beautiful brown eyes His recent STD tests were negative. He worked at a health food store, did not drink alcohol, and he had not been with a woman in over six months. And yes, he was really into older women. It all sounded good, so I invited him over.

I stood in my kitchen, plugged my speakers into my cell phone, and put on some blues music. Tommy came up behind me. He put his hands around my waist. He leaned forward and his soft lips met mine. Instantly I felt wet in my pussy and weak in the knees. I started moaning and leaned into his kiss. My entire marriage I thought men didn't like kissing, but all the men I had met so far seemed to love it.

Tommy's erect penis pressed against my groin. I pulled away a bit. I liked a man to warm me up with kissing, then finger fuck me or touch me in some way, before I touched his penis. While we kissed, he reached his hand in the back of my tailored pants, inside my thong panties, and my slippery wetness. He gently pushed his finger deep inside, and finger fucked me nice and slow.

"Oh my god, fuck, that feels sooooo good," I whimpered.

I loved discovering these new feelings in my body. Why had my husband never finger fucked me? Oh yeah, I remembered: because he used my pussy as an ejaculation device and finger fucking me didn't give him orgasms.

"Let's go in my bed," I suggested when I caught my breath.

We hurriedly took off our clothes. I gasped at the sight of his lean muscular body, especially his toned abs. His curved cock was erect and almost touched his stomach. He was rock hard, even though I was old. Maybe I was sexier than I thought.

"Oh my god, you're so hard!"

He smiled proudly.

"Your body is amazing," I told him. "Your legs, wow, they're so strong."

"That's from skateboarding," he said.

I loved giving compliments. I didn't say it so he would tell me I was hot too. I already knew I was.

Tommy got in bed with me. He kissed me tenderly and I whimpered at how gentle he was. I fell back on my pillows, and he got on top. Tommy's head moved down between my legs. He sucked my outer labia and then sucked and stretched my long inner labia, which was sexy as hell. Most men ignored my labia during oral. His tongue flicked across my clit, flicking and sucking. I spread my legs wide apart.

"You're really good at that," I told him. "Do you like doing it?"

"Yeah." He had a huge smile on his face. "I love it!"

I wrapped my legs around his head just like the women in some porn pictures. *I deserve this,* I repeatedly told myself. But I really didn't think I did so I stopped him.

"Here, come lay on your back," I invited him.

He moaned the second my tongue made contact with his balls. I was so gentle. I loved hearing a man moan, and being the reason for it. I inhaled deeply into his sweet musky smell.

"You smell good!" I whispered and looked at him. He was watching me too. I wished Brad had looked at me during oral, instead of keeping his eyes shut.

I sucked gently on the head of his penis, imagining it was my clit, and suckling on him the same way it would feel good on me. I licked my left hand to make it wet, wrapped it around his shaft, and stroked him up and down with that hand while I sucked on his cock at the same time. He gasped. I felt satisfied that I knew how to please a man.

I put a condom on him, and he held me tight as I rode him. His penis sent waves of pleasure through my body. I moaned louder. I felt safe in Tommy's tight embrace. He moved slowly and deliberately inside me, for my pleasure, not just for his own.

My heart opened to his masculine strength and sensuality. I surrendered to him and myself and the moment, and immediately I felt my pussy relax from deep inside and release more lubrication. A few more thrusts, and my pussy gripped his cock. I was not doing Kegels. My body was just responding. This is what I had started to feel the night I told Brad I loved him and he told me to stop saying that. There was definitely a connection between my heart and my pussy.

The pleasure was intense and my moaning turned to wails. I didn't care if my neighbors heard me moan. I hoped our deepening pleasure would last forever. Tommy gently turned me on my stomach, and entered me slowly. His warm strength on me, his hands on mine, his breath in my ear, and his curved hardness gently pushing inside me felt like being with God in the womb.

"Yeah, just like that…like that…wow, that feels sooo good."

He was younger than my eldest child, yet he handled me like a man. I was completely his. He thrust his penis slow and deep inside me. I stretched my arms out, and I was wide open, giving myself to him completely. I was making love.

Tears of gratitude and pleasure rolled down my cheek. Brad usually got mad when I cried so I assumed men did not like a woman to cry. I no longer cared what men wanted. I wanted to feel, and men just needed to get used to it and handle their own discomfort about it. I just had to tell him I wasn't one of those girls who was overly emotional for no reason and needed his comfort, or that I cried out of feelings for him.

"Don't worry, I'm fine, I just want to cry," I said softly.

"Let it out….let it out…let it out," he whispered into my ear.

Wow, I didn't expect that. My heart welled up with emotion. I had dreamed of this type of love making, where a man wanted and encouraged my emotions instead of disregarding them or pushing hem away, especially in the throes of passion. Tommy pushed deep against my cervix, where I felt the pleasure reach maximum intensity. Then he flipped me over.

"I'm close to coming," he said, as he looked in my eyes.

"Where do you want to come?" I asked, hoping he would choose inside me.

"In your mouth."

He wasn't amazing anymore. The lovemaking was replaced with pure lust and his MILF fantasy. I adjusted emotionally to our new scenario easily. I was glad I did not feel hurt. Tommy sat on the edge of my bed and I kneeled on the carpet at his feet. He looked relaxed, so I knew he wasn't about to come right then. I took my time.

I loved being at his feet, submissive like that. He looked right at me. Slowly, while we looked each other in the eye, I licked the shaft of his cock and circled my tongue around its ridge and head. At times he squinted in pleasure, or closed his eyes briefly, then he opened them again and looked at me. It was erotic. I sucked on his cock as he grew harder and harder, and I knew he was about to orgasm.

"I'm going to come," he whispered as he looked in my eyes.

His eyes had a faraway look. His body tensed and his breathing quickened. He maintained his gaze on me. How daring of him. I was incredibly turned on, and looked at him. I continued sucking him with his eyes deeply lost in mine. He moaned and I felt a rush of warm liquid in the back of my throat, and a sweet taste on my tongue. I loved his open eye orgasm. It seemed ironic that my hookup buddies were giving me the kind of intimate sex my husband had constantly refused.

I swallowed quickly. I wanted to love the taste of semen, but I did not like the mucous-like texture so I always took it in the back of my throat and swallowed quickly.

Tommy's body relaxed. He got up and looked around for his clothes and it seemed like he wanted to leave. Then he paused as if he realized it wasn't fair for him to leave without me having an orgasm also. I was really horny.

"What about me?" I asked.

"Yes, right," he said in a flat voice.

I was disappointed. I was faced with the same predictable routine I hated in my marriage and with other men: intercourse as foreplay for masturbation. I almost felt used, but maybe it was my fault for not insisting on coming first.

"Do you want to watch me masturbate?"

"Yeah I do. I've never seen a girl do that."

I masturbated and his enthusiasm made it easy to let go. My orgasm flowed and pulsed like a wave and when I looked at him I saw he was hard again. I felt happy and satisfied, and snuggled up to him.

I fantasized that Tommy and I would start dating and maybe fall in love. I had dated older men when I was his age, so the age difference may not be a problem for him either. It was close to 10pm, and time for him to leave before my son came home.

"Will you spend the night next time?"

"Sure, I will," he said, and got dressed and left.

I PAID FOR A ROOM

October 31. Jeremy, 35, construction worker.

The day after I met Tommy, I was on a high. On my trail run I noticed a large oak tree. Its silvery leaves fluttered in the breeze like a symphony. Was the tree speaking of love, showing me I had finally found it? Or was I just high from the previous night's intoxicating hookup?

Want to come over? I texted Tommy after my run.

No

My heart sank. I wanted more of this good sex, and why wouldn't he want that too? Maybe he feared our intimacy and passion, or the stigma of dating an older woman. I let myself cry. Then I went online to look for new opportunities because I was horny. That's when I met Jeremy, a single father of three.

Jeremy said he could meet for coffee after trick or treating with his boys. All the coffee shops were closed by the time he was done, so we met at Denny's. Jeremy was 5'11", lean, with a chiseled face and a sensuous manner. I definitely wanted to fuck him. Neither of us could have sex at our homes. His roommate was home and watching his boys and Oliver was at my place.

We needed a hotel. Since Jeremy seemed broke from paying all the child support and alimony for his three children, I paid for the room. A few years earlier, I could not have imagined being so horny, I would pay for a hotel just to have sex. We spent two hours together at the hotel. I gave him an A+.

The next day, I kept thinking about Tommy. He opened my heart to an intoxicating flow of love. I kept replaying the scene where he had me on my stomach, pushing deep inside me, while I was engulfed in his tender strength. I longed for more of this tenderness and hard masculine cock, and since he was the only man who had given it to me, I longed for him. I allowed myself to cry and sob.

Tommy didn't reply to my many texts. I would win him over the same way I won over my husband and children when they were distant: love and reassurance. I sent him several texts to tell him how wonderful he was, how great the sex had been, and how much I wanted to see him. He still didn't reply.

THE FUCK LIST (NOVEMBER)

I was horny and I couldn't think of a single reason to be abstinent or wait for some boyfriend to come along. The problem was finding men for sex. I needed to create a harem of sorts, a stable of men I could call when I got horny. I got out an envelope, and on the back I wrote down the names of all the men I fucked in the past months. I had a dozen names on the list. The older men I met were not on the list. I had no interest in fucking old men anymore. I rated each man's sexual performance: A = rocked my world in bed, B = sex was okay, C = sex totally sucked. I did not rate the women, because I no longer wanted sex with women.

The "A" men were passionate and dominant, had hard cocks in a shape that felt good, stayed hard as long as we both wanted, could thrust and keep the energy going, put me into a deep state of surrender and submission, got me very wet and aroused and engorged, wanted me to come first, and orgasmed in my pussy in a condom in a frontal position because they liked the intimacy.

The "B" men were good, but not worth repeating. They withheld their masculine strength in bed.

The "C" men had at least one of these turnoff characteristics: submissive in bed, bad breath, neglected my orgasm until the end, poor erectile function, premature ejaculation, could only orgasm doggy style or in positions which made me an object.

I texted the A men. Justin was tired from work. He was weird to be too tired for sex. Scott said he was at a basketball game with his mom and sent me a snapchat. I thought he was strange to prefer a sports game to sex. Jeremy had his boys. Tommy and Nate didn't reply.

I texted the B men. Martin did not return my text within the hour. That left the C guys, and I didn't ever want to fuck any of them again.

I went online again and looked at more profiles. It wasn't about needing to feel desired, or wanting attention, or a man to hold me or buy me things. It was about being horny and wanting to fuck, and satisfying my intense sexual curiosity. How would he fuck me? How would I feel? Can he make me orgasm during oral sex? Could I have a vaginal orgasm? Could I get attached? What determined how attached I got? What will he do to my pussy and how will he kiss me? Could I have open eye orgasms? How much emotion could I put into it? Did I dare do all the things my husband never let me do, like play romantic music, look my partner in the eyes, rub my pussy on his legs, and cry during sex?

The attachment problem seemed hopeless. I had developed huge crushes on Jenna, Justin, and Tommy after just one encounter. I had cried over them, even at work, and I didn't have a single coping tool. Maybe reliving pleasant memories was the problem. Or was it my love of those memories? Or was the problem creating pleasurable memories in the first place? Was I a weak needy woman who didn't love herself enough? Was I seeking love? Was it the eye contact? Or was it normal to feel this way? I had to fuck more men to find out.

TWO MEN ON THE SAME DAY

A young man caught my eye. Kevin was 28 and smoking hot. He was a successful entrepreneur, tall, handsome, fit. Kevin said he liked older women for the sex. We set a coffee date for Thursday evening. Then he texted a penis picture. If he hadn't been so hot, I would have cancelled the date right then.

The next day, I got a text from Nate, the 23-year-old Marine. He asked how I was doing. I remembered his young hard body on mine, how he called me "Ma'am", and it really turned me on. Nate said he was no longer a Marine. He worked in a warehouse and went to the gym several hours a day, to be in top shape for his modeling shoots. I forgot my sadness over Justin and Tommy. Maybe the way to not get attached was having multiple lovers. I asked him when he could come over. Nate said he was free Thursday after work and would come over on his way to the gym. I didn't like that. I liked a man to get showered and dress up for me, and the gym comment implied he wouldn't stay long. Also, Thursday was the same day I had invited Kevin over.

If I wanted them both, I needed to have them the same day. I debated whether it was appropriate to fuck two men in one evening, because in the past, some had objected.

"I don't want sloppy seconds," a man had once said.

"I use a condom," I replied.

"I don't want to have sex with you after you had some other guy in you."

"Why?"

The men never had an answer. However, it turned on other men.

"That's so hot! Let me be your second date. Let him come inside you, and don't wash up after him. I want to eat you out.."

But because of my beliefs, I put men like that into the swinger category, and men who wanted to be the only one, into the relationship category.

Yes, I could fuck two men, three men, four men, as many men as I liked in one day. I was single, and had no obligations to anyone. I just had to be respectable and shower and brush my teeth between men.

Nate, 23: "Your Pussy Is So Tight"
November 4, afternoon. Nate again (23, Marine).

I left the office early for my date with Nate. I put on a sexy dress, heels, and my favorite perfume. I opened the door and there he stood and I blushed. He was wearing his t-shirt, plain jeans, and work boots, which were ordinary, but he was tall, strong, and handsome, just like I remembered.

"Hi, how have you been?" he asked in his soft deep voice, and smiled at me.

"Great. It's so good to see you."

"You look amazing!" he said, as he came inside and shut the door.

I walked over and wrapped my arms around him. I pressed into his strong muscular stomach and held him tight.

"Wow, you feel so good!" I looked up at him.

His warm lips met mine. I moaned softly and felt myself getting wet. My vagina was so beautifully responsive from nothing but a kiss. Maybe it took me a long time to orgasm, but I got wet in an instant. Nate reached behind me, under my dress. He put his hand down the back of my panties, and slid his fingers easily inside my wet pussy. I moaned louder. We were still standing inside my doorway.

"Oh my god, that feels so good!"

I lost my balance and he held me with his other arm and his fingers probed deep inside me. I didn't want him to ever stop fingering me. I writhed my body to meet his probing fingers. My heart and pussy relaxed and softened, as I surrendered to his strength. I felt more wetness deep inside. *Deeper, deeper, don't stop, please.* Brad could have so easily had my surrender like that. He totally missed out by letting me go.

Nate scooped me up and walked toward my bedroom.

"Aren't I too heavy for you?" I giggled. I had asked him that before.

"No," he laughed.

He put me down gently on my bed and got undressed. I noticed his colorful large tattoos and strong lean body. I had not noticed the tattoos the first time. I didn't have tattoos, but I loved them on men. Nate's cock was hard as a rock. I couldn't wait to feel his hard penis inside me, and maybe I would have a vaginal orgasm because his cock was hard for a long time and he was so tender with me.

He put his head between my legs and I spread them wide with anticipation. His lips gently tugged on my outer labia. Then everything changed. My mind was no longer on my pleasure. I became preoccupied with my performance and value. Did I smell fresh? Did Nate enjoy my pussy or was he just doing it as a favor to prove he was good in bed? Did he think my pussy was beautiful despite the stretched opening from my three vaginal births? How long would he be down there before his tongue tired? Did he have a time limit like Brad, and had he checked the clock? My arousal wasn't building. Was it his technique? What did Aiden and Martin do with their tongues and if I knew, could I tell Nate and could he do that also and get me off? How many additional men needed to give me oral sex, before I felt deserving? Two? Ten? 100? Would it be different in a relationship, or was I the problem?

I tried to let go of all the thoughts in my head and gave myself permission to receive pleasure. My friend Allison once said every Marine she knew loved eating pussy. *Relax, Schahrzad, enjoy it, he's a Marine, he loves pussy.* Or does he?

"Do you like doing that?"

"Yes!"

His tongue settled on my clit, and then he sucked gently. I liked the sensation. I didn't recall him sucking the first time. I rose up on my elbows and our eyes met. We looked at each while he sucked tenderly on my clit.

Yeah, I definitely wanted to date him. Maybe he liked me too. Is that why he came back and looked at me while he suckled my clit? I imagined he was my boyfriend who loved going down on me, tenderly pleasing me, and doing all the things Brad never wanted to do. It didn't matter if it was real or not.

"Damn, you're so good at that," I said, still looking in his eyes.

He smiled.

The intimacy and having it all about me for so many minutes made me uncomfortable. I didn't feel deserving. My thoughts about my performance and value were ruining everything. I got up and asked him to lay down. I scooted down to between his legs and pleasured him with my mouth while I looked him in the eyes. I brushed my face against his hard cock and he liked that and smiled.

"Did you bring a condom?"

"No."

Again? He probably never used a condom. I had many in my nightstand. I slipped a condom on and started riding him.

I liked being on top. I could angle my hips so his cock hit different places deep in my vagina. Nate thrusted slowly and deliberately from the bottom. I was mesmerized by the sensations. I became the girl who just lay there because it felt too good to move.

"Your pussy is so tight!" he whispered.

"Really, I'm tight?" Damn, that turned me on!

"Yeah, you're really tight."

Wow, I had a tight pussy. I had not heard that before. I asked Brad once if my pussy was looser after childbirth and he said he didn't know, since he wasn't sure how it felt before. Nate was used to fucking young women. Did he mean I was tight like young women, or tight compared to how he thought I would feel for my age, or compared to other women who had given vaginal birth? Maybe all those Kegels had paid off.

Nate gently flipped me on my back, without slipping out. His competent move put me into a deeper state of trust and surrender. My surrender and submission to a man felt spiritual, because it was a trust and a letting go to the unknown adventure ahead of us. That's why I picked men I trusted, so I could let go like that. Nate held me tight and moved purposefully inside of me. I kept getting wetter.

In porn, women sometimes looked at cocks going in and out. I knew it turned men on to watch the penetration, and to know the woman liked seeing it too. I tensed my abs and raised my head to watch his hard cock sliding in and out of my pussy, the condom shiny with my fluid, my long inner labia wrapped around his cock. It didn't really do much for me though. What really turned me on was seeing the V line above his lean hips as he thrusted.

"You like seeing my dick move in and out of your pussy, baby?" he asked.

"Yeah, I do," I exaggerated.

"Can I come inside you? Without a condom?"

"I love a man coming inside of me! But I can't do that with you without a condom. Why do you like coming inside a girl?"

"It's more intimate."

"Yeah. Well, come inside me, with a condom."

Nate held me tighter, thrusted a few more times, and then pulled out and lay down. He didn't hold me close and kiss me and try to give me an orgasm. At least he didn't get up right away like last time, but it was lame. I knew men could perform better.

"It's really better to let the woman come first."

"Yeah, I know," he replied.

I masturbated to orgasm with him right next to me, yet I felt all alone. Maybe he would open up more if we dated. I used all my courage to ask.

"Can we go out sometime, maybe to the beach or something?"

"Then it would mean something," he said. "I don't want to be in a relationship."

While he got dressed, he told me about his calendar shoot in Dallas, and then he was gone. I felt deserted. I didn't feel used. Nate was sweet to me, and I enjoyed myself. But I longed for a deeper longer connection, and I was just a pit stop between work and the gym. I let myself feel sad and then I sobbed. When I finished crying, I sat down and played piano. The tender music of Chopin filled my heart in all the places he had opened up and left behind.

I had to cheer myself up for my date with Kevin. I showered and put on a pretty dress. I was still wondering if it was appropriate to fuck Kevin right after Nate. Since Nate had ejaculated in the condom and I had washed his scent off, it seemed perfectly fine.

Kevin, 28: He Was A Stud

Later that evening. Kevin, 28, entrepreneur.

I arrived at the coffee shop on time. Kevin was seated. He was one of the best looking men I had ever seen, and he put on all his charm. He rose to greet me, and shook my hand, and we went up to order our coffees. I let him pay. Sometimes I paid for the coffees, because it didn't seem fair that the man always had to pay and the woman acted so helpless; however, recently my sister and some friends convinced me that men enjoyed paying for a woman. I let myself receive. We sat down and the conversation flowed, so after a half hour of talking, I invited him over.

At home, in my bed, I surrendered to his kisses, embrace, strength, passion, and gorgeous hard cock. He had two orgasms, I had one, and we joked and laughed. Maybe I found a good hookup buddy at last. I gave Kevin an A+ and added him to my fuck list.

After that, I gave myself permission to fuck more than one man in a day. My friends admitted they did it too, because, as one said, "sometimes schedules require it". I liked having sex with two men in one day. It felt freeing, like breaking out of prison - the prison of my beliefs and upbringing. I was taught to fuck only one man at a time, because men expected that of women. I had gone along with a monogamy dating standard my whole life, not questioning it at all. But I wasn't anyone's property and I was single and had no monogamy agreements. Men at the polyamory retreat liked me regardless of how many men I fucked, and they were my new standard. I was done repressing my sexuality to please some future husband, society, and future employers.

BORED AND DISTRACTED AT WORK

I had been at my company over two years. We were growing. My company was pleased with my work…..specifically my curiosity, loyalty, and intelligence. I got involved in new projects and had more responsibility. I asked for an increase in my hourly rate, and got it. My flex-hours and independent contractor status made a vibrant personal life possible. I had time for meditating, running, leisurely mornings, relaxing evenings, and sex, because I worked only 25 – 35 hours a week, and I could come and go when I wanted.

Yet, despite the opportunities and wonderful colleagues, I was bored at work. I was doing work anybody could do and I felt trapped being indoors all day. The large windows and light streaming into my office didn't help. I yearned for something creative, where I wasn't stuck at a desk. Sometimes I updated my resume and looked online for other jobs, but I never went on any interviews, because I did not find a job that seemed worth trading my part-time flex hours for a standard life based on productivity at a desk, long commutes, and all the stress-related illnesses that went along with it.

I took frequent breaks to browse my online dating sites, and this lowered my productivity. I felt guilty for staying at the job, when I was not committed to it.

My tingly genitals also distracted me. A few times when everyone was out of the office, I masturbated, just to get some relief. I liked being so horny.

LONELY, YET UNAVAILABLE

I had been single and in my apartment six months, and had not met a single prospect for dating. I went everywhere alone: movies, restaurants, coffee, running, and walks in nature. I liked all my walks, except for the nighttime walks alone on the Oceanside pier, which brought out in me a romantic longing to be with a man. Maybe I shouldn't walk alone in the moonlight? I thought of taking a vacation, but not alone. Vacations required a lover. I didn't like traveling anyway.

I still staid up until I was thoroughly exhausted before I went to bed. My friends had offered suggestions.

"Get a body pillow."

"Get a bedtime routine that comforts you, like reading a good book with hot tea."

"Make your room and bed a place you long to be."

I pictured fluffy pillows, candles, and large teddy bears. I didn't want pillows or stuffed animals. I wanted a man who gave me everything I didn't get with Brad. I yearned for a man who loved me, held me at night, and brought out more feelings in me, a man who made love to me and didn't bolt after he came.

Usually people gave me words that did not help:

"You'll meet someone when you least expect it."

"You should be happy in yourself before you get a boyfriend. I met my boyfriend when I wasn't even looking."

Did that mean I had to stop wanting a boyfriend, in order to get one? Why didn't they dump their boyfriends and get happy in themselves, because some of them were not always happy either? Besides, maybe they were happy single because they were relieved to finally get out of their unsatisfying relationship. I had times like that in my life too, where I was happy to be alone. But I had been in a loving marriage, and I knew what I was missing.

I imagined a boyfriend but got stuck immediately by two factors. First, I had no idea what age I wanted. A man in his 20's was appealing. He was at the same stage of life I was: childless and developing a career, and his young hard body was erotic. A man in his 30's or 40's with children at home had similar life experience and could give me a do-over on family life and my failed marriage. My boyfriend and I could take the kids to soccer, have family dinners, and make love all night. A man in his 50's seemed scary, because he reminded me of lost vitality and death, but he would have time for me.

Second, I felt guilty for wanting a boyfriend at all. I believed relationships were for weak needy people who could not be happy without them. Why would anyone need a relationship unless they were in their 20's and wanted children? Why would anyone need a relationship after the children were gone? Wasn't that just being needy? I considered getting a temporary relationship, so I could experience passion and intimacy, without the baggage of it needing to last forever or feeling needy for wanting it.

Thanksgiving was only a few weeks away. After work, I drove over to Brad's house. I was glad he had the house, so he could deal with providing turkey dinner for the kids. I hated holidays anyway. I parked on the street instead of my old spot in the driveway. I turned the key in the lock, and opened the door, and our black lab ran up to greet me. Why didn't Brad ask me to return the key?

I went into Oliver's room. "Oliver!" I said happily.

Oliver smiled when he saw me. "Hi Mom."

I sat on his bed and petted his cat, Tabby. "When are you coming over again, honey?"

"Sunday. I'm so busy with school, homework, and gym on school days, and it's so much work to carry all my things over."

"Yeah, I know. Would it help if we got you a second set of books from school, so at least you didn't have to bring all that?"

"No, that's okay. The other thing is that since you live further from my school I have to get up 20 minutes earlier and spend double on gas."

"I'll give you gas money," and I handed him $60. He smiled.

He wanted to come over. He was just trying to make it all work too. I missed him, but at the same time I was glad he was gone because I could have sex whenever I wanted.

"Where's Chandi?"

"She's at work."

"Ok., honey, I'll let you get back to your books and I'll see you on Sunday."

On my way out the door, I ran into Brad.

"I'm making Thanksgiving dinner. You can join us if you like," he said.

"That's really nice of you, but no thanks."

On the way home, I wondered why he was so nice to me, and why I couldn't stand him. Usually the person left behind was angry with the spouse who left. Our situation was flipped. I figured my resentments would disappear with time.

The next morning, I felt happy. I didn't want a relationship. I wanted temporary passionate encounters and the freedom to fuck any guy I liked. If I had not been so horny and curious about my sexuality, I would have been abstinent and buried myself in career, piano, reading, children and friends, volunteer work, and exploring San Diego solo.

KEVIN, 28: RAIL AND BAIL OFFICE SEX

November 8. Kevin again, the 28 year old entrepreneur.

I was late at work, editing a report at work, when I saw a text from Kevin.

What are you doing?

I'm at work.

Can I come by?

I had often fantasized about having sex at work, because I had a fetish for businessmen in suits and was constantly horny. In my fantasy, I pulled up my skirt, sat on my desk, and spread my legs for a handsome man in my office. He unzipped his pleated trousers, pulled out his cock, and fucked me with abandon.

Kevin's timing was perfect, because everyone else had already left for the day. I gave him my address. He arrived within a half hour and I unlocked the door to our suite and let him in. Kevin followed me into my office. He stood against my desk, and stripped from the waist down. He had not even kissed or touched me. I debated sending him home, but I wanted to try office sex and maybe he would warm up. I knelt at his feet because I liked being submissive. I licked and sucked his cock and within two minutes, he came in my mouth. I expected him to pull me up, kiss me, and pull me close.

"I have to go to the bathroom, " he said.

He took his clothes and went down the hall. I knew he could get hard again immediately, and I was excited to have him fuck me on my desk. A minute later, he came back to my office. He was fully dressed.

"I have to go," he said.

Seriously? What a loser.

"I didn't agree to have you come and ignore me completely. I feel a little used," I said, as I walked him to the door.

He grinned sheepishly and said goodbye. After he left, I got mad. I texted him, *You went from A+ to D. What a loser to come over and not care about my orgasm. Fuck u. Don't ever contact me again.*

I liked how I could show my anger.

Is your daughter good in bed? He texted an hour later.

What a loser, to bring my daughter into it. Maybe that was his way of getting back at me for telling him off. I became fascinated by his behavior. How could an man deteriorate from A+ to D from one encounter to the next? Was he afraid of showing his feelings so he had to treat me like an object the second time? Is that why he worked so much, to avoid closeness with a woman? Is that why he was still single and not dating in his late 20's? I locked up the office.

"HE'S ALWAYS ONLNE"

On my drive home, I called Mary and told her about Kevin because I really needed to vent.

"He sounds lame."

"Yeah, his nerve. I couldn't believe it."

Remember that guy I've been seeing, Tom?" she asked.

"Yes. The 55 year old sales guy."

"Yes. I've been exclusive with him now for 3 months, and each time I go on OKCupid, he is showing as being online."

"I'm sorry."

"Can you go online and see if he's on there?"

"Yeah, when I get home. I'll call you back in 10 minutes."

When I got home, I looked him up. Sure enough, he was online. I called Mary.

"Tell me his screen name again."

She told me and I looked him up. "Yup, he is online."

She sighed. "That makes me so sad. Why is he on there, when he can have me? We have so much fun together."

"DI know. I've had that happen a lot. Did he say he would be exclusive?"

"No, and I didn't want to ask, but we have so much fun together and I don't want to date many men. I want just one man."

"I'm sorry."

"I'm really horny."

Mary was always horny.

"Go online and find a hot guy for hooking up," I advised.

"I get attached though."

"Have sex with guys you can't fall for. Get a young guy."

"I want a relationship. I don't want just sex."

"You're not finding a relationship and you're always horny, so find a fuck buddy."

"No, I don't want to get naked with a man unless I know him. And I was just getting comfortable with Tom."

"Well, at least you're dating. I just fuck men."

She laughed. "You want to come over Friday night? I'll make you dinner."

"That sounds wonderful. See you then."

Everything she said made sense. I compared myself to her, and women I knew, and women I read about and saw on TV. I didn't know anybody who hooked up as much as I did and with men so much younger. Why didn't other women pursue sex for its own sake? Women were just as horny as men, but they didn't go around fucking at random, unless they were drunk.

Some people said I gave myself permission because I was from Germany, a country where people were more sexually open and did not have shame or guilt about enjoying sex. Maybe they forgot I had a Persian father, who taught me women should never give men sex, unless they were married.

My only problems were finding men for sex, and motherhood. Oliver was with me every other week, and that meant no sex. Most young men in San Diego lived with roommates and parents, due to the high cost of housing. They did not want a girl over for sex and moaning. I had to do all my hooking up at my place, on the week I did not have Oliver.

FEMALE CONDOM

I sometimes used a female condom, because it gave the man more sensitivity. The female condom had a closed end with a ring that hooked around the cervix like a diaphragm, and a wide open end that stuck out by several inches from the vagina. The man would put his penis inside the condom and start thrusting. Men liked it because it wasn't tight around their shaft like male condoms. The problem was that the condom had a large failure rate. It shifted easily without my knowledge, and the man's ejaculate was inside me.

Here's a rundown of the next two weeks:

Nov 9. Tommy, 21 again, female condom slipped, A+
Nov 10. Tony, 32, B
Nov 16. Tommy, 21 again, A
Nov 17. Brett, 19, D
Nov 18. Jose, 27, B

Caden was a 6'3", skinny, 19-year-old Marine from Oklahoma, stationed at Camp Pendleton. He didn't show up for our coffee date, which was odd. I wrote him off as rude and a flake.

TWO MEN IN ONE DAY AGAIN

Justin, 20: Trying Out Taboos
November 22. Justin.

I was glad when Justin texted me. I had hoped we could go out before sex, but he just asked to come over. He was probably embarrassed to be seen in public with me because of my wrinkles. I was a little hurt about it, but it made sense and I was horny. We made a date for the next evening.

He stood at my door, wearing that same long coat.

"Hi Justin," I smiled at him. "I forgot how tall and strong and handsome you are."

"You look great too! I'm glad to see you again." He beamed a smile at me.

I flirted with him as I wrapped my arms around him and snuggled up against his chest. I felt relaxed, and warm in my heart and pussy.

"Do you want anything to drink?" I offered.

"Let's drink a glass of red wine, and sit and talk," he suggested.

I did not want to drink alcohol before sex, but I also wanted to be flexible and not rigid, and open to new experiences. All my sex had been sober. Why not try sex on wine?

"Sure, that sounds great!"

I poured two glasses of cabernet sauvignon, and brought them to my dining room table. I lit candles. We sipped our wine and talked and he kept his eye contact with me. His calm confidence was impressive. I wondered if I could have pulled that off at his age.

"Do you still like older women?" I asked.

"I don't think it's something that ever goes away," he said, looking right at me.

Fuck! That was hot. I walked over and kissed him. His lips were warm and soft. It felt like he yielded to me, and then I yielded to him. A warm feeling arose in my heart. Did that mean I was becoming attached?

"Here, let's go in my bedroom."

I lit two candles and the lamp on my nightstand, and quickly took off my clothes. I turned around and saw he was naked too. His cock was rock hard. He had a thin lanky build and was only 20 years old, but inside he was calm and had a strong presence. I trusted him. He lay on top of me in bed, and we kissed, sensuous and deep.

"I want you inside me," I whispered while I looked him in the eyes.

He got up and took a condom out of his pants pocket. Good, he was responsible and came prepared. He got on top again and pleasured me deep inside with his penis. I clutched him tight, lost in my moans and the intense pleasure inside my body. His cock took me to places I wished I could take myself so I wouldn't need a man to take me there. He felt sweaty. It was October, but it was in the high 50's that night. I offered to turn on the A/C. He didn't want me to get up. He said the temperature was fine. I wiped the sweat off his forehead. I loved how hard he worked to fuck me. I raised my head and looked at his cock going in and out of my pussy.

"Do you like watching?" he asked.

"Yeah."

I didn't know what else to say. I wish I could have said something really sexy, but I wasn't that comfortable or experienced with hot talk. What if I said something that sounded weird or turned him off? I wrapped my legs around him and pushed my hips up. I didn't care that he was sweaty and dripping on me.

"Do you want to come on my face today?" I asked.

"Yes!"

He turned me around doggy style. I had to make sure he didn't ram me, because it hurt when a man went too deep right before I was fully engorged.

"Easy, easy, easy, start out easy, let me get warmed up first."

He slid in and out slowly, very slowly, and I relaxed and my body opened up and I took him in. I loved how my body opened like that. I imagined he was looking at my ass, although I had no idea. I couldn't see him.

"Yes, yes, yes," I moaned louder, pushing my hips back to get him deeper. I gripped the sheets to hold on and pushed back harder. It was turning him on and he moaned.

I wanted to try something new with him, something I'd been curious about. I turned around and looked at him.

"Some of my friends call their lover 'daddy'. Do you like to be called 'daddy'?"

He smiled. "Yes!"

I said it, just quietly at first, and then in a normal voice.

"Fuck me daddy, fuck me daddy."

He thrust deeper and his cock felt harder. I turned around. He had a big smile on his face.

"You like me saying that?"

"Yeah, I do. Say it again."

"Fuck me daddy…fuck me daddy," and I gripped the sheets and pushed back.

He moaned and pushed deeper. His moaning was hot.

"I'm close to coming."

"Tell me where you want me, so you can come on my face," I said.

"Just here on the bed is fine, just turn around."

He gave a few more thrusts, and then pulled out and I quickly turned around to face him. He positioned his cock a few inches from my face. I was excited to be so close to his cock that was about to orgasm. I looked at his face so I could watch him come. He stroked himself three times, then his face grimaced and he moaned loudly and several squirts of thick creamy liquid shot out of his cock and onto my face, neck, and hair. He beamed proudly.

My face was full of cum. I did not feel degraded when he did it, but it didn't turn me on either. It seemed that men thought that women loved their ejaculate or at least they wanted women to do so, but there was nothing sexy or arousing about the ejaculate itself. I was more turned on feeling a cock pulsing or hearing a man moan or watching his face as he climaxed. I rubbed the creamy liquid in my face. He smiled at me.

"Wow, that was hot!" I said.

"Yeah, that was amazing."

He lay down on the bed and I rested my head on his stomach. The dry cum pulled my skin tight, like a facemask. I left the cum on my face while we talked. After about ten minutes, I washed it off. My face felt smooth, like after I used a face masque.

"I need to go," he said.

I did not want him to leave. But of course he was free to go, and I wasn't going to put a guilt trip on him. I walked him to the door.

"I'll see you again soon," he said and gave me a kiss.

My heart felt a little tug when he walked out the door.

Billy, 19: Professional Skateboarder

Later that night. Billy, 19, professional skateboarder.

Shortly after Justin left, I had an incoming message on OKCupid from a 19-year-old professional skateboarder name Billy. He sounded tipsy on the phone and he wasn't as tall as I liked, but his skating pictures and his hot body turned me on. It would mean two men in the same day. He didn't have a job or car, because he skated over 8 hours a day and all his money went for competitions.

Going out at 10pm and fucking a 19-year-old professional skateboarder seemed like an adventure far removed from my good girl persona. I drove 40 minutes to his friends' house to pick him up and brought him back to my place.

Billy had a beautiful hard cock and was extremely skilled at oral sex. His cock felt extremely good. I started out on top and then he turned me around doggy style.

"Fuck me slowly," I whispered. "Go slowly from this angle until I get warmed up."

He did as I asked. I imagined my pussy was stroking his cock to climax, while my round ass gave him a visual feast. He came in the condom. The only downside was that he was very tipsy and kept smoking cigarettes.

The next day when he was sober, he was socially awkward and eager to get home. On the drive back, I tried to make small talk. I asked him why he liked older women. Billy said they were better in bed. After I dropped him off, I went home to shower and get ready for work My dad was wrong to think my life was only good because of Brad. My life was good because of me.

TWO MEN IN ONE EVENING

Caden, 19: He Did Not Make A Sound
November 23, afternoon. Caden, 19, Marine.

It was Sunday. Caden, the Marine who stood me up for coffee, texted me to apologize for standing me up. He said he just got his phone back. It was taken from him during an inspection when they found whiskey in his barracks. They also gave him three days of house arrest. I thought it was hilarious. I still wanted to meet him because he looked so sexy in his pictures, so we set up another coffee date for that afternoon.

Caden arrived on time. He looked just like his pictures, except he had a lot of acne and his blond hair was completely shaved. He did not make eye contact and he only talked to answer a question. He told me he had never had sex sober. He had always been drunk. He seemed like a sweet kid who was not yet comfortable with himself or in social situations. I admired him for having the courage to meet up with me at all. He was probably just super horny.

He looked in dire need of love. I could get him to relax and open up, show him how good sober sex could be, and inspire him to cut back on the drinking. All he had to do was give me a hard cock to ride for a long time. I invited him over.

In my kitchen, he just stood there. He didn't make any moves on me or say anything, so I invited him to sit down. He sat upright like a statue at my dining room table, and did not say a word. It was really awkward. I needed to initiate, that was clear. I walked over to him and leaned over to kiss him. He refused to kiss me. He just sat there. Whenever a man refused me in some way I would keep an upbeat mood.

"I usually like to start out with kissing. It's fine you don't want to kiss. You are always at choice."

I was trying to figure out how to get myself turned on and start some kind of sexual interaction. He did not answer.

"Would you like to lie down and I can give you a massage?"

I thought the massage would arouse him enough to take charge. He agreed to the massage. He removed his clothes while I got some oil. He lay on his stomach and I sat on his buttocks, spread the oil on my hands, and slowly rubbed his back. I loved giving massages. He was completely quiet, so I could not tell if he enjoyed the massage.

I asked him to turn over to see if he was aroused. He rolled over and his cock was rock hard. He lay on his back, his arms out to his side, eyes closed, perfectly still. He was rock hard, otherwise I would have thought I was looking at a corpse. There was no way I could ride him like that. And he had not even tried to touch me once.

I decided to give him love by giving him a blowjob, and show him a taste of sober sex. I knew I was amazing the way I licked his balls and cock, savoring and teasing, but he still did not make a sound or look at me. I lingered at the ridge. Most men let out a moan when I did that. I listened for a reaction. Nothing. I wondered whether he was alive. His penis was erect, so probably yes. His chest barely rose and fell. I thought back to my nurse aid days. I looked at his neck artery. Good, he had a pulse.

I wanted to just get him off and get him out of there. I sucked his cock. He came suddenly in my mouth, without warning, while he lay perfectly still with his eyes closed. There was no moaning, no quickened breath, no clenching of legs, no flinching. Immediately after he came, he said he had to go. He got dressed and left in a hurry. We never talked again.

Rick, 24: He Loved Rimming Me
Two hours later on November 24. Rick, 24, accountant.

That night, I had a coffee date with Rick, a 24-year-old accountant who was into older women. Unlike the other men I met, Rick did not work out. He had a belly, sallow complexion, and no muscle tone. But he was tall, nice, and so eager about me, that I invited him over anyway.

He helped me undress, and when I pulled down his pants, I gasped. He had the widest cock I ever saw, and he was above average length. He asked me to turn around while I held on to my sink counter, and then he got on the floor and licked my rosebud (ass). He was moaning really loud. Licking my ass was turning him on, but I just felt awkward, and a bit embarrassed, mostly because he was on all fours on the ground.

We went to my bed, and right away he stroked his cock. His timing was off. A man should be turned on by touching the woman. I put a condom on him, and since the girthy part of his cock was in the center, the condom rolled all the way down his shaft and fit tight. Once he entered me, I was in heaven. I had never enjoyed penetration so much in my life. I gave him a B, since he didn't make me come, and I did not like his body.

I went to bed at 1am, and masturbated, like I did every night. I felt relaxed and tired before I climaxed. I rolled over, and within seconds, I was asleep.

The rest of November looked like this:

Nov 25. Tony and Keith (a threesome I did not enjoy), D
Nov 26. Rob, 37 C
Nov 27. Mitch, 27 (turned out to be alcoholic, took him to detox), A on the first night, C for the duration because he spent 3 days with me and we never fucked again.
Nov 30. Jordan, 20, oral only, D

CAN A WOMAN ASK A MAN OUT? (DECEMBER)

It was early December, and the Christmas buzz was on. The kids and I talked about whether to go to the Nutcracker, Handel's Messiah, or both. Brad called and asked what I had planned for Christmas. I had no plans. I didn't want any plans. I had never enjoyed the heavy holiday meal or shopping for more stuff. Sending out cards was a chore. All that was left were the tree and decorations, and I didn't want the hassle. I told Brad he could have the kids for Christmas. I didn't want Christmas. I wanted an orgasm from a man.

Dec. 1   Danny, 27, Marine officer, C
Dec. 3,5,7 Rob, 24, C
Dec 9   Tony again, A++

The online dating sites were time consuming, and I had seen the same profiles over and over. I wanted to get away from it all. I closed my online dating account and trusted I would meet men in real life.

I started looking at the men I saw at my Crossfit gym. One Saturday, I noticed a handsome man in his early 40's. He talked to me often during the class and encouraged me in the workout. He was nice, and a perfect dating prospect. After class, I looked for a chance to talk to him. He walked out to his car. Nice - a new BMW. Very classy taste. I caught up to him, just as he had opened the door to his car.

"Hey, do you want to get a coffee sometime?" I asked.

"I'm married," he said and smiled.

He wasn't getting in his car to leave. He just stood there. Had I subconsciously chosen a married man because he would be unavailable? I looked at his finger.

"Oh you weren't wearing a ring."

"Thank you for the compliment," he said.

"Well, I'm single and looking for nice guys to date, I didn't know you were married."

I did not apologize, because asking a man out was not wrong, and I didn't like people who always went around apologizing for their own existence.

"Thank you again for the compliment," he said, and then he got in his car and drove off.

Darn. Almost all the Crossfit guys I had seen at three different gyms looked unhappy, tense, or very overweight, and all the hot ones were married. I walked back to the gym to stretch.

I told my friends about asking the man out. Almost all my male friends thought it was hot. Some of my female friends encouraged me, while others disapproved, "Men are hunters and women are prey," they advised. "Let the man make the first move." That went against every grain in my gut. I didn't want to become prey or go through life as an observer, hoping someone would begin a conversation.

Besides, the Crossfit guy was flattered. Why did men always have to go out on a limb and face rejection? Maybe they liked being desired and approached. Who came up with these dating rules anyway?

I was ready for the next step: asking out a man I had just met. I scouted out the men at Starbucks on my way in. A man in a dress shirt and tie was working on his laptop at a table by the door. He was a good target. I ordered my coffee and then I nervously approached his table on my way out the door.

"Hi. Can I sit down?" I asked.

"Yes, sure."

The man eagerly moved his papers aside to make room.

"I'm Schahrzad."

"Scott." We shook hands and he kept moving papers around.

"I am looking for men to hookup," I told him.

"Oh, really?" he said, and handed me a piece of paper. He fumbled for his pen. "Here, write down your number."

I wrote down my number. That was easy. I felt bold. I waited for Scott to call me, but he never did.

I did this again a few more times. Only one man called me, and that man didn't ask me out.

GHOSTING

Meeting men in person was fun, but not useful for getting sex. I got out my Fuck List and browsed it for men for a hookup. I texted some men to invite them over. They did not reply. They just blew me off. It made me mad. I didn't like being ignored, especially by a man who was once in my home and my bed. A gentleman would tell a woman he wasn't interested.

I was puzzled that men turned me down. Didn't men get horny and want sex 24/7? Weren't men watching porn and hiring escorts and buying girlie magazines and have a high sex drive? Maybe those guys got into a relationship, preferred hookup variety, or did not like my passionate intimate sexual style? Was sex low on the priority list compared to work and hobbies? Were they tired from work? Did they prefer hanging out with friends over having sex with a woman they had fucked once after coffee?

Were environmental contaminants lowering men's testosterone and their sex drives? I wished more men would reply to my invites, rather than blowing me off so I could learn about human sexuality, but that's how it was.

When I told other people that men ignored me, I learned it was happening to them also. I googled this and learned it was called ghosting. It meant disappearing because the person lacked courage to say "I am not interested".

Simmering and icing were versions where a person kept a prospect around, stringing him or her along for some time in the future. The most powerful dating communication was called power parting, where someone was authentic and said, "I'm no longer interested".

Sometimes men who had ghosted me, texted me out of the blue. It was when they were horny. If I liked the guy, I saw him anyway, because I wanted a good cock more than I wanted to take a stand for a man not replying to my texts. So whenever Tommy asked to come over, I let him, because I still had feelings and was crying over him, and I had not learned how to let that go.

CO-PARENTING AND MY EX

I worked, paid my bills, kept my apartment clean, and arranged my dates. I went to my son's swim meet and my "ex" was there too. He greeted me with a smile, and still I couldn't stand him. I was nice anyway. I admired Brad for being so kind to me, when I was the one who left. We sat next to each other on the bleachers and made small talk, because that was good for the kids.

"YOU SHOULD BE SATISFIED"

Jeremy, the man with whom I shared a hotel on Halloween, called to see how I was doing. He felt more like a friend, so I asked him about my sexual inadequacy.

"It's hard for me to come from oral sex. Most people are bad at it or too rough or don't do it long enough."

"Tell the guy what you like."

"I can't do that. I just don't feel comfortable."

"Do you think a guy is going to kick you out of bed if you tell him what you like"? he asked.

"Haha, not really, but maybe he'll think I'm weird or demanding," I said. "Besides, it's not fair of me to ask a man to spend 30 minutes making me come when he doesn't even know me or love me," I said.

"Men are lucky to get pussy. You're giving a man something very valuable. Of course you should be satisfied!"

"Really? I see it the opposite way, that the man is giving me something very valuable. I'm lucky to get a good man with a hard cock that delivers good sex! That's hard to find."

"Most guys have no idea what they're doing down there and would like a little input anyway," he continued.

That made sense, except I didn't know what I wanted him (or her) to do different. I couldn't see what the man was doing with his tongue on my clit, so I couldn't correct him. Men who needed direction often lacked sensitivity on their tongues and all the direction in the world could not bring passion and sensuality into someone. I decided that going forward, if I liked the man's tongue action, I would ask him what he was doing, so I could teach the next man.

It had been over a week without sex. I yearned for physical touch and affection, not just a cock. I called my favorite hookup guys. Jeremy was good in bed, but he could only get turned on enough to orgasm when I gagged on his cock, and I didn't like doing that. Jose had stopped replying to my texts even though he had been a regular fuck buddy with an A+ rating. Sometimes I wondered if he secretly had a girlfriend.

I got out my fuck list and texted my favorite men. One man said he couldn't make it and gave no reason. Other men replied and said they were still at work, or exhausted from work and had to get up early the next morning. The rest never replied. They were weird to be too exhausted for sex or blow me off. I had no idea it would be so hard to get sex. I had more sex when I was married.

I went back online, and that's where I met Doug, a 31-year-old retail manager. We made a lunch date for the next day. Two hours before our date, he texted to say he had a work emergency. The roof was leaking at his store. He was really sorry and would be in touch when he had that solved. That evening, he rescheduled for two days later. The morning of our date, he called to say his dog was sick. He wanted to see me the following day. Right as I left to meet him for lunch, he texted to say he was called in to work. I understood things coming up and because he stayed in communication and rescheduled instead of cancelling, I went along with it. I looked forward to meet a man who was so into me.

Rick texted and asked to come over on Thursday, his day off. He wasn't my favorite guy, but he would do.

PORN CAUSED HIS ERECTION PROBLEM
December 12. Rick again (24 year old accountant with the large cock).

On the morning of my sex date with Rick, I wore my Ann Taylor silk blouse and midi pencil skirt to work. I felt sexy and classy in my tailored business attire. I stayed at the office only five hours, because I had to get home for sex. Sex was more important than doing a company's job for an hourly wage. Why did so many people got their satisfaction out of work and scurrying around to meet company deadlines, when at the end of the day they were too tired or grumpy for sex? Maybe one day I would understand and get satisfaction from work and not sex.

Rick arrived shortly after I got home. He took off his clothes and sat on the sofa and stroked his cock. Why did he strip and why was he masturbating, instead of getting turned on doing things to me? I went over to kiss him, and he stopped touching himself long enough to put his arms around me. I liked his kisses.

I undressed and we went to my bed. He immediately stroked his cock, just like last time. It finally dawned on me, he was trying to get himself hard. Despite all the attention he gave his own cock, he wasn't getting hard. Rick was only 24, he should have a stiff erection. I had to bring it up, without scarring him for life.

"Why don't you get hard?"

"I don't know. I think I masturbate too much."

We tried to have sex, and Rick never got hard enough for penetration. I gave him a hand job and I masturbated to come. This was lame. I wasn't worried anymore about his feelings. I had to be honest, and maybe that would motivate him to step it up.

"I don't want to have sex with you anymore if you don't get hard."

"I understand. I'll stop masturbating and then I'll call you again."

After Rick left, I went online and read about men, masturbating, and porn. The articles said that porn's high stimulation was addictive, and men who masturbated frequently to porn had brain changes, making difficult to become aroused by a real woman who required interaction. The solution was going cold turkey and abstaining from masturbation for weeks. After a few months of no porn, the man's brain was normalized. I texted all this to Rick, because I really wanted to help him.

Doug, the man who kept rescheduling, called and we made a lunch date for the next day. If he cancelled again, I was out.

"SPIT ON MY COCK"

December 13. Doug, 30, retail store manager.

Before work, I went in for my quarterly STD tests. Doug had not cancelled, so I went to meet him for lunch. He was strong and tall, about 6'4", kind of muscular, just like in his pictures.

He seemed extremely interested in me. He leaned forward across the table and kept telling me how beautiful I was, how much he liked older women, how he could not wait to just be with me and have great sex. Would a man who was so interested in me, be better in bed? Could he give me an orgasm? I had to get back to work, so we planned a second date for hooking up.

After several attempts and some rescheduling, we finally set a second date. I left work early and met him at the beach. On our walk, he kept grabbing my ass.

"I love nice asses. Wow! Your ass is just beautiful!"

And then I ran in the water and back to him and hugged his waist.

"What a nice ass! I love anal sex. I can show you a really good time," and he smiled at me.

I liked his touch and flirtation, and I felt playful. I wasn't sure about the anal sex that day, but it was something I wanted to explore more and if he was good at it, maybe I would do that with him. I invited him over.

Back at my apartment he changed a little bit. His eyes became serious and lusty. He no longer wanted to touch me. He wanted to be serviced. He became a little more determined, a little more sexually aggressive. He took off his pants and sat on my sofa. I went over and licked his balls and penis, thinking that was how he liked to start things off. I did not set my own agenda, because

I was curious about different men's sexual styles. I wondered how he would take charge of me and what he would do to me. Doug didn't take charge. He sat still and became verbally demanding.

"Spit on my cock, spit on it," he whispered in a low voice, his pupils small.

It seemed hot, although I was a little uneasy of his demanding tone. I spat on his cock a few times. It turned him on, as he got harder and moaned, and the look in his eyes became more lusty and distant. I suggested we go to my bed, thinking we could change the energy. Maybe he would want to go down on me or have penetration sex. He agreed, so we went into my bedroom.

He sat up in my bed and demanded me to suck on his cock, to keep spitting on it. I couldn't tell if it was my spit, or the sound of my spit that got him so turned on, so I spat louder and added a slurping sound. The louder I did my spitting and slurping, the harder he got, and the more he demanded me to keep sucking him. His pupils were just slivers.

I felt a little afraid and my pussy was dry, but my curiosity kept me servicing him. He kept being loud and demanding and asking me to spit on his cock and suck him. He came in my mouth with a loud moan and then he immediately got up and got dressed. What about me?

He walked to the front door. I had to express myself.

"Hey, I just want to let you know, this was really one-sided. This was just all about you."

He looked over at me. "Next time, it will be all about you."

And then he opened my front door and he was gone. I opened my windows and washed my sheets to get Doug's scent out of my house. The encounter with Doug sucked. His interest in me did not improve the sex. I wished I had asked him if he watched a lot of porn. Going forward, I would only meet men who told me they loved giving oral sex. Then I went back online.

JACKSON, 22: "I LOVE FACESITTING"

Jackson, a 22-year-old economics student, sent me an online message saying 'I love eating pussy'. He was 6'1", with a bright smile and blond hair, so I was definitely interested. We set a coffee date for the following afternoon.

December 14. Jackson, 22, economics student.

Jackson was waiting for me when I arrived at the Encinitas Starbucks, and I liked that. He was handsome, just like in his picture. We ordered lattes and he paid. We sat at a long table to talk. I spoke softly, because we would speak of sex and I did not want anyone eavesdropping on our conversation.

"So, you like older women?"

"Yeah, I do. I don't like girls my age."

That's hot," I told him.

He smiled.

"Are you into giving a girl oral sex?" I asked.

I wanted to hear him say it. I would only invite him over if he loved it.

"Yeah, I love going down on women, having a girl sit on my face. "

The face sitting part got my attention. I didn't feel comfortable sitting on a man's face, but it sounded really erotic. If he loved face sitting he was probably good at oral sex and I had a safe space to ask for exactly what I wanted.

"It takes me a long time to come." I waited for his answer.

"Oh, I love doing it. I could do it for hours."

Hmmm....I imagined him licking my clit for hours and I got turned on.

"That sounds amazing. What else are you into?"

" I don't like intercourse," he said.

"Well, how do you like to orgasm then if you don't like intercourse?"

"Oral sex."

"I see."

"I have fantasies. I'm into BDSM and kink," he continued.

"Oh, I'm not into that."

"I also like sensuous play, like being bathed in a tub and then toweled dry."

"Oh, that arouses you?"

"Yes, it doesn't make me hard but it turns me on."

"I don't understand being turned on but not hard."

"It's hard to explain. It just sets the mood for me."

"Wow, that sounds amazing and fun. I miss giving my kids baths, and I miss having hugs, so your timing is perfect. Would you like to come over?"

Jackson followed me back to my apartment. On the drive, all I could think about was sitting on his face. I was aroused and wet, thinking about straddling him with my pussy rubbing on his face. I didn't have to worry about him doing me a favor, because licking pussy to orgasm was his turnon.

At my place, I gave him a glass of water and we sat on my sofa. We didn't kiss. Neither of us wanted to.

"Take off your skirt and panties," he instructed, and lay on the floor in my living room. I did as I was told.

"Come here, sit on my face," he instructed.

My clit throbbed. I walked over to him, stood with one foot on each side of his face, and lowered myself down on him.

"Here, position me where you want me," I said, because I didn't want to smother him.

"You're fine right there."

He stuck out his tongue and the second it hit my clit I shuddered. He licked me softly, all over my labia, rolled his tongue alongside and over my clit and I started moaning. He flicked his tongue lightly side to side and my arousal built quickly. I sat down with just a bit of pressure on his face, and stuck my swollen hard clit in his face, in his mouth.

Could he tell how turned on I was, by how big and hard my clit was? Is that how men felt when they pushed their hard dicks into my mouth? Sometimes when I masturbated I pretended I had a penis and it was big and hard and all the girls could see how turned on I was. Clits were smaller and we women didn't go around exposing our swollen clits, but why not? I wanted my arousal to be seen. Dare I tell him about that? Could I ask him to suck on my big hard clit? No, I was embarrassed…it was small and maybe he would think I was silly to say it was big and hard. Maybe he didn't notice, because it was small. But I was hard and swollen. Could he tell?

His technique with face sitting was amazing. I didn't want to expend any thoughts or energy in keeping myself upright.

"I want to lay on my back, my legs are tired."

He laid me on my back and kept licking my pussy and clit with determination. I heard my breathing quicken and my moaning got louder. Jackson focused more on my very hard ridge. He held my legs tight. His breathing picked up and he circled his tongue slowly around the most sensitive part of my clitoris: the little button, or pearl. He could tell I was close to coming, before I even knew it myself. He read the signals in my breathing, warmth, lubrication, and engorgement.

Then I felt it imminent. It started deep inside me. My legs trembled, it built up, my breathing quickened, my nipples got harder, my toes curled, and then I let my orgasm explode out my pussy, up my body, and out of my mouth with a loud roar. I came all over his face. I didn't have anything coming out like a man did, but I imagined myself coming all over his face and it excited me.

I looked at Jackson. His cock was hard. That was hot.

He didn't want to fuck. He wanted oral sex too. I gave him a blowjob while I looked him in the eyes and he came in my mouth.

That was fun! I couldn't wait to try bathing him. We made a date for him to come back the following week.

All my STD tests came back negative.

The kids came over. I told them about Jackson, like I had with other men before him. My boys listened intently, and my daughter squirmed. I persisted in the conversation despite her discomfort, because it was my job as a mother to educate her properly, and sex was a proper part of life.

December 18. Jackson again (22, economics student).

Jackson came over for the bubble bath. I looked forward to the closeness and cuddling as much as I looked forward to the sex.

He took off his clothes and got into the hot water filled with bubbles. I washed him gently with a washcloth. I felt warm inside, pampering a man like that. He smiled. I washed him, washed his hair, squeezed out the washcloth and let the warm water run all over him. I wished I had a rubber duck. Did he like toys too? Did he maybe have a fantasy of being in a diaper, because I had heard of that too, or was I giving him all he wanted?

"Here, I'll dry you off."

He got out of the tub, and I wrapped a towel around him and dried him off. His penis was soft. I didn't understand how it turned him on exactly.

I went down on him first, so he could get off right after his bathing fantasy. Then he went down on me again and afterward we talked for about an hour.

"I just don't like intercourse," he told me.

"I see," I said.

I didn't know what else to say. Did he have an emotional issue? Was he abused or molested as a child? I did not want to judge him or make him feel wrong for his preference.

"I'm really into kink," he said and took out his phone. He showed me pictures on tumblr of penises pinched by safety pins and tightly bound with rope and other painful images. I was shocked by what I saw.

"Oh my god, that looks painful!" I gasped.

How did people get turned on by being in all that pain, and wasn't it dangerous to their genitals? They could cut off circulation.

"Yes, and that's the turn-on. Once I pinched myself for so long and I cut off my circulation, but it came back."

It seemed like so much effort had been put into creating the pain. Why? It was interesting and it wasn't up to me to understand.

He showed me images of women sitting on men's faces, which turned me on immensely. In one image, a man lay on the floor and a woman in a red dress and high heels just sat on his face, so dominant, like she totally deserved it. Damn, I deserved it too. Why had I gone all those years never doing that?

"Oh my god, that is so hot! I want to do that!!"

I felt flushed and my clit started throbbing, which surprised me because I had just come. I made a tumblr account and subscribed to those pictures.

Jackson and I hugged and he left. We never saw each other after that.

The next few weeks looked like this:

December 19	Rudy, 23, C
December 20	Cory, 27 (A++), dinner and a sleepover
December 22	Cory and I went to the shooting range, sleepover, A++
December 25	Warren, 34 and Tony again

INNER PEACE

Maybe I would never again meet a man who felt the same attraction to me that I felt for him. I had to be content alone.

It seemed a necessary human experience, finding comfort and solace in oneself. A voice from inside spoke to me. *I want to be completely self sourced in my finances and love before I get into another relationship.*

If I was happy inside, it would not matter if a man returned a text. I would be free to speak my truth to him, instead of withholding it out of fear he wouldn't like it and leave me. I could completely surrender and open to him because I wouldn't lose myself since there was nothing to lose. I wouldn't have to worry about him dying or leaving, because I was already full and made my own way in the world before I met him, and could do so again.

My next relationship would be an addition to my life, not the source of it. It would not be a man's responsibility to give me love or security I was unable or unwilling to give myself. I had no idea how long it would take to reach this goal, nor how to get there. But I wanted it more than anything in the world.

I sought this peace in meditation and nature. Fortunately, near my home I had a choice of trails, eucalyptus groves, and of course the beach. When I felt lonely, I went to these places, sometimes with a coffee, other times with just a water bottle. Sometimes Chandi went with me.

I often admired my toned curved body (but not my face) in the mirror. I had liked my body all along. I didn't even have a scale. I went by how I felt and how my clothes fit and how I looked in the mirror. I noticed that the more I looked in the mirror, the more I liked myself. I took more selfies. At first, I took them in private, but then I challenged myself to do it in public. It was difficult at first because nobody took a selfies of just themselves, probably because we were taught admiring ourselves was sinful. Then why did it make me so happy?

I tried to love the unloved parts of me, starting with my face. I had wrinkles and my eyes sometimes looked puffy. I knew mentally it was just in my head, and many men thought I was beautiful. They took me to dinner, beach walks, or coffee, so they were not embarrassed to be seen with me. Once I asked a 19-year-old man if he thought I was old, and he kissed me in a busy parking lot and said other men were just jealous of him and wished they could have me. The age issue was mine: I had to see my wrinkles as beautiful. I loved how my face showed my emotions. I was beautiful when I cried, laughed, or showed tenderness. I had trouble loving my wrinkles. I put loving my wrinkles on my to-do list, along with forgiving Sarina for having sex with Rudy, and focusing more at work.

I took the self-improvement courses I had dismissed decades earlier, when they did not fit, because it would have complicated everything to move forward when my husband was standing still.

It was a start, but results were not immediate. My mood was easily ruined when a man did not reply to my text.

"ARE YOU A SEX ADDICT?"

Over the holidays, a good friend from Phoenix came to visit. She had been married 25 years and she was surprised at my many sexual encounters.

"Why do you have so many men? Are you a sex addict? Maybe you switched your addiction from pills to sex."

I laughed, but it was a fair question.

"Addictions rob people of themselves, make them smaller. What I do is making me bigger, more alive. And both I and the men I meet are better off as a result of our interaction. Touch and sex are nourishment for my soul and my body."

"Well, I can sort of see that," she replied.

"There's more. People are usually ashamed of their addictions. They hide them. They don't want anyone to know. I put myself out there. I'm proud of what I do. I'm discovering myself."

"Yeah, but I just couldn't do that, have sex with all those men."

"I guess I just give myself permission to do it. I don't know any other women who do what I do. I'm not sure. "

Secretly, I gave myself two years to fuck whoever I wanted. It would all run its course and I would tire of the meaningless hookups and want a relationship.

DANNY, 28: FALLING FOR A MAN I NEVER MET

I had heard of people who fell for each other online without ever having met, and women who were swindled out of money by men who lived in faraway places. The ploy was to get the woman emotionally hooked, then say he (or she for lesbians) needed money to get out of whatever country they made up to be stuck in. Usually the sum was thousands of dollars. Men from other states sent me messages telling me I was beautiful, and how they couldn't wait to meet me. I always deleted these messages and blocked the man. I always shook my head. I was a logical grounded woman. There was no way I would start an online conversation or search for any man outside of my own city.

I certainly would never fall for someone online, someone I had never met. I didn't even message much. I went right for the coffee meeting, so I could get to know the man in person.

I met him online one morning in early December, browsing online profiles before work. He was a 28-year old blond haired man, tan, with a big smile and broad strong shoulders. I was smitten, so I clicked on his profile. His name was Danny and he lived in Orange County, about an hour away. He was outside my search radius, but the site had placed him in the side bar.

His picture melted my heart. I loved blond haired men. He looked just like Brad when we met. He lay on a beach in his bathing trunks. His toned calves, firm stomach, aviator glasses, and dimples were hot as fuck. Warmth rushed through my heart and vagina. I pictured myself riding him. Looking at his photos touched a place inside me where my dreams and fantasies lived.

My entire body got so hot I ripped off my sweater. It was interesting how arousal heated up my body.

I sent him a message, mentioned the distance, and held my breath. He replied within minutes.

"Well, hello there beautiful. You're not that far away. I'd love to come see you."

My heart skipped a beat. I asked him how tall he was and what he did for work. Danny said he was 6'1" and worked for the Navy. He said he was looking for a relationship and would come see me in two days. I was so excited!

He texted the morning of our meeting. Something came up at work and he would not make it. We texted each other for days on end, rescheduling our dates. I alternated between hopeful and sad, depending on what he said to me. He had a second job on the weekends so he could make his alimony and child support payments, so he had little free time. Sometimes we talked on the phone.

He was a gentleman in all our conversations. Had he mentioned sex, I would have blocked him, but he was nice and that made me like him more. I fantasized about him, mostly about riding his cock, but also that he kissed me tenderly and told me I was beautiful. I looked at his pictures over and over. His sensuous face and blond curly hair evoked images of romantic novels and brought a warmth inside my heart that I liked feeling. Within weeks it was clear I had fallen for him. Days went by without any texts from him. I kept checking my phone. I went online to see if he was online. He was. Why was he online and not texting me? Why couldn't he make time to see me after work? Why didn't he let me come to see him? I was heartbroken and I cried.

"THE KEY FOR SCHAHRZAD IS TO SEEK CONNECTION WITH HERSELF"

I was no better than other women who chased love and dreams spun out of thin air. I hated losing my inner peace again. It was bad enough crying over Brad, Julia, and Justin, people I had actually met. This was the last straw. I had to get my power back. I turned to my friend Deidre who channeled, and asked for advice. The next time she sat down to channel, she asked about Danny and sent me this email:

Q: I would like to ask about Danny for Schahrzad. Do you have anything you would like to tell me for her?
A: The answer for Schahrzad has nothing to do with Danny or with any other man or woman she is seeking. The key for Schahrzad is to seek connection with herself. She spent many years in that place of depleted giving we just discussed. And this is now a time of recovery for her. A recovery from this depleted giving. As such, Schahrzad is seeking pleasure and fun in external circumstances.

As if she could suddenly fall for the 'right one'. Though there is no right one out there. We do not believe in one match for one person. There are multiple possibilities for people to find love and connection. The world is constantly in flux. You could meet the love of your life in one moment in time, and the next, if you change one element, miss that bus or decide to stay home, you could never meet them. We do not see predestined paths for people. You are all creating your realities through the exchange of energy.

As such, there is nothing that Schahrzad needs to worry about. Tell her that she does not need to focus on Danny or anyone else. Try to bring the focus to herself. She mentioned intuition. That is the key to peace for Schahrzad to develop her intuition more by doing her daily meditations and being more connected. The more she is connected to herself, the more she will attract people who will fulfill a loving connection with her. The more she is disconnected and seeking outside of herself, the more she will feel starved for what she does not have.

There is no such thing as 'the one' out there. The one is you. You are the one. And as such, you are the one with source and with every human being on this planet. Thank you. You are loved.

I read that again. And again. A relationship with myself. What did that mean exactly? Maybe I could get that relationship with myself today and then Danny would come over tomorrow and we would start dating. I laughed. That wasn't what they meant. I had to be genuinely happy from within, without feeling a man could make it all better.

I wanted this happiness that didn't depend on getting a text, but I wasn't there. I wanted Danny with all my heart.

Danny and I texted and talked a few more times. Our almost-relationship had two disagreements that we patched up. It felt so real. Then right before Christmas, it all sizzled out. He stopped contacting me. I was devastated. The pain in my heart was unbearable. Sometimes I cried because I felt the real connection between us, and other times it felt like I cried over a fantasy.

I spent Christmas with my friends, and the kids went with Brad. I was glad he was giving them the holiday experience. I didn't want the hassle.

CHAPTER 12

I WANT A RELATIONSHIP

I asked my friends to set me up on blind dates, but none of them ever found a match for me. Maybe I would turn into a cat lady, a woman who gave up on men and was satisfied with gardening, travels, friends, writing, and her multiple cats, and whose pussy shriveled up from lack of use.

Whether I wanted a relationship along with the sex, or just sex, depended on how horny I was. When I was very horny, I felt a warmth and tingling in my genitals and wanted to fuck with a hard cock. A dildo would not do it. I wanted to wrap my arms around a man's body, kiss him, smell him, and moan in his ear. I wanted to be on top and ride him hard, long, deep, to fill every craving and desire deep inside my body. When I was less horny, I wanted sex in a dating situation, involving dinner, an interest in each other, and a sleepover.

But something seemed off. I was pursuing men in their 20's, because they gave me passionate sex without the baggage of a house and a garage full of stuff. If I really wanted a relationship, wouldn't I date men my age?

Christmas Day., Matthew came over with all the ingredients to make me a vegetarian dinner. I felt satisfied I had raised my boys to be thoughtful and enjoy cooking. His dinner was delicious. Afterward, he cleaned up the entire kitchen. Was he an overachiever, or was he just doing what he enjoyed?

BILL, 49: IT WAS JUST PHYSICAL

December 26. Bill, 49, district sales manager.

I was excited to meet a handsome man my age, because I was curious how a man that old would be in bed. Bill was a 49-year-old executive recruiter who lived downtown. He was 5'10", fit, with an active lifestyle and twin boys in middle school. I still didn't have that relationship with myself, but maybe that could be overlooked and we could date. We set a date for coffee.

I immediately felt comfortable around him. The way we acted at coffee felt familiar. We both had been in long marriages and had children. He grabbed our coffees, I took the napkins. He threw away the cups, I pushed in the chairs. Each of us knew it took two to make something work. I was really curious how the sex would be. I followed him in my car back to his condo.

He offered me wine. I didn't like that, because I liked to have sex sober. Why did he need wine? He set his glass on the coffee table and invited me to sit on the sofa. He turned on the TV. Why did he need the TV? I didn't come over to watch TV. I came over to connect and kiss and fuck. Why did he sit there and watch TV? Why didn't he put on music and look at me?

Bill kissed me. His kisses were motions he made with his lips, devoid of passion. I was curious though. He was a single dad my age. Maybe the sex would be amazing. He took off my clothes in the living room and we sat again on the sofa. His touch seemed mechanical. I wasn't turned on. Why didn't he invite me into the bedroom, where we would have soft sheets and a warm blanket and room to romp around? The sofa was narrow. What about our juices? Wouldn't they stain the sofa? And how many other naked women had been on that sofa, and did he clean it regularly?

Bill went down on me, and he was a little too rough so I asked him to stop. Maybe I could liven things up with my good blowjob. I went down on him, but since I was a bit turned off by the loud TV and the sofa, I wasn't really into it. I didn't ask him to turn off the TV or take me into the bedroom, because I wanted to experience how different men had sex. If the sofa and TV were his way, then let me have it. I had already ruled him out for dating, so I stayed for the experience.

He fucked me on the sofa with his penis going in and out, in a mechanical way as if we were two blowup dolls. I considered he had been single several years and had probably had his share of heartbreaks and disappointments in love. Even if at one time he was open hearted and passionate, all those disappointments over time could have shut him down. Sex could have become just physical for him, just another routine. One woman tonight, a different woman a different night.

I suddenly realized I could be on the track to turn out just like him! If I kept having sex with so many men, a day would come where the next guy would be just a motion to me. How long could I be innocent and playful and fresh in my hookups, if I did that for years? No, I had to end my hookups or cut back. I had to leave periods of time in between, so each man felt new and special, and not like another body for the night. And I thanked him for that lesson.

December 29. Alex, 23, Saudi Arabian student. Role-play.

HIS LIMP DICK: "I MASTURBATE TOO MUCH"
December 30. Rick again (24 year old accountant with the wide cock).

Rick picked me up and took me shopping for lingerie at the sex store near my apartment. He bought me a gorgeous white bra and matching panties. Back at my place, I put on my outfit and I was absolutely stunning.

"You're so beautiful," he said.

He wasn't hard that time either. We did mutual masturbation, which was a pleasurable sexual activity for me, but I didn't like his soft dick. When we were done I asked him about it.

" You did not get hard. Do you watch a lot of porn?" I asked.

"Yeah, I do, but I don't think it's the porn. It's the masturbating."

"I doubt it. I think it's the porn. You're probably so used to getting off on images, you lost your ability to enjoy sex with a real human."

"Maybe."

"Try stopping the porn, see what happens," I suggested, wondering if that was really possible.

"I've thought of that before."

"Good, because honestly, I don't want you to feel bad, but I don't want to have sex with you if you're not hard."

He really needed to figure this out, not just for me, but for himself and any woman he dated or married.

WHY ARE MEN ALWAYS LEAVING IN THE MORNING? December 31. Edward, 21, spiritual coach.

On New Years' Eve, I went to a party hosted by my polyamorous friends. I noticed a young man in an armchair, absorbed in a book. He wasn't paying attention to any ladies. I liked his contentment, lean fit body, and blond hair.

I introduced myself. He said he was Edward, a vegan and spiritual coach. He was only 21. He said he had been to many polyamorous events, but had never had sex with any of the people.

We kissed and I liked his passion. We went into the family room and made out on a sofa. I invited him over and he initially said no, because he didn't hookup. I almost had to convince him to come over.

At my place, I put on music, and the first song that played was the Passenger song, "Let Her Go". We both liked the romantic mellow feeling of the song. It was perfect for a cold night, for two single people. He had a gorgeous hard cock, and he made love to me with the same passion of the music. We fell asleep in each other's arms. Edward was a relaxed sleeper. I didn't like sleeping with men who were fidgety, snored, or had insomnia. I woke up a few times in the night, noticing his quiet, peaceful sleep. I debated waking him to fuck, but maybe he needed his sleep or would be mad if I woke him for sex. I could wait until morning.

His phone rang at 6am. It was his roommate, saying he had to go into work early, and they needed to return their rental car earlier than planned. I hated that men were always leaving when I wanted morning sex. It would be great to do something besides coffee + fuck, or have a guy ask me to breakfast instead of rushing out the door in the morning. I scheduled a healing session with Edward for the following week.

HE LIKED ME

Sarina called on New Year's Day. I let it go to voicemail. She told me she was sorry about Rudy, and wanted her sister back. I wasn't mad at her anymore, but I didn't want to have people in my life who so nonchalantly put their own gratification above my feelings.

January 5. Jerry, 34, programmer.

Jerry invited me to lunch, and then we went back to his house. His neighborhood looked old and the houses were not maintained and it reminded me of death and decay. He bought the house about a year before. His house probably cost $300k because it was San Diego. I could not imagine myself ever living there, so dating was out.

He made us tea and told me about his prior marriage. He seemed content to talk forever. He moved too slow. I needed more action.

Finally we got into this bedroom. He was slow in bed too and he did not excite me. After sex he asked when he could see me again. I told him I did not want to see him again. He put his eyes down and I thought he was sad. I wasn't the only one getting dumped.

BOOTY CALL

Doug, the man who demanded me to spit on his cock, called at 1 am. I let it go to voice mail. He asked to come over. I didn't want him to think I was an option, so I returned his call.

"Hello?" he answered quietly.

"You're a bad memory and I never want to see you again," I yelled.

"Let me come over. I'll make it up to you, I prom….."

"You're an idiot and a loser. Don't ever call me again," I interrupted.

"I really just want to see…."

I hung up on him. He was a loser to get off at my expense, promise to make it all about me next time, and then make a 1a.m. booty call. I wondered if he was possibly married.

Booty calls were demeaning., and not for me. A man needed to be a gentleman and schedule a date in advance. Besides, I liked sex in the morning and daytime when I was horny and awake, not at night when I was tired.

January 6. Jose again

Jose texted me out of the blue. He was free that evening. Since he was so good in bed, I let him come over. We sat on my sofa and talked for half an hour and then we had amazing A+ sex. I liked that he didn't just fuck me. Neither of us had feelings for each other, which made us perfect fuck buddies.

CHRISTOPHER: A FAMILY LIFE FANTASY

January 9. Christopher, 44, executive recruiter.

Christopher was a successful father of three. He had been a fighter pilot in the military and had his own recruiting business.

He was divorced for several years. He was attractive and fit, totally my type. I liked this man in his 40's who was building his career, instead of men in their 50's who wanted to wind it all down.

We met at the beach in Carlsbad. I liked that he was already there, waiting for me, when I arrived.

"Do you date a lot?" he asked.

Why did he ask me that, right off the bat? It wasn't his business. Did his ex wife cheat on him?

"Yes I do."

Christopher shuffled his feet. He said he had not dated in months, because he had his kids 50%, and the rest of his time was spent on expanding his business. I invited him over, and he hesitated, citing the rash ointment on his leg. I talked him into coming over.

He was passionate in bed, and extremely skilled at oral sex. I stopped him, because I did not feel deserving. He got up to get a condom out of his pants pocket. I liked that he was responsible.

He fucked me quite well and came inside me in the condom, and afterward I masturbated for my orgasm. Then we got dressed and had tea. He made some comments about not liking that I had sex with so many men.

Before he left, he asked me out for the following Wednesday. I was thrilled to finally had a man who was hot and wanted to see me again.

I texted Christopher the next morning when I got to work. All day, I waited for his reply. I fantasized about making dinner for him and his children, and being a part of their lives. I liked this man for a relationship, not just sex. I checked my phone all day for a reply. By the time I left work he still had not replied, which indicated his lack of interest and broke my heart.

After work, I stopped at Brad's house to see the kids because I didn't know how to be happy alone when I longed for so much passion.

That evening, Christopher called to say his kids had been sick all day and he was swamped caring for them. Furthermore, I should not be texting him, because his kids often checked his phone, and he didn't want them to know he had a lady friend. He said I could use email, and reminded me he would see me on Wednesday.

He no longer seemed hot. What kind of man could not have phone privacy and had to hide his dating? But I was needy, so I wanted him anyway.

Right after I got off the phone with Christopher, Rick called. He said he cut back on the porn and masturbating, and he wanted to see me, and possibly date me. I didn't want to date him, but seeing a man who wanted me for more than sex sounded healthy. I would definitely see him again, but I was turned off because he did not move the action forward and schedule a date.

WALTER, 35: COMFORT

January 10. Walter, 35, massage therapist.

I was really distracted at work. I wanted Christopher to hold me. Was I a bad person to want his arms around me? It wasn't bad when I was married. Maybe single people should not need touch, but married people could.

I decided to go for a massage. I was still filling out the paperwork, when a muscular male massage therapist in his mid-30's came out. He was around 6'1", burlier and bigger than the type I usually went for. He looked like a cuddly bear. He smiled at me and looked back at his forms. I could sense I was about to get playful with him. Anything could happen in our massage room. I smiled under my breath. He called my name and said he was Walter.

"Wow, you're really muscular," I said as I followed him down the hall. I felt sexy and powerful to flirt with him so openly. He turned around and flashed me a smile.

What I Did For Sex

In the massage room, I got under the sheets and waited for him to come in. He pulled down the sheet and put his warm oily hands on my back. I had an intense feeling of pleasure. He moved his hands up and down my back in firm strokes. He asked what I wanted massaged in the one hour we had, or if I wanted 2 hours.

"Can you increase my massage time to 2 hours?" I asked him.

"Yes, let me let the front desk know," he said.

When he came back in and shut the door, I let go into a deep relaxing massage. I fell asleep. He worked on my entire body with his strong hands. I forgot all about Christopher.

"Your skin is really soft," he told me.

"Oh, thank you."

It was a huge compliment. I didn't put on any lotion. I used to years before because it often felt dry, but since I started taking cod liver oil, I no longer needed the lotion. After the massage, as he walked me back to the front desk, I stopped him and whispered so nobody could hear

"Hey, do you want to go out sometime? Can I have your number?"

"Sure, hold on," he said quietly.

He went into the staff room and came back with his business card. His cell phone number was written on the bottom. He didn't want any of the staff to know he gave his contact info to a client. I texted him as soon as I got out to my car. He called back right away. I invited him to come over for dinner. I actually wanted company, not just a fuck. He said he would bring a bottle of wine and be there by 9pm. That just felt really good. I was even in the mood for a sleepover.

Walter arrived with a bottle of cabernet sauvignon. He told me funny stories over dinner and wine. I felt comforted. Sitting across the table from a nice man who liked me and didn't want to just fuck, reminded me of my dinners with Brad, our happy times together, and my divorce, which was about to be final. I drank a glass of wine and he drank the rest of the bottle.

Walter kissed me as we cleaned up after dinner. He was so passionate and he turned me on with his kissing. I loved getting lost in his big burly arms. Maybe he was my type too, because I sometimes liked teddy bear guys when I was younger. We left the dishes for later and went in my bedroom. Walter went down on me because he liked a woman to come first. Like most men, Walter wasn't super good at oral on me, so I masturbated to orgasm. I was super wet and still turned on. I put a female condom inside me, making sure the end was sticking out, and climbed on top. Walter held me real tight and kissed me sweetly while I rode him.

We fell asleep in each other's arms. I didn't have feelings for Walter, but he nourished me deeply. The next morning we had sex again. He left after breakfast and said he would be back.

I didn't care about Walter. I was excited for my date with Christopher.

GIRLFRIEND ADVICE

I ran my man stories by my friend Tina at lunch. She was a divorced mom of three and dated often.

"Oh my God, I invited my massage therapist over and he spent the night. He fucked me so good!"

"You're hilarious. You should write a book."

"No. I don't want to write a book. What have you been up to?"

"You know that guy I met on the camping trip, Jack? He and I are really hitting it off. He's amazing in bed," she said.

"I wish I had good sex. It's so hard to get good sex as a single woman. I meet all these guys for coffee and I give them great sex and they blow me off," I told her.

"That's because you haven't established a relationship first. I always wait to have sex until the third date," Tina replied.

"I always have sex on the first date, because if the sex isn't good, there's no reason to have a second date," I explained.

"But the sex gets better with time."

"I'm afraid to count on that. I don't want to have feelings for a man who is terrible in bed. I need to check him out in the bedroom first," I insisted.

"The sex gets better. And they won't blow you off if you get to know them."

That actually wasn't true. Tina was reciting a mythical dating model, not her actual experience. Men blew her off all the time even though she waited to have sex, and sometimes she got too horny to wait and gave a guy a blowjob in the car on the first date before they ever got home.

She wasn't much help, so on my drive back to work I called Mary.

"Mary, I'm so tired of guys blowing me off. I really wanted to date Tommy."

"You'll never get into a relationship if you have sex with so many men," Mary told me. "Men don't like a woman who sleeps around."

"But I just want sex. Why can't we start with sex?"

"A relationship is more than just sex," she explained.

I didn't want the parts that were not sex. What were those parts anyway?

"I also like good conversation and sleepovers and cuddling," I defended myself.

"Maybe, but a man in his 20's will never get into a relationship with you. The age difference is too great. If you…."

"You have no idea what is possible," I interrupted. "Are you a fortune teller?"

"Listen, you can argue if you want but I am just pointing out something. The young men just want you for sex. If you want a relationship...."

"You have no idea. Tommy made love to me."

"Sex is not love, Schahrzad. I'm saying that because I am your friend. If you want a relationship, you need to go to at least age 45."

I wanted her to be happy for me liking younger men, and pray to the gods to send a younger man my way, instead of lecturing me that I was doing it all wrong. I wanted to keep my cool, but I was furious.

"I can create anything I want!" I said, and hung up.

Why did my friends give me advice based on what <u>they</u> wanted, which was someone who took them places, comforted them, gave them advice, and shared their life. I could get those needs met myself or with my girlfriends.

I wanted a man mostly for the sex. If the sex was good, I could be interested in dating or a relationship. The relationship would be mostly about lots of hot sex, sleepovers, good conversation, and sometimes spending time outdoors and going to dinner or shows. There was no way I wanted to meet someone's friends, watch his home improvement projects, or learn about his hobbies. Maybe I was selfish to treat men as sex objects. Could a relationship really never come from that?

MY DIVORCE (JANUARY)

Brad and I had a noon appointment at the courthouse to finalize our divorce. It was over one year since I had filed. We didn't have court orders because we agreed on everything. Oliver would keep coming and going as he liked, hopefully every other week with each parent. I kept my last name. A few days later, my divorce decree arrived in the mail.

A CANCELLED DATE

I had looked forward to my date with Christopher every day since we met. On the morning of our date, he still had not contacted me with details, and I didn't like that. I felt powerless, at his mercy. That afternoon, he sent a long text. He apologized. His mom had been sick the past week, and it was getting worse and he had to fly to the East Coast immediately. He was really sorry. He didn't reschedule. I was devastated. Maybe God was punishing me. All my prospects evaporated.

I had to learn how to have sex like men: by compartmentalizing and not getting attached. Maybe I was too needy. I cried for a half minute, and set my hopes on seeing him when he got back.

On Friday after work, I got ready for Oliver. I stopped at the grocery store to stock up on pasta, frozen chicken breasts, and fruit. I washed his sheets and cleaned his bathroom. I did what he could do for himself, because it was the only remnant I had of being a mom.

HE MET ALL MY SEXUAL NEEDS

January 18. Steve, 45, math teacher.

I had a date scheduled for that afternoon with Steve, 45, father of 5, who was looking for a relationship, according to his OKCupid profile. He would have his own place and could invite me over. I felt guilty leaving my son to go out, but I wanted sex more than I wanted time with my kid.

Oliver came over around noon. We caught up on our lives and then I had to tell him I was leaving.

"Honey, I have a coffee date this afternoon."

"Ok, Mom, will you be home for dinner?"

Darn it, maybe not. I didn't know. I sucked as a mom. What was the point of having Oliver over, and then leaving him to go out?

"Honey, I don't know. "

"I don't like coming over here when you just leave."

"I know. Leave your laundry out. I'll wash it for you when I get back. And here's $60 so you can get gas and something to eat."

"Thanks, Mom!" He smiled and looked happy.

"We can do something tomorrow."

I drove to Carmel Valley to meet Steve.. He was over 6' tall, fit and strong, and he was funny, but I had trouble overlooking his white hair, because it reminded me of canes, wheelchairs, nursing homes, and death. Since he did not color his hair, it meant he was a better person than I, because he could overlook such things. He told me he recently quit his demanding corporate job because it required too much travel and time away from his kids. His new job as a teacher gave him time for his children, but it meant less responsibility and a cut in pay. He picked up his kids from school, made dinner for them, and attended all their sports games. I liked his fatherly commitment, yet it didn't excite me to be with a man who wasn't growing his purpose and mission. Dating was out. Sex, however, was a possibility.

"I'd love to invite you over, but my son is over at my place," I said.

He hesitated. "Well, you can come to my house. It's a total mess, since the kids just left this morning."

How bad could it be?

I followed him to his place. His entry way had two large bins overflowing with shoes, his living room was littered with toys, and on his refrigerator were school calendars, pictures of his kids, and scribbly drawings saying "Dad I Love You". It all was super cute.

He kissed me and I melted into his strong arms. He lifted my dress, took off my panties, and sat me down on his sofa. I fell back on the cushions, fully aroused and trusting. He spread my legs and licked my pussy. He was still wearing his clothes. This turned me on a lot, because it meant he loved my pussy so much, that he forgot to undress. He was really good at oral. It didn't take long, and I came hard, my moans filling his house.

After my orgasm, he suggested we go to his bedroom. I followed him down a hallway littered with toys. I caught a glimpse of the kids' bathroom, with towels on the floor, a hamper overflowing with clothes, and a counter of miscellaneous brushes, hairpieces, and Barbie dolls. It wasn't dirty, just messy. I couldn't picture myself living with him in this house. Dating was definitely out.

He undressed and that's when I saw his 7" long extremely hard cock. He put on a condom and he held me tight, kissed me deeply, and took charge in bed. He moved me all around and I enjoyed it a lot. By the time he orgasmed, he was drenched in sweat.

I didn't like his sweat on me, so I asked for a towel and took a shower. On the drive home, I decided I could never date this guy because of his messy house, old bedspread, and white hair, but he could be a good hookup buddy. I gave him an A+.

SQUIRTING WAS A DISAPPOINTMENT

January 20. Walter again (my massage therapist).

Walter, my massage therapist, came over for dinner. It felt comforting to have a man in my home, in my kitchen, at my table. This was much better than just sex. I had a glass of wine, and he drank the rest of the bottle. I didn't like all the drinking, so he was definitely out for dating. Over dinner, he kept talking about squirting. He found it so hot, as most guys did. Since I never had squirted, I was defensive about it.

"I've never squirted, and I don't want to. It seems like a messy thing that guys want women to do as a performance function to prove their competence in bed. No thanks."

"I love a woman squirting", he insisted.

It meant I could never satisfy him or other men, because I could not squirt, and maybe something was wrong with my body. But I honestly had no desire for it.

After dinner, we put the dishes in the sink and went straight to my bed. I was glad he wasn't like Brad, who would have insisted on washing dishes, because he liked that more than fucking.

I liked Walter's kisses. He grabbed me tight and kissed me, while he put his fingers deep inside me. I got lost in his touch. I didn't want him to ever stop. He started doing it faster and faster, and then it no longer felt good. I was about to tell him to stop.

"You're squirting," he said.

I looked up. Streams of liquid flew out of my vagina. He kept fingering me, and the liquid continued squirting, flying out of my vagina and landing several feet away.

"Oh my god, I squirted," I cried out, in complete surprise.

Walter smiled and looked pleased. But wait - what was the point of squirting? I didn't have an orgasm with it and I made a mess.

"Please don't do that again," I told him.

"Why not?"

"It did not feel good, I did not have an orgasm, and we made a mess. That's why!"

We had intercourse and he felt good. Walter spent the night. I felt comforted by him, but I wasn't interested in him for a relationship.

The next morning, Walter said he wanted to date me. I didn't like him that way and I hoped he would not fall for me. But I knew men did not fall for women that easily. We made a date for Wednesday.

Walter texted me good night. I knew he wanted more, and I should end it, but I felt comforted by him so did not tell him, and I kept the date for Wednesday.

PEGGING

January 22. Walter again (my massage therapist).

Walter texted me good morning. I hoped he was not falling for me. Before I went to work, I went online and found a good prospect. Blake was 42 years old, 6'1", with blond hair and blue eyes. Since we both liked outdoor activities, I suggested a beach walk near my office for the following morning.

That night, Walter came over for dinner that night. I had one glass of wine and he drank two bottles. I didn't like all his drinking, but he acted sober so I let him stay. I was very turned on and wet when I rode him, so when he put his finger near my ass, I didn't stop him. He inserted his finger slightly, and I moaned louder, a signal to him I liked it. He stuck his finger deeper in my ass. I moaned more and pushed against his hand. I felt unbounded, wild, and free. His finger in my ass heightened all the sensations.

I wanted to do that to him, so I climbed off him to go down on him.

"Can I put my finger in your ass?" I asked.

"Yes, I love it."

I liked his playfulness. I got some lube out of my nightstand, put a generous glob on my finger, and rubbed it near his rosebud until my fingertip felt his tight opening. I sucked his dick before I entered him, so it would feel good. If it hurt, he would likely ask me to stop. Men weren't like women: they didn't put up with pain just to please us.

I sucked his cock, leaving my finger near his rosebud, slowly pushing in past the sphincter. He let out a moan. Slowly I slid in further, deeper in to his ass, my finger moving up into his rectum, while I sucked on his cock. I felt myself getting wetter. Fingering his ass felt arousing, like a man would feel fingering my vagina. Walter was moaning really loud.

"I have a strap-on," I said. "I bought it to use on a woman, but I've never used it."

"Use that on me."

That surprised me. Many men loved a finger in their ass, but they didn't go around asking to be penetrated with a dildo. He was more fun than I thought.

"Yes! Awesome. I'd love to," I told him.

I wasn't aroused by the idea of fucking a man in the ass, a technique called pegging, yet also excited to try something new and finally get a chance to use my harness. I got my Aslan leather harness out of my closet, put it on, and adjusted the straps to make sure it was snug. Then I pushed the dildo through the opening of the harness. I admired myself in the mirror.

"Look at my cock," I said, as I admired and stroked my dildo.

Walter sat up in bed, and by the time I reached the bed, he was on all fours. I knelt behind him, my dildo at the level of his ass. I got myself into my male energy mindset. I imagined the dildo was my cock. I looked down at my cock and Walter's round bottom, and in that instant, realized the importance and significance of what I was about to do. I had to make sure I delivered.

He trusted me with his vulnerable ass. I could not let him down by hurting him or making it feel ordinary. I would impress him with my sexual abilities. I would use my cock as I used my finger: sensuously. I would make love to his ass. Was this the responsibility and performance pressure that a man felt when he made love to a woman?

I rubbed generous amounts of lube on my cock and his bottom so he would feel pleasure as I slid inside. I pressed the tip of my cock gently against his asshole and once I found the entrance, I pushed a little harder until the tip of my cock penetrated his rectum. He let out a moan. I felt powerful, pleasing a man in that way.

Slowly, I pushed my cock in a little deeper, and he let out another moan. He began rocking back and forth. I pulled out slowly, and he moaned again. I penetrated him again, this time going about one quarter inch deeper. I debated just going for it, but his rocking indicated he wanted thrusting. I pulled back out. Each time I penetrated him, I went one-quarter inch deeper. He moaned loud, rocking back hard on my cock. I got more excited, the deeper I got. Finally I let him have all of me, filling his bottom with my long thick cock. Then I started thrusting.

My heart flowed with love as I slid my cock in and out of his tight asshole. I wasn't fucking him. I was making love. My eyes welled up with tears. I wanted to make him feel even better. I thought of what else I could do. His pleasure seemed to be completely in my hands. I reached around to stroke his penis, sliding my hand up and down his hard shaft. He moaned even more, and I wanted to keep doing it, but my back hurt when I leaned forward, so I rubbed my hands on his bottom and focused on the penetration....in and out, in and out, giving him pleasure, nice and slow. He still moaned and rocked with my motion.

"Come here," he said.

I pulled out, took off my harness and dildo, and lay under him. He held me tight and kissed me passionately. He was so hard. I put on a female condom, making sure the end stuck out. He fucked me with his beautiful wide cock for about ten minutes and then he came. When he pulled out I noticed the female condom had slipped, so his ejaculate was inside of me also. I saved sex without a condom for men who I thought could turn into a relationship. I had to be more careful next time I used a female condom.

Walter spent the night. He kept saying he liked older women and wanted to date me. I hoped he wasn't falling for me. The next morning, I made him coffee and then he left for work.

ORGASM DURING PENETRATION AND LADIES FIRST
January 23. Blake, 42, VP of engineering firm.

After Walter left, I showered and confirmed my beach walk date with Blake. Then I went to work. I left the office just after

11am to meet Blake at the beach. He walked up to me nervously, his hands in his pocket. No confidence, not hot at all! I debated just telling him I changed my mind and wanted to leave, but there was a chance he would be completely different a few minutes into our conversation. I had met enough men the past year to see their transformation after they relaxed. Men who showed their nervousness at coffee, laughed and talked easily within five minutes. In my bed, after climax, these men glowed and chatted. I would give Blake a chance. I was also curious about sex with a man that age.

We walked barefoot on the sand. He told me about his children, marriage, career, surfing, and running. I liked his story. This was much better than men in their 20's. The wind picked up and I said I was cold, so he gave me his jacket. It didn't mean anything, but it was nice. He became more relaxed around me, and I noticed he was handsome. He seemed interested in me, despite my age and wrinkles. I was surprised. TV ads and society had convinced me that youth was 'in', and women my age were having plastic surgery, Botox, and skin peels to look younger. I recalled his profile has specified women up to my age range.

"Don't you prefer younger women?" I asked.

"I like older women because they know what they want. Also, younger women want children and I don't want any more children."

We finished our walk and he wanted to touch me under my clothes. I let him. He put my hand inside his pants and I felt his hard erection.

"I can stay hard for hours," he said.

We laughed, but I didn't like him touching me under my clothes on a beach in broad daylight. I did not want him anymore. He asked to come over and I told him I had to get back to work. I returned his jacket and went back to work and forgot all about him.

January 24. Blake.

Blake pursued me with text messages about coming over. It had been so long since a man pursued me instead of blowing me off, I forgot pursuit was even possible. I really was not interested in Blake, but since he was so insistent, and I had no plans that evening and was curious about sex with a man that age, I invited him to my apartment.

Blake arrived freshly showered, wearing a black V-neck cashmere sweater, his blond locks showing off his handsome chiseled face, and I just about melted. His cologne turned me on too. I could have looked at him for hours.

"You're so handsome!" I looked up and flirted with him.

I was completely smitten. Over a snack and hot tea at my dining room table, he told me about his kids, work, and the last woman he dated.

"I looked at your Facebook," he said.

So he was interested in me? Or just curious? I had not thought to look at his.

I put the dishes away. Blake followed me into the kitchen. He grabbed me tight and kissed me. A feeling of warmth and surrender rose up my body and I melted into him. We kissed and when I opened my eyes, my heart expanded in wonder at his beauty. I could have looked at him every day for the rest of my life.

He lifted my dress, unsnapped my bra, leaned down, and circled my nipple with his tongue. I surrendered to him.

"Oh my god….oh my god….," I moaned.

He leaned down and sucked gently on my nipple. He smelled so good too. Then he reached into my panties and my very lubricated cunt. I went weak in the knees and held onto him. What was he doing to me?

"Let's go in my bedroom." I could barely get out the words.

I quickly went into my bedroom, and for some reason, I pulled back my down blanket. I always had sex on top of my covers, but

Blake felt like a man to be with under the covers. I jumped in bed and watched him undress. He was gorgeous. His body was lean and toned, just the way I liked, and his cock was hard. He got into bed on top of me, and kissed me tenderly and nibbled on my lip. A moan escaped my mouth. *Take me, take me, I'm yours.* I leaned up and lustily pushed my tongue into his mouth. He returned my hungry kisses and fingered me soft and deep. I pulled him closer on top of me and clutched my arms tightly around his neck, while he kept fingering me.

Blake moved down to my pussy. I raised my head off the pillow so I could see. He put his mouth on my vulva, sucked my labia, and flicked my clit with his tongue. He spread my outer lips apart with his thumbs so he could get really close. Damn, it felt amazing! He could definitely make me come if he kept going long enough. I still didn't feel I deserved it, so I stopped him and went down on him.

His penis was long and thin, which was definitely not my favorite shape, but he was extremely hard. I gave him good head, and then I laid on him and kissed him while grinding on him.

He looked at me tenderly, the way a man in love would look at his woman, and the way I always wanted Brad to look at me. My heart melted. I wanted him inside me. I put a condom on him, and then he turned me over into the missionary position and entered me slowly, like he was making love to his wife. I had never felt that way with a man. I didn't think Blake had feelings for me, and he probably treated all women the same way, but I liked it anyway.

"I can stay hard for hours," he whispered.

He told me that once before. I liked hearing it again.

"Yeah, that sounds amazing," I said.

He started thrusting. Did he expect me to come from penetration, and that's why he told me he could stay hard a long time?

"I have to confess and tell you that I don't come from intercourse," I announced, wondering what he would do about it.

"Here, let's do this," he said, and gently moved me on top.

When he said *let's*, a warm feeling come over me. He created an "us" and offered to take me to new places, sexually. I had longed for Brad and other men to take me to new places sexually, but none ever had, so I gave up on that dream, concluding I was too demanding, and should not count on another person to give me things I should be giving myself. But deep down, secretly, I longed for a man to take me to new places, open me to new experiences, and show me parts of myself I didn't even know existed. Could Blake be such a man?

"Some women can come by riding on top and rubbing their clit here," and he pointed to his pubic bone.

"Wow, I want to try that!" I moved around, not sure what to do. "How do I position myself?"

"Every woman fits differently."

We moved around on the bed and experimented. I lay on top and rubbed my clit on his pubic bone while I rode him. My clit was not rubbing on anything.

"Can we move into a position so I can masturbate while you're inside me?"

"Sure. Here, I have an idea."

I loved that he had so many ideas on how I could come. Blake got up and stood on the edge of my bed.

"Scoot down," he whispered.

I got on my back and scooted toward him until our groins touched. My legs were hanging off the bed. I stretched them and supported my feet against the wall behind him.

Blake slid his hard cock into me, and went in and out slowly. I rubbed my clitoris with my fingers while he watched. I had a few problems with it. First, his thrusting felt better than my rubbing and was distracting me from masturbating, and second, his cock sliding in and out pulled on my inner labia and moved my fingers off its spot. I needed him to stop thrusting and remain hard. It seemed like a lot to ask.

"Could you hold still?" I asked.

"Yes," he looked at me tenderly.

He stood still and barely moved. He looked at my legs, while I looked at his high cheekbones, blue eyes, blond hair and tan face, and rubbed my clit in circles. He whispered some words and remained still. That was his mission, being still so I could take my time. Looking at his face aroused me. I didn't have to fantasize. I kept my eyes on him as I rubbed myself, getting more and more turned on, with his hard cock perfectly still inside me.

I felt my pussy grip his cock. It meant I was closer to coming. I felt my wetness sliding down my upper thighs. Would he lose his erection and slip out since he wasn't moving, or get so turned on by my pussy clenched on his cock that he would orgasm right then? He whispered more hot talk that I couldn't make out, which turned me on even more. I looked at his gorgeous face as I rubbed my clitoris, and an orgasmic wave grew from my depths and it was powerful and couldn't be stopped.

My pussy gripped and pulsed on his cock and I erupted in a long loud moan while I looked at him. His eyes were on my legs. I hoped he felt every throb of my vagina engulfing his cock, and was impressed with my long and tight contractions. He let himself feel a few contractions, and then moved inside me and filled me with his hardness while I rode my orgasm to the end.

"Wow, thank you," I whispered as I looked at him. "I have never come with a guy inside me, except maybe once a long time ago. That was awesome, thank you."

He smiled. I liked him. I was all wet and warmed up. He got on top of me and penetrated me hard until he came.

"Thanks for making sure I came first," I told him.

"Ladies first," he answered.

"I love that! It makes so much sense for the woman to come first."

He held me while I laid on him and we talked. After about half an hour, he got dressed and then he left and said he would be in touch. I went to sleep happily.

My encounter with Blake was amazing. I kept thinking about him. I built him up in my mind as I relived the key sexual moments, specifically his gorgeous sensuality and leadership in the bedroom. I wondered about his interests and personal life, and imagined myself making dinner for him and his children.

The next day, I texted him, but he didn't reply. I was heartbroken. They said a girl should wait for a reply before sending another text, but I couldn't wait that long because I had so much to tell him. I just wanted him to hold me. Maybe God was punishing me because I didn't have that relationship with myself.

POWER PARTING

January 25. Walter again (massage therapist).

Walter and I had dinner at my place. He drank three bottles of wine that night. I didn't like being around all that drinking, and I didn't want to date a massage therapist because I liked successful and professional career/family men like Christopher or Blake. We had sex and it was good.

"I really like you," he kept telling me, after we had sex.

I hated to hurt his feelings, but I could not string him along. I had to tell him.

"I don't feel the same way about you." I forced out the words.

"Wow. Oh wow," he said, and looked sad.

"I have to be honest," I explained.

"I was looking for a reason to stay in San Diego. I thought you could be that reason."

He spoke softly. I remembered the sadness of wanting someone who did not want me. But I didn't feel sad. I just wanted him to leave.

"Look, I like you, I want to keep seeing you, I thought we had something here," he said.

"I'm sorry, I just don't feel the same way."

Walter looked sad when he left that day. I left it up to him to deal with his own experience.

The next day, on Saturday morning, Oliver bounced up the stairs to my apartment. I heard a key in the door, and there he was.

"Mom, look what I brought!"

In his arms was our family cat, Tabby. I still had not hung my pictures, but I had a pet. Chandi came over after work. I texted Matthew to join us. He said he was busy, which meant he didn't want to come over. Matthew kept his distance not because of any disinterest or animosity, but because he needed space from his parents so he could individuate. I knew he loved me. He had his own place, his girlfriend, his part time job, and his 4.0 GPA. Oliver, Chandi, and I sat around my dining room table with tea and cookies and stayed up late into the night, talking and laughing. I was finally handling motherhood and dating like a boss.

At the end of January, Rick, the 24-year-old accountant who had erection problems, called. He had been liking my Facebook posts and texting me occasionally, so when he called, I picked up the phone.

"I'm in Oceanside visiting a friend. Can I stop by? I'd really like to see you."

"My son is here this week, so I can't have anyone over."

I didn't want to see him anyway. His limp dick was such a turnoff.

"Okay. I'll try you again when another time. By the way, I stopped masturbating. It was the masturbating, not the porn, that made me not get hard."

"Oh, I didn't know that could happen."

"Yes, I was masturbating too much."

"Well, I'd definitely like to see you again if you're hard. I just can't today."

"Let me check my work schedule and I'll get back to you on another day I can come over."

I liked that he pursued me out of want, not need, and made himself vulnerable about his sexual issues. I wished Christopher was the one doing the pursuing. I invited him for dinner. I did it via email so his kids would not see my text on his phone. Maybe that was fine, because it was faster to type on a keyboard than on a cell phone. He emailed ; he wanted to see me as soon as things wound down with work and his kids' sports teams. Why was it so hard for this man to get a few hours to himself and see a woman he liked, who lived only 20 minutes away? He probably was not that into me.

BEDROOM PERSONA
January 29. Blake again (42 year old VP with the gorgeous face)

I was at work and it was 9pm, and I got a text. It was Blake, the man who let me orgasm on his cock. He asked if he could call. Yes, I texted back. I was beyond excited. Maybe he missed me too. And calling instead of texting was hot! My phone rang and it was Blake.

"This is Schahrzad," I answered.

"Hey, it's Blake. How are you?"

"I'm at work. It's nice to hear from you."

" I'm at a friends' house. We just finished playing tennis. Do you want to come over?"

"I do, but I don't want just sex. I want more. If I come over, I want to spend the night."

"Sure, you can stay the night."

I took that to mean he also wanted more than sex. But I really didn't know, because I didn't ask.

"Alright, let me go home and grab some things then I'll come over."

"Perfect. I should be home in half an hour. I'll text you my address."

His townhome looked like a bachelor pad. He had no toys laying around. His ex-wife had kept the house, which made sense because of the children, and he was renting his place. When I arrived, he was in the middle of washing the dishes from his kids who had left that morning. He offered me some leftover chicken he had made them the night before. He was cute, offering me leftover chicken and nothing else with it. He sat next to me on the sofa, while I nibbled on his bachelor pad chicken. I liked how it was all so real. This family man thing was nice. I put the plate on his coffee table and straddled him. I liked this man who did not push me away when I wanted sex. We kissed on the sofa and he unbuttoned my blouse and lightly touched my nipples and drove me wild.

Blake asked me to follow him into the bedroom. I used the bathroom first, and when I came in, he was naked in bed. He seemed too lazy about it. He should seduce me. I rebooted my attitude. Maybe he was just being real. I came into the bedroom with a smile, and lay on top of him and we kissed.

"Sometimes it takes me a long time to come," I said.

"A woman's orgasm is a delicate thing," he said.

I immediately relaxed and trusted him. I liked that he knew a woman's body and I could be myself. I put the female condom inside me, making sure the ring was around my cervix and the end stuck out. Blake entered me from the top, and slid his penis inside the female condom. He moved gently and slowly. His strong body on me felt comforting. A new feeling appeared. It was in my heart. Was I falling for him? Did he feel it too?

"I'm afraid I could be falling for you, and I don't want to," I said.

"That is always a risk. Thank you for telling me how you feel."

What did that mean? Did he like me too? I pushed those thoughts aside and focused on his thrusting cock, and then the feeling in my heart was gone. I looked if the female condom was still in place. I no longer saw it stick out, which meant it had slipped and was not serving its purpose. Sometimes that happened with the female condom. We needed to use a regular condom or none at all. I asked Blake about his sexual history. He said he was been STD-tested a month ago and had sex only with one woman since, and had used a condom.

I removed the female condom out and slipped his cock inside me. He felt so much better skin on skin. I got on top. The room was semi dark and his eyes were closed.

"Let's turn on the light so I can see," I requested.

Blake turned on the lamps on his nightstands. His eyes were closed as I rode him.

"Here, look at me," I whispered.

He opened his eyes. He was so handsome. I sat up on him and rode him so he could see my beautiful body. He got more turned on and flipped me over into the missionary position, his heavy breathing in my ear. His erection felt strong and demanding, pushing deep inside with each short thrust. I liked those short pulses deep inside, pushing next to my cervix.

Blake got up and asked me to touch myself. He obviously wanted me to come first. I rubbed on my clit in circles. He brought his cock near my mouth, and I sucked on his head like a lollipop. I didn't care how weird it looked, because it was deeply arousing. As I got close to coming, Blake quietly and slowly moved off the bed and slowly inserted his cock into my pussy. It was a brilliant move. The problem was I wasn't progressing to orgasm anymore. He noticed and brought his cock back to my mouth. I closed my eyes and masturbated and sucked on his cock as he watched.

"You're so sexy," he whispered.

Those words released my inhibition. My orgasm built and I came within minutes. I was soaking wet. I looked at his penis and he was rock hard. I liked that he was turned on by me.

"How do you want to come?" I asked.

"In your mouth," he said.

I went down on him. His breathing became louder and faster and almost scared me a little. I liked that he wasn't quiet like Brad and other men. I just needed to get used to mens' sex sounds. His legs tensed, and finally I felt his contractions and warm liquid shoot in my mouth. He moaned a long time, and fell back in exhaustion. It took him well over one minute to catch his breath.

Blake tried clumsily to hold me. Didn't he know how to hold a woman, or did he not like me? Did he wish I would leave?

I wished I was with Christopher. I got up to check my phone. Wow, I had an email from Christopher. I wished I had him, not Blake. He wrote lentil soup and sex sounded amazing. Why was he emailing me, when he lived only twenty minutes away? And why didn't he move the action forward on my dinner invitation?

I went back to bed. Blake was turned with his back to me. Could he feel my heart was with another man? Was that why he didn't talk to me or touch me ? There was no way he could read my mind. Maybe he was just clumsy with intimacy. He lay perfectly still, which was awkward. I debated leaving, but it was late. I made myself the big spoon and held him because he didn't hold me, and we fell asleep.

I woke up with daylight and felt aroused. I pressed my body against his and rubbed on him and after about one minute, he turned around. I saw he was hard. He kept his eyes shut and let me ride him. He reminded me of Caden, just laying there with an erection and wanting sex but not touching me. It was boring and awkward. I tried to get myself and him excited by changing positions, but nothing helped. Finally, he had an orgasm. I just wanted to leave.

Blake didn't say anything. He got up and went into the kitchen. I heard the coffee grinder. I made his bed and when I came out, he had coffee ready. He had that post sex happy glow.

"I'd like to see you again but nothing exclusive. I still want to have sex with other guys," I said.

"Keep me as another horse in your stable," he smiled.

Was he glowing because he liked me, or was it the post-sex hormones? Was that 'horse in the stable' comment a good thing to say and what did he mean exactly? I probably said it to put up a wall, letting him know he was just another fuck. There wasn't a need to have said anything at all.

We drank our coffee in silence. There wasn't anything to talk about. *Would I see this man on a date where there would be no sex? No, I didn't like him for dating. I just liked him for sex.* I just wanted to leave.

When we finished our coffee, Blake grabbed his jacket and walked me out to my car.

"I'll be in touch," he said.

"I won't call you. If you want to see me again, you call me," I told him.

The next day, as I kept replaying the lovemaking scenes in my mind, I liked him more and more. I knew he didn't have his kids that weekend. I changed my mind on not contacting him first, because I wanted him and I liked to go after what I wanted. I grabbed my phone and sat on my bed to send him a text.

I really like you and I'd like to see you tomorrow.

He replied within minutes.

Busy tonight, but looking forward to seeing you again

Busy? I was devastated. How could he be too busy for me?

I needed to talk to someone, because it hurt too much to deal with alone. I called Mary and told her everything that had happened the night before. Mary said the 'horse in the stable' comment was a bad sign and made him think he was just another fuck. Should I be ashamed of fucking so much? I didn't like her advice so I ignored everything she said and texted Blake a few more times to make sure he understood he could have me anytime he wanted. Then I replayed our hottest sex scenes over and over in my mind, until I felt so sorry for myself, I cried. Damn it, why was I always crying over men?

I got some tissue to blow my nose and wipe my tears. Then I went into the kitchen to make tea. I sat on my sofa, sipping my tea, looking at the majestic trees outside my window, and fantasized about Blake. I forgot about his clumsiness, how he kept his eyes closed and wanted me just for sex, that I wanted to leave when the sex was over, and that he did not reply to my texts. All I could think of was his gorgeous face and his tenderness, strength, and leadership in bed. Thinking about him was better than my boring job and my life that lacked passion. Maybe I would end up moving in with him, and I would have my career and we would have family dinners with his kids and go to soccer games. Maybe I would have a do-over on my sexless marriage.

Maybe the universe was withholding a relationship from me, until I had built that relationship with myself. I had meditated and introspected for decades, but I still didn't know how to have a relationship with myself.

Oliver came over that evening.

"I met the most amazing man, but he is ignoring me," I said.

"Don't tell me about anyone unless you're serious about him," Oliver said.

He had a point. I was always mentioning the latest guy I was into, instead of getting excited about him. One day, when I was no longer depleted, I would no longer need to blurt out my latest romance prospect. I didn't know how long that would take.

January 31. Tommy again (young surfer).

Tommy texted me for a booty call on my way home from work, and because I was horny and longing for affection as well as a hard cock, I invited him over. The sex was not that satisfying, because he did not know how to be emotionally present for the duration.

THE BAR FLY AND WHISKEY DICK

February 1. James, 43, programmer.

Saturday night, I went out with the goal of picking up a man. Although I liked my men sober and bars were not a place to meet men for dating, they held potential for hookup sex. After all, I wasn't an alcoholic and I sometimes went to clubs. I went out with Mary to a club in Encinitas catering to middle aged people.

James was a handsome 43-year-old man seated at the bar. He had planned an elaborate party for his young son's birthday the next day. We talked about an hour. He bought me a drink, and intermittently went outside to smoke a cigarette. He seemed responsible and fairly sober. I overlooked his smoking and invited him over.

James couldn't get hard. Whiskey dick. I fell asleep, hoping for sex in the morning. He got up at 6am, and said he had to leave to get his house ready for his son's birthday party. It was probably an excuse for his permanent whiskey dick. I was on the right track to not meet men at bars. I would never make that mistake again.

Tommy was still sending me snapchats. Initially his snaps had been hot, when they involved surfing or work, but they were getting sillier, with pictures of his open mouth full of ice cream, or hanging out with kids his age at the skate park. I was done with that immature kid for good.

I LOVE ANAL

Rick, the accountant who masturbated too much, asked to come over on his next day off. I liked that he planned ahead and wanted to see me in the daytime, instead of calling late at night for a booty call. I considered it.

"Will you be hard?"

"Yeah, I haven't masturbated in a week, and I stopped watching porn 3 weeks ago."

Since he liked me as a person, not just for sex, and he felt so good when he was hard, I said he could come over in the morning. I would go in to work at lunchtime.

February 3. Rick again (24 year old accountant with the wide cock).

Rick came over around 9am that morning. That time, he was really hard. He wasn't stroking his cock. That time, when he liked my rosebud, I loved it. My bottom felt loved and warm, and I felt my body open to him.

We hurriedly put on a condom. He lay me on my back and entered me. His cock felt so good when he was hard. I was dripping wet and engorged and so turned on, I asked him if we could have anal sex. I had done that only a few times in my life. I was worried about the anal sex because of his size, but I asked for it because I wanted it.

I turned around doggy style and Rick penetrated me slowly. It didn't hurt. It felt good. Soon, he was all the way in and he moved in and out slowly. It felt sooooo good. I was moaning and wailing with pleasure. Damn, I liked anal sex. Why did he feel so good, and other men hurt me with just their finger? It really was about technique. When I had enough, I turned around to tell him.

"That felt so good, but I've had enough."

He pulled out his cock and I saw there was no condom.

"What? Why did you take off the condom?" I asked. I wasn't mad.

"I thought it was fine to go bareback, since it was anal," he said.

"You didn't ask me, and you didn't say anything." I struggled to understand.

"I'm really sorry."

"It's much easier to pass an STD through anal penetration because there isn't any lubrication in the ass."

"I'm so sorry, I'm sorry."

I had a part in it too. I decided from then on, I would check for the condom every time we changed position. But it would have been better to be with a man who had the maturity and integrity to not blindside me by taking off the condom when I wasn't looking.

Rick left and I updated my Facebook status with "I got fucked in the ass." I got dressed for work. I stopped for coffee. I noticed my gait was more confident, bold, and secure. Anal sex had changed my entire demeanor and brought out my power.

The next day, I expected my ass to be sore. Usually it felt sore, even if a man had just inserted a finger in it. But there was no reminder of the night before, except my pleasurable memories. I learned a huge lesson: anal sex is pleasurable when the woman is warmed up and engorged, and the man enters her properly. Too many men think they can enter an ass like a pussy and are too rough, and no wonder women want little to do with it.

February 9. Walter again (my massage therapist).

I went in for a massage to say goodbye to Walter. He was moving to the east coast. After my massage, I turned around on the table and sucked his cock until he ejaculated in my mouth. I did it because he had been so nice to me and I wanted to give him something in return. Then we gave each other a long hug goodbye.

THE BAD GIRL MYTH

Just like in high school, sex was all I was getting from men.

"I don't date men, I just fuck them," I told the lady at the makeup counter.

"Oh my god, you're so cool," she gushed back.

"I just fucked a 24 year old guy earlier today," I told the waiter when he asked me how my day was.

"Wow, I love how open you are," he said, hopeful perhaps I would take his number.

After telling hundreds of people about my hookups, including every man I met for coffee and took to my bed, I still had not met one person who said I was dirty. All those bible quotes about premarital sex being bad were just words meant for other people. I felt alive after hooking up, not used, depleted, or regretful. The men respected me, probably because I respected myself. Maybe women who were bullied or harassed for fucking were disrespected because they were needy, drunk, manipulative, angry, or cheated, factors having to do with their personality and not sex itself. My parents were wrong too. I was furious I had allowed myself be deceived like this. My love of fucking was just as natural as my love of meditation, coffee, motherhood, and watching the news.

The only time I had shame about hooking up was around men I wanted for a relationship. The kind of men I liked, respectable family men, would want nothing to do with me if I had a lot of penises in me. I had to question the assumption. If the woman was dirty for having had another man's penis in her, did that mean all penises were dirty, or just all penises except that of the man who was judging me? My logic didn't even make sense. Regardless, it was so entrenched in me, and if men believed this, they could still disrespect me for fucking so many guys. It was my own inner work to do.

Whether I was a bad girl wasn't even a factor, because no man ever said he could never date me because I fucked so many men. The problem was I rarely saw a man who intrigued me or with whom I felt synchronicity, or mutual attraction for a relationship.

MY NEEDINESS

I longed for a passionate successful man and a dynamic relationship based on personal growth. Did these men not exist, or were they turned off by my neediness?

I was needy. I admitted it only to myself. In public, I had a roving eye for men, hoping to find "the one". This magic man would be instantly drawn to me, and approach me to start a charismatic conversation.

When I had sex, I got lost in the man, instead of getting lost in myself.

I longed for men I could not have. I fantasized about them endlessly. Maybe I was still depleted.

I had a long way to go in that connection with myself.

The following week looked like this:

Feb 14   Samuel, 44, single dad, B
Feb 17   Jeremy again, he never gave me an orgasm, he only liked oral if I chocked on his cock which I hated, but he felt super good during penetration, B

DWIGHT, 53: "I HAVE SUCH A HEADACHE"
February 21. Dwight, 53, biotech consultant.

Dwight and I met for coffee at a Starbucks near my office. He was extremely attractive and fit, with a flat stomach, and a successful career. His kids were in college. Maybe my friends were right, that sex should be saved for the second or third date if I wanted a relationship, so I didn't have sex with him on the first date.

For our second date, he asked to meet at an upscale lounge in Carlsbad for a drink. I liked his spontaneity. It was 7pm and I was about to leave work, so his timing was good. Yet I hesitated. A date for drinks conjured up images of plastic-surgery-faced divorcees in skimpy dresses and men with stale cigarette smoke on their pressed shirts, who stumbled home at night and woke up in random beds in the morning. I did not want to meet for drinks.

"Let's meet for coffee or a walk on the beach instead," I suggested.

"No, meet me for drinks. Just one drink."

I wanted to be flexible and open to new experiences, so I agreed to meet him for a drink.

Dwight was already seated at the bar with a martini when I arrived. He looked dashing: a suit and tie, and most likely expensive shoes. I greeted him with a hug. We both ordered cabernet sauvignon and a cheese plate. We chatted about our work and children, and he told me about his travels. The whole time, I tried to imagine myself riding him. I wasn't sure I wanted to fuck him. Even if I wanted to, could he perform?

"Do you have ED?" I whispered, so nobody could overhear.

"ED?"

"Yeah...erectile dysfunction. My husband had it. I'm just wondering, in case we have sex, because I don't want to have sex with men who have it."

"Oh, you have nothing to worry about in that department," he assured me.

His gray hair made him seem old and thus more likely to have ED, so when we walked out to my car, I asked him again if he had ED. He reassured me he did not.

"Well, do you want to come over? You can spend the night," I invited him.

"Sure!"

At my apartment, Dwight asked for more red wine. Why did he need to drink, when he finally had me all to himself? I poured him a generous glass of cabernet sauvignon. He sipped his red wine in my kitchen, and told me he had several women for hooking up. I could imagine women sought him, but why was he talking about his other ladies, when he had me right there and could talk about me, or just come closer and kiss me? By the time he finished his wine and tales of other women, I was really sleepy. He didn't turn me on, but I was curious to try sex with a man his age.

We took off our clothes and lay on my bed. I had my first look at his penis. It was completely flaccid and soft. I didn't like that at all. I wanted him rock hard so I could ride him. He was useless. Maybe I could get him hard. I licked his balls and licked and sucked his penis until eventually he was a little erect and then he came in my mouth. He never was hard enough to ride. We fell asleep together. The next morning, I wanted to have sex so I reached over and hugged him.

"Oh, I have such a headache!" he said.

I didn't have any medication at home, not even Tylenol, since I didn't get headaches.

"I'll go to the store and get you some ibuprofen," I offered.

"No, no, I'll go home," he said.

"Why weren't you hard last night?" I asked.

"It was the red wine."

He hurriedly got dressed and left.

If he knew red wine caused him to have ED, why did he drink so much of it? And since he seemed to know this was a problem, why did he lie and say he had no problems with his erections?

We texted a few times that morning. He wanted me to come over later that day. He said he would be hard and we could try again. I texted him to ask what time would work, and to be sure to pick a time when he could be hard for sure. He did not reply to that text and I never heard from him again.

I was really out of integrity at work. I was online constantly, and more interested in fucking or being outdoors in the sunshine, than working. I had never been so horny in all my life. I was constantly wet, engorged, and turned on. Everyone was out of the office. I closed my office door and masturbated.

"LEAVING THE OFFICE FOR SEX MAKES A BAD IMPRESSION"

February 25. Steve again (math teacher).

I left the office mid morning to go to Steve's house. I wondered if my colleagues knew I was leaving the office to fuck. Steve gave me an orgasm from oral sex and he turned me on a lot in the penetration. That time, when he lay on me all sweaty, I didn't mind. I held him tight and let his sweat soak on my body.

"Do you want to get a coffee?" he asked, as I got dressed.

"Yeah, that sounds amazing."

We drove in my car to the Starbucks. I liked his strong body standing behind me in the Starbucks line. Did he think he should pay, because he was the man? He had been a rock star in bed, a definite A+++, so he deserved whatever he wanted.

"I've got this. You totally deserve it, after your performance this morning," I said, loud enough for others to hear. He smiled.

We sipped our coffees outside, in the warm February sunshine.

"Do you want to come for a sleepover?" I invited him.

"That sounds wonderful. Let me check my schedule with the kids and sports and I'll let you know in the next day."

I was getting a little attached, but I still couldn't see myself dating him.

When I got back to work, one of the associates pulled me aside.

"Schahrzad, can I talk to you?"

"Sure."

He came in my office and closed the door.

"When you leave the office during the day to have sex, it gives the appearance you are not serious about your work."

I was not that serious about my work, but my hours were not his business. He was not my boss. Was this sexual harassment, telling me I wasn't allowed to leave work to have sex? Could I leave the office for my son's swim meet or to have lunch with a friend? Was it the sex that bothered him or my playfulness? Maybe he secretly wished he was me.

"Well, I am an independent contractor, which means I set my own hours, and I like that perk and will continue to use it."

He had some nerve, seeking to damp my sexuality, which had been dampened my whole life. I didn't work there to impress people with my career ambitions. I was there to contribute and have an intellectual outlet, as well as an income to support myself, but none of that could interfere with my primary goal of discovering my sexuality.

DICK PICS AND MY RELATIONSHIP TO MY PUSSY

I stayed late at work that day, to make up for the time at Steve's place. That evening, I took a break and browsed profiles on POF, a dating site. Sam, a nice man in his late 20's, asked for my phone number. I was sure he was a good prospect for meeting for coffee, so I gave it to him. Immediately, I received a cropped photo of his penis.

I was furious and wanted to slap him. I sent him a text and blocked him online.

You're a lame loser. No game. Gross. Don't ever contact me again!

His penis was repulsive because the poor lighting made its skin tone look corpse-like, and where was his face? I always was angry when men sent me dick pics. I went into the fight part of the fight/flight mode. I was in no actual danger. I was sitting in my office holding a phone.

I didn't want to go through life reacting, so I took a deep breath, closed my eyes, and asked why I was angry.

My true feeling was hurt and disappointment, because sending him my number was an invitation for friendship, and he had reduced my offer to body parts. The dick picture said, "My heart is off limits. You're just a fuck so all you get is my dick." He didn't know I needed his heart, to want his cock at all.

I texted Rick and Jose to ask them about this. They said a dick pic guy was socially immature, but did not intend to upset or repulse me.

I had to think about the man's motives. Maybe he hoped for a pussy picture in return, and maybe some women sent them, and then the man would masturbate to the picture because he did not need the whole woman to be aroused. Maybe he imagined I was so aroused by his picture, I finger fucked myself furiously while looking at it, like the actresses in porn.

I sat again and thought about it. Maybe these men could teach me something, despite their lack of social skills. Why did men send dick pics and women did not go around sending pussy pics? I imagined sending a man my pussy picture, proper etiquette and standards aside. I cringed at the thought. Its many colors and enlarged opening from childbirth were gross.

I could show my pussy to a man in my bed, because he already liked me and was turned on and could overlook such things, but baring it all to a stranger, that I could never do. I knew I wasn't

What I Did For Sex

the only woman who felt that way. I had seen a documentary about the book Petals, a sepia photography collection of women's vulvas. The women in the movie didn't like their pussies either. Pussy hate had led to labiaplasties, and a general numbing of our sexuality. It all started because we idolized the vulvas in the magazines, not knowing they were photo shopped.

I wanted to get over that and love my pussy. I texted Rick again, because he liked me.

Do you think my pussy is ugly?
No, it's beautiful.
Really?
Yes.
Can I send you a pussy picture?
Yes, of course.
I sent him the picture. He replied, *Beautiful.*
You don't think it's ugly?
No, your pussy is gorgeous.

I sent my pussy picture to a few more of my hookup buddies, and they all liked it. I wanted to like it too. Since the only thing wrong with my pussy were the thoughts I had about it, I just had to change my thoughts. "My pussy is beautiful," I told myself. I didn't fully believe it yet, but it was a big shift.

If my pussy was beautiful, could I really send its pictures to men without being labeled as trash? Would I still be respected and considered a lady? I knew the pussy social rules. Men could talk about their package, make innuendos on TV, say they had blue balls, and rap about fucking their bitch, but I never heard women talk like that. We did not have pet names for "down there", admit our lust on national TV, or sing with abandon about riding hard cocks. Men could sit with their legs spread wide, but womens' pants were not sufficient to hide our pussies. It also required crossing our legs. We were not to share our pussies with anyone, except in private by men we loved, preferably men we had married. Women who showed their genitals in porn or to many lovers were called sluts, and certainly could not garner future employment in many organizations, especially as teachers in elementary schools.

I still didn't like men sending me dick pics. Men never flashed me in person. They just did it online. Sensual men, who knew how to arouse a woman, never flashed me at all, or mentioned sex in our messaging. These were the men I met for coffee.

"MOMMY, WHAT IS SEX?"

I was making friends with younger people. My new friend Lauren was only 24 years old. She invited me to a hip new spot, Lofty Coffee in Encinitas. We grabbed a table outside and ordered coffee and yoghurt with fresh fruit. A group of women, a couple with their toddler, and a single man sat nearby. Lauren and I caught up on our personal development work, friendships, sex, and dating. I told her about the polyamory retreat I had attended two months earlier, Kevin's rail and bail at the office, the skateboarder, two men in one day, and Caden who did not make a sound.

"I'm so tired of bad sex," I complained.

"What do you consider bad sex?" she asked.

"When a guy is not hard enough or he doesn't care if I have an orgasm, or he won't go down on me or he is too submissive in bed."

"Teach them what you like," she suggested.

"Is that what you do?"

"Yes, I like telling a man how to go down on me and what I like."

"Wow, that's awesome. I need to do that, but I'm still not sure what they're doing when it feels good and what I want them to do instead. Most men suck at oral sex. I'm good. I get every woman off. It's not that complicated."

"True, some are better than others."

I walked Lauren back to her car.

"Did you notice that couple with the toddler?" she asked.

"Yeah, they sat next to us."

"Did you hear the little kid?" she laughed. "He kept asking "Mommy, what is sex? Mommy, what is sex? What is sex?"

"Really? That's hilarious. I didn't even notice." I paused. "What did the parents say?"

"They didn't say anything."

"Did I do something wrong? I mean, they could have moved to a different table or asked me to lower my voice."

"I think they were listening too."

"Oh my god, that's hilarious. I guess most people don't talk about sex so it can grab the attention. I'm just in my own world. I don't even notice anyone when I'm talking."

"You're funny, Schahrzad. It was great to see you again."

She got in her car and drove off and I went to work.

STEVE: "WE NEED TO END THIS" (MARCH)

It was March. It was just one year ago, that I left Brad's bed. Birds chirped in the morning, and the days were longer. I yearned for a man in my home, someone for whom I could cook and snuggle with, after I did the dishes. Was the universe punishing me, not because of my sexual proclivities, but because of some inherent badness?

March 1. Steve again (44, math teacher).

Steve came for a sleepover. Maybe I couldn't date him, but I liked him in bed.

March 5. Steve again (44, math teacher).

I left the office early afternoon to go to Steve's place. His kids had left their toys all over, but I liked he was keeping it real. I liked that he always made me come, and made me come first. I liked his penetration.

The next day, I felt a happy glow. I felt like I was the sun. It was my gratitude. It was from Steve.

March 10. Steve again (44, math teacher).

Steve felt super good. Maybe I was getting attached. I texted him a few times that night to let him know how good he felt, and that I couldn't wait to see him again. I still didn't want to date him, but I definitely had more feelings.

That night I was cooking with Chandi, when I had a long incoming text from Steve. He said he had a responsibility for the feelings we created together. He wanted a relationship, but not with me, because I didn't open him up the way he needed to be opened. He said we shouldn't see each other again. I was devastated. I needed an outlet, so after dinner I joined a gym so I could start swimming. Swimming calmed me.

March 13. Blake again (42, VP).

I got a text from Blake. He wanted me to come over. I had forgot all about him, but I was curious how I would feel when I saw him again, so I went over.

"Hey, it's great to see you," and he gave me a quick hug.

"Thanks."

He invited me in.

"I'm watching a show. Only five minutes left, just have a seat," he explained.

He sat in front of the TV, glued to the screen, while I sat alone on his sofa. Zero people skills. After his show was over, he asked if I wanted to watch a movie. He sat next to me on the sofa and we watched a show. I didn't even like TV.

Finally, he invited me to his bedroom. I liked the sex with him. Then I held him and tried to sleep, but he was stiff in bed. It all felt awkward.

"I can't sleep," he said.

"I'll get up with you," I offered, because I knew how be part of a team.

He got up and poured himself a drink, and one for me. We sat on the patio, sipping our drinks, and then he wanted to watch more TV. This man had no idea how to get comfort from a woman.

The next morning, I fucked him while he had his eyes closed. Maybe he had intimacy issues. Maybe that led to his divorce. He made coffee while I made the bed.

"I need some egg whites to get my strength back," he joked.

I looked at him, so handsome that he made my heart melt. But I had no desire to be with him at all once the sex was done. Nothing pulled me to his insides, his core. I was sure I would never cry over him again.

Blake walked me to my car. On the way back, I had my post sex happy glow, and by the time I got home, I was fantasizing about him and couldn't wait to see him again. It was obvious he didn't feel that way about me, since he had never asked me out, and could not get comfort from my presence. He needed the TV, a drink, and his eyes closed.

On March 23, I had a sleepover with Jeremy at his place.

THE MAN I FELL FOR ONLINE

I showered and went to work. That day, when I browsed online profiles, I thought of Danny, the man I fell for and had never met. I messaged him off the dating app to see how he was doing. He said his work schedule had freed up and he wanted to come down to San Diego. We set a coffee date for later that month, when he had a day off.

March 24. Danny, the man I fell for online.

Danny and I met for coffee in Oceanside. He was heavier than in his picture and not as handsome. My fantasy had been all for nothing. He said he gained weight. Our conversation did not flow as I had imagined. I invited him over anyway, just to have sex with my once-fantasy-man. He sat on my sofa and we had nothing to talk about. I invited him to my bedroom, where he was clumsy and came in 2 minutes. I didn't even want to masturbate for him. I told him to leave and I never heard from him again.

DOMINATING A WOMAN
March 29. Ruth, 36, bisexual mother of two.

I attended an all-girls sacred snuggle party. Ruth, a beautiful married bisexual woman, caught my eye. I wanted to be like the man and have a woman open and surrender to me. I lay on top of her and kissed her. She moaned. I felt powerful and aroused, making her moan. I put my hands on her body and between her legs and felt her soft swollen lips. I slipped inside her lubricated opening and pleasured her with my fingers, while I kissed her. She moaned harder and writhed in pleasure. I loved opening a woman like that. Men were lucky, getting us women to surrender and open to them, to moan for them. I got her close to an orgasm and then she lost her buildup and we both felt let down.

I kept having sex, mostly because I was horny. The beginning of April looked like this:

April 5   Jeremy, sleepover, A
April 18   Lance, 28, oral only, C
April 19, Chris, 27, mechanic, lunch, very passionate, A++

"I REALIZED I WANT A WIFE AND CHILDREN"
April 24. Jonathan, 31, pension fund auditor.

Jonathan met me for coffee at a quaint coffee shop in Encinitas. He told me about work, hobbies, and his childhood. He was sensual, attractive, and his beard was hot. Maybe this was a man I could actually date. We had been sitting for two hours and he had never mentioned sex.

"I like younger men," I told him.
"I like older women."
"For dating or for sex?"

"For dating. I'm looking for a relationship. Girls my age are so immature."

We had been sitting for a long time. I stretched my legs.

"Do you want to go for a walk?" he invited.

"Yes, that sounds amazing."

We walked to his car and he opened the door for me. Being a passenger in a man's car felt like a date, not just a fuck. He drove a few blocks to Moonlight Beach, and he took his flashlight so I could see where I walked. He held my hand so I felt safe. We walked in the dark night, and he led me to a secluded spot. I liked that he took charge and led me, but I hoped he wasn't going to try for sex in the sand, because it reminded me of sex in the car. A man who cared for a woman would bring her to a comfortable private bed.

Jonathan kissed me. My mental resistance melted away in the strength of his embrace and the passionate tenderness of his lips. Since I liked how he kissed me and he wanted more than sex, I bypassed my dislike of public sex and being outdoors and getting full of sand. I agreed to sex at the beach. He lay on me, and my entire heart and pussy opened wide in love and surrender. It was his energy, his interest in me, and his passion…. I got more wet than I had in a long time. Afterward, he drove me back to my car and asked when he could take me to dinner. I gave him an A+++.

April 25. Jonathan again (31, pension fund auditor).

On our second date, Jonathan and I met for sushi at a hip restaurant in Oceanside. I noticed an uncomfortable silence at dinner. Maybe it was the age difference. I invited him over anyway.

The sex was completely different that night, very mediocre. He didn't hold me as much or kiss me as deeply and he kept his eyes closed.

After he left, I texted him and asked why he was so distant. He apologized. He had realized over dinner he wanted to date a woman his age so he could have a family, and he didn't want to tell me when he was there. I thanked him for taking care of himself. I wished he had ended it over dinner, instead of withholding in the bedroom.

He was the second man who went from A+++ to a D, not because he was tired, but simply because he no longer wanted a connection.

CHAPTER 13
PURPOSE AND MISSION

In May, I flew to Sacramento for a facilities funding conference, bought some spring dresses, renewed the lease on my apartment, and went in for my STD tests. All my test results came back negative.

I reviewed my life. My ex-husband was in a committed relationship and all I had to show for my first year single was a long fuck list. It was time to forge deeper connections, and a good place to start was my family and friends. I needed to forgive Sarina. I dialed her number.

"Hello, Schahrzad?" she answered.

"Yes, Sarina, how are you?"

"I'm so glad you called!"

"Yes, I want to get past our disagreement."

"I'm so glad. I really missed you."

"Yeah, I missed you too. Tell me what happened with you and Rudy. Did you ever end up seeing him?"

"Yes, I did. " She paused. "I invited him to see me, because I thought you and Rudy were done. He said he wanted a relationship and he would consider moving closer if we had a connection."

"What?"

"Yeah, he really led me on!"

"I can't believe he lied to you like that, and that you believed him."

"Yeah, you know I don't hookup. I only have sex in relationships and I wait months to get to know a man before I have sex."

"Yeah, true."

"He convinced me about a relationship. He talked about skiing together and trips and our children being friends. I really fell for it."

"Damn! What a player. Did you at least enjoy the sex?"

"It was alright."

"Really? Just alright?"

"Yeah. He came out for a 3-day weekend. The sex was mediocre the first time and went downhill from there. On our last day together, we didn't even have sex at all. We sat on the sofa watching TV and didn't even talk. I was so glad when he left."

"Oh my god, that's so funny."

My STD test results came back: negative for everything

I signed up for some personal development courses, talked myself into staying at my job, and kept exploring my sexuality. Some of the men I met for coffee were not attractive enough to invite over. The beginning of May looked like this:

May 2   Dave, 24, nice wide cock, he did not care if I came, B
May 10   Alex, 38, brewery manager, I came on his cock while I masturbated, B
May 15   Jeremy again.

MORMONS DON'T MASTURBATE
(MAY, ONE YEAR SINGLE)

May 17. Scott, 34, realtor.

Scott met me for dinner at an upscale restaurant in Carlsbad. He lived in Orange County, and had come down to San Diego for our date. The hostess showed me to his table. He had a good table, overlooking the entire restaurant. He wore a nice shirt and tie, and got up to greet me. I liked his manners.

"Order whatever you want," he said.

I relaxed into his presence. When the waitress came for our drinks, I ordered red wine and he ordered water.

"You don't drink?"

"No, I'm Mormon."

"So you never drink?"

"No. I've never tried alcohol, caffeine, or tobacco."

He told me about his education and his coastal property listings as a realtor. He didn't say it to brag, but to impress.

"I love older women. I'd definitely like dating you."

"Oh wow, that's hot."

After dinner, I invited him over. He followed me in his sports car.

In bed, he just wanted to please me, but he could not make me come, so I masturbated to orgasm. Then it was his turn.

"How would you like to come?" I asked.

"Oh, I don't need an orgasm."

"You don't want to come?"

"No, I just like to please the girl."

"Do you masturbate?"

"Not really. The last time I masturbated was 5 months ago."

This was strange. He didn't feel deserving or did he think sex was bad? I had no interest in a man who did not masturbate or want an orgasm. He changed his mind on spending the night, because he said it was hard to sleep at someone else's house. He gave me a long hug goodbye and left.

The next day, when Chandi came over, I asked her about it, because her high school had a large Mormon population. Chandi said one of her classmates was caught masturbating, and he had to go to confession in front of some Mormon elders. I googled it and learned Mormons viewed masturbation as selfish, and since we ought to be God-like and selfless, the only acceptable sex was directed toward the spouse. I didn't know religion required people to hate themselves.

SEX EDUCATION, GOVERNMENT, CHURCH, AURAS, AND LOTS OF FEAR

Mormons were not the only people repressing their sexuality. Our entire society had constructed an elaborate web against enjoying sex. It is this author's opinion that the repressed lust fuels the demand for online porn featuring mostly forbidden and grotesque scenarios, avoidance of open discussion about sex, avoiding sex or certain acts even after marriage, and suppressed pleasure. Combined with anger, the suppression also led to molestation, child sexual abuse, and sexual harassment. Combined with other repressed emotions, suppressing lust leads to reluctance for men to dominate and reluctance for women to surrender.

Suppression starts at home, where sex education usually consists of silence. The government contributed to it by withholding safe sex information. In 1994, Dr. Joycelyn Elders, surgeon general, spoke about distribution of contraception in schools and teaching children about masturbation, both as a way to reduce the spread of the AIDS virus. She was forced to resign within weeks of making her comments, and nobody has dared broach the subject ever since.

Middle school sex education focuses on the disease model or abstinence. The curriculum warns against pregnancy and STDs, and avoids teaching about the pleasure of sex, a woman's right to pleasure, and the nature of relationships. The medical supplies required to avoid pregnancy and STDs, namely condoms and birth control, are usually banned from free distribution.

Religion warns against lust and premarital pleasures, a sure road to hell. The fear is that sexually empowered people would have sex all day long and abandon their work and social obligations. Many religious people feel shame and guilt for their natural sexual desires. They push their lust and desires away, and hope to resurrect it all after marriage. Often this does not work, because beliefs are difficult to undo. Many religious women feel shame around sex their entire lifetimes, and can not masturbate or enjoy sex with their husbands.

Spiritual people warn against the dangers of mixing auras. In this theory, sexual intercourse causes auras and karma to overlap, which is bad because the sexual partner always has a lower vibrational energy. Oddly enough, the sexual partner's vibrational energy is never higher. It is recommended to cut the energy cords or cleanse the aura after a sexual encounter.

With all these fears and shame, it remains a wonder people have sex at all. It is this author's opinion that much of the sex that is happening is shrouded in guilt and shame, and requires fantasies, forbidden settings, and avoidance of deep intimacy and feelings that are a natural part of sexuality that is fully embraced and loved.

A BLACK MAN

It was time to try black. I had never been with a black man, mostly because I liked white guys. I longed to expand my heart and not judge people on skin color. I was also curious to see what all the fuss was about with black guys. I had heard "Once you go black, you never go back", and "black guys have huge cocks".

I offered to meet Max halfway between our homes, because he had such a long commute and he was nice. I met him after work at a Starbucks in Mira Mesa. He was freshly showered and wore a beautiful expensive looking shirt and gold chains. He was quite attractive. And big. Overweight. While we drank our coffees, I invited him over. He made several excuses, which made no sense. I never had encountered a man so into me, making excuses about sex. Brad at least said no and never had excuses. Did Max run out of Viagra, or did he have a wife at home?

"I can come over tomorrow evening," he said.

May 20. Max, 35, prison guard.

Max arrived at my apartment after work. His hug and kiss were ordinary. His touch and scent were repulsive. We took off our clothes and he lay on my bed, unable to move because of his big size. His penis was flaccid, and despite all my efforts, I could not get him hard. I licked his ass, sucked his cock and kissed him while I moaned, and let him finger my wet pussy. His penis remained flaccid.

Was his weight the problem? I had once read something about excess belly fat on men causing more estrogen. Or was it poor blood flow?

He didn't say anything, which made me think it happened frequently and could be the reason he did not want to come over the night before.

He was not able to orgasm and I did not want to orgasm. His limp penis, and how he just lay there in bed, were a turnoff. I was glad when he left.

DAVID, 32: INSPIRATION

May 24. David, 32, chemical engineer.

I noticed him right away: a lean man, about 6'2", in his early 30's. His tall strong body and handsome face melted my heart. He wore a plain T-shirt and jeans, nothing fancy. We were at an event held by my friends Chelli and Dave, a married couple in their early 30's who were in an open relationship. The event would feature eye gazing and vulnerable authentic communication exercises.

He saw me too, and came toward me. I looked up at him flirtatiously. His eyes twinkled and my heart melted in an instant.

I rarely saw a man with joy that lit up his eyes. This man could be dating material.

"Can I give you a hug?" I asked playfully.

"Yes," and he smiled at me.

I grabbed him tight and buried my head in his chest. He put his arms around me. Damn, he was strong. He was lean, which meant he had real strength created from exercising outdoors, not pushing objects up and down in a gym and accumulating bulk. His strength aroused me. I felt protected. I didn't worry if he liked older women. I just assumed he would, since he had come over.

"You're so strong! I like tall lean guys, and I love younger men!" I beamed him a huge smile.

"Oh, you do?"

'Yeah. I'm Schahrzad by the way."

"I'm David."

I liked how our attraction and interest developed naturally, instead of the result of an online encounter. Over the next few hours, we sought each other out for some of the exercises. They developed our intimacy and closeness. For decades I had wanted to do these activities with a romantic partner.

David handed me his business card and pointed to his phone number. I liked that he was making moves on me. When the event ended, he went in the men's restroom. Maybe he forgot about me. I stood outside and waited for him.

"Do you want to go out to dinner with me and my friends?" I asked when he came out.

"I'm so tired. I'm just going home to sleep."

But he wasn't leaving. He just stood there and looked at me. I felt arousal mixed with hope.

"Do you want to come to my house for dinner and a sleepover?"

"Really? That sounds awesome."

I gave him my address. I hoped he wouldn't change his mind on the way over. It seemed too good to be true. This felt like romance, not just a fuck.

Outside my apartment, David grabbed me in a tight embrace and kissed me. I wiggled out of his arms. I wasn't sure it was proper to kiss hookup guys in front of my neighbors. We put the overnight parking permit on his car and then we were finally alone in my apartment.

It felt good having a man in my kitchen. I put on my apron. He would probably consider me girlfriend material, all womanly like that. I heated up the lentil soup from the previous night and offered him something to drink. He said he didn't drink alcohol. Good. I liked how I picked sober conscious men.

Over dinner, he talked about his parents, career, long distance cycling trips, and volunteer work with men. There was something special about men who bonded with other men. I liked how his eyes twinkled when he talked. His voice was deep and soothing, his words warmed my heart. He was totally my type for a boyfriend. Maybe he would want to date me. Since I liked having sex without a condom on occasion, to give myself a more intimate experience, I asked him about his STD status. He said he had been abstinent for 8 months, and his STD tests from a month before were negative for everything. He also told me he had to be somewhere at 9am the next day. I hoped he would like me enough to ask me to go with him the next morning.

After dinner, he sat on the sofa, legs apart, his eyes twinkling, exuding confidence. I playfully straddled him and that's the first time I felt his erection. It pressed up on my groin. I wrapped my arms around his neck and looked with awe into his sparkling brown eyes. His energy made him so attractive.

"You're so handsome!" I beamed at him.

He didn't say anything back to me. I wished he had. Maybe he didn't give compliments to women he was just fucking. Our kissing started slow and heated up, and right when my panties felt damp, he picked me up and carried me into my bedroom. I giggled when he put me down because I felt so happy.

David slowly took off my clothes. I liked the tender attention of being undressed. He went down on me and he was really good because he didn't go right for my clit – he started with my labia. Then he sucked on my clit and made circles with his tongue.

"Wow, that feels amazing!"

I still had that thing about men going down on me too long unless they totally loved it, and we had just met and he probably wanted some attention too, so after five minutes I stopped him and returned the favor and played with his balls, asshole, and cock.

When I was ready for his penetration, I scooted up and kissed him. His hard cock pressed on my pubic mound. I looked into his eyes as I ground on him, and since I didn't feel anything in my heart, my mind drifted to an extremely attractive man in his early 50's I had seen in my apartment complex. That man would know about the needs of a woman my age, children, compromise, and picking up the dry cleaning.

David was on the bottom. He looked deeply into my eyes while he s-l-o-w-l-y pushed just the tip of his cock inside me. My body quivered in response. I had never been entered so slowly and deliberately. His eyes were intently on me, as if searching for signals to the pleasure he gave me down below. Just as s-l-o-w-l-y, he pulled out. He repeated this slow in and out motion, pushing deeper with each thrust. He was totally in control. It was the hottest thing I had ever done. By the time he was all in, I was moaning loud and my pussy was soaking wet.

He stayed in deep and pushed against the end of my pussy. He was barely moving, yet the sensations were intense. I liked this slower sex. I moved my hips too and rode his cock the way it felt good for me for what seemed like at least ten minutes. I was soaking wet. I wanted more of him.

"Stick your finger in my ass," I begged.

A deep wave of pleasure washed over me from my bottom and I rode him like that, with his finger in my ass. He was sweaty from all the thrusting and that was hot.

David picked me up gently and turned me over. He lay next to me, brought my knees to my chest, and hugged me with one arm. I was turned on by the novelty of it all, and how he took charge. He slid his cock inside and fucked me in the cradle position, while he looked at me. I felt safe and surrendered to him completely. Maybe that's what they meant with the spiritual parts of sex. It was like surrendering to God's will in my prayers. I felt a little guilty for just being able to lay there while he did all the work, but it all felt so good and I liked how he took charge. He was really sweaty by then.

"Let's give me a break," he said, and slowly pulled out.

His cock glistened with my pussy juices. David slid his fingers deep to where his cock had just been, and pressed without moving his fingers. Damn, that felt good!

"You should touch yourself," he said sweetly.

I closed my eyes and rubbed my clitoris. He licked his fingertips and slid them across my nipples, sending boosts of stimulation to my clit, while he fingered me and played with my nipples.

"You're such a good girl to touch yourself for me."

That turned me on even more and I felt something building deep within my body. I looked at him. And then it came, from deep within. My orgasm swelled out in a big wave, in which my moan became a roar, and my roar became a long exhaling scream, lasting at least thirty seconds. It was the most intense orgasm I ever had. I looked at him and saw he was rock hard.

He got on top, and since I was wet and could take it deep, he gave it to me harder. I grabbed his ass with both hands and pulled him rhythmically toward me, and back and forth. I wanted him as deep inside as I could.

"Deep, deep, deep," I whispered to him. "Let me have it deep!"

That turned him on, and since he wanted to take his time, he slowed his thrusting. He didn't want to come yet. He kissed me tenderly and then he nibbled on my ear lobe and pressed his warm tongue inside my ear. It drove me wild! I didn't even know I loved having that done!

"Go deep again, let me have all of your cock, deep."

Then he was ready. He went faster and then it all felt better so I knew he was harder and close to coming. He moaned and stopped thrusting and held me tight. I felt warm liquid drip out of me. We held each other and fell asleep together. He got up during the night to get something out of his car while I slept. He could have just left then, but he came back to my bed. We had intercourse again in the morning, and then I hoped he could stay.

"Do you want some coffee?"

"No, I have to be somewhere at 9am," he replied.

Darn it, he didn't invite me along.

"I'll see you again," he said.

"That's what they all say."

He left without making another date, just like the other men before him. David texted me that he got home safely. I didn't ask him to do that, and no other man had done that.

David texted me the next day and asked if he could see me a few days later. I felt respected that he set our dates up ahead of time, and didn't just call at the last minute when he was horny.

May 28. David again.

He came over again, and the sex was good. He liked me to come first and he stayed hard a long time and was passionate with me.

"What do you like about older women?" I asked after we made love.

"They know what they want."

He said he couldn't stay the night. He texted me when he got home.

From then on, I replayed key moments of our time together, and I grew more attached. Whenever I thought of him, I imagined he felt it and was thinking of me also. I probably fabricated a connection that didn't exist. I sent him a few well-positioned poses with my derriere nicely exposed. He said they were distracting him at work, and asked when I was free again.

I invited him over for the following Tuesday, and cancelled the two hookups I had planned in the interim, because I wasn't sure if it was appropriate to fuck other guys when I liked him and he wasn't fucking anyone else. I still wanted to fuck other guys, but I also wanted to follow dating protocols, whatever those were.

June 4. David again.

David came over and he was good in bed. Unlike other men who started with an A+ and often became a B or C, David consistently gave me A+ sex. I was super wet and turned on while we were fucking. David moved me into the cradle position again. Our eyes were locked together, and my heart melted when I looked into his twinkling eyes. He gently and slowly pushed his cock against my vulva.

"Do it," I said, waiting for his cock in my pussy.

"Yes?" he asked and moved his cock toward my ass.

Did he think I wanted him to fuck me in the ass? I didn't ask for that, but I was going to let him if that's where he was headed.

"Don't we need lube?"

He kept looking at me and slowly slid his cock further in my ass. I was so wet, he slid around easily.

"We don't need lube?"

He didn't answer. He looked at me tenderly. Slowly he pushed his cock against my ass, without going in, and he looked at me, just pushing there, waiting for my reaction before he took it further. I felt safe and loved. I was willing to surrender to whatever he wanted to do to my ass.

"I trust you," I whispered as I looked in his eyes and surrendered to him.

As soon as I spoke those words, my entire lower pelvis relaxed and opened up. My ass, my pussy, my heart, it was all one and it was open.

We looked into each other's eyes. Nobody blinked. He pushed his cock slowly into my ass. David slid about half an inch further with each thrust. I was soaking wet. We didn't need lube.

His cock was all the way inside my ass, and he moved in and out while I moaned with pleasure. My moans were deep and guttural. He thrust sensuously inside my ass, and then slipped his cock out of my ass and back into my vagina. It was supposed to be a no-no to go from anus to vagina without washing first. But I trusted him and I didn't want to break the flow of our connection by getting up to wash.

I had my orgasm and then he had his and we laid and cuddled.

"I noticed I came first every time we were together. I liked that," I said.

"I love giving women orgasms and I like the woman to come first," he said.

He left and an hour later he texted me that he was home, and may not have time to see me again before his vacation. Over the next few days, as I replayed key moments of our time together, I grew more attached to David. I liked him for more than sex. He was perfect: a man who moved through life with purpose, and whose happiness derived from his integrity and actions. I wanted what he had and I wanted him. I thought of him constantly. Did David want me too? I had to find out.

I really like you and can't wait to see you again, I texted.

Kiss me and let me fly, he replied.

Wait - what? Did he mean fly away for good, or fly away and come back for more kisses between flights? What did he mean? I fought back tears. I texted him and he sent a long text back explaining all the characteristics he wanted in a woman. It seemed he was describing me. So why fly away?

I made a bold move. I called him and told him I had feelings. David said he didn't feel the same way. He said he was sorry he hurt me, and his focus was advancing his career and finding a wife. He wanted a family.

"Why did you come back to see me if you only wanted sex?"

"The first time we were together, I said I would come back and I wasn't sure I would, but when you said 'That's what they all say', I decided I couldn't do that to you. And then each time I came back, I grew a little more attached. That's why it's best to end it now."

He also said he had some advice for me.

"When you meet a man you like, date him for 4-6 weeks before you have sex. Get to know him. It makes the sex so much better."

I was definitely out. I was the girl who fucked him the first day. That's not the kind of girl he wanted. He didn't date girls like me….girls who hooked up when they felt like it and had a long list of lovers. He just happened to meet me and like me. Getting a good man like David meant I couldn't go around having sex whenever I wanted. But how was I going to hold off on sex for one date, let alone dates spanning 4 – 6 weeks, when sex was the first thing I wanted?

ABSTINENCE

I couldn't hookup anymore. I was too sad. David and I practically made love. I felt secure around him and trusted him. Men like him, and sex like that, were hard to find. If I couldn't have him or someone I felt that way about, I didn't want to have sex at all. I decided to go abstinent again.

I was crying constantly. I thought ghosting was the reason I cried over men, but it wasn't. David spent thirty minutes on the phone in a power parting, but it didn't make the ending any easier or stop my heart from breaking. I understood all his reasons for not wanting me, yet I held out hope he would change his mind, because our connection had been so awesome.

I hated being sad again, in the pit of misery, and powerless over my own joy. My sadness made no sense, because I didn't even know him - I just liked how I felt around him. Maybe it had to do with that relationship with myself. I had an idea. The feelings I felt around David, were my own. What if I could create those same feelings, without needing him at all? I sat on my sofa and closed my eyes, to remember how I felt around him. Slowly the feelings came to me: awe, joy, and inspiration.

I could feel awe and joy admiring my own body instead of his. I started taking more selfies, and looked at myself in the mirror when I danced or showed my feelings, even when I cried. I was beautiful when I showed my feelings.

His cycling turned me on. Cyclists and their long lean bodies had long aroused me. What if I cycled, instead of longing for cyclists? I borrowed Chandi's bike to try it and took a few 30-mile bike rides down the coast. I felt free and powerful with the wind blowing through my helmet, my body drenched in sweat, my strong legs pushing the bike forward. Yes, this was good. I bought a bike and a bike rack. I started cycling on weekends and I liked it. Men who passed me were amazed by my speed.

I was inspired by his purpose. David's life was full in all the places where mine was empty. I became obsessed with finding a purpose, my mission. Maybe a mission would make me forget about wanting a man.

"YOU SHOULD WRITE A BOOK"

I was doing all that, but I was still crying over David. It was hard to be happy when I longed for so much passion, and he had seemed so perfect. It had taken a year to find someone like him, and it could take forever to have it happen again.

I told myself to trust life, and be open to what it gave me. And I cried. I told myself to let myself cry, and I cried. I told myself to stop thinking about him, because I knew I was a bad person for being sad and not happy. But I didn't know how to be happy when I longed for so much passion, so I cried.

I had to pull myself together. Maybe I could be happy if I found my mission. I needed a mission. What was my purpose, post-mothering? I sought deep inside myself for answers. I prayed. I meditated, went in nature, sat in silence on the sofa. I asked my friends. Some people said nobody needed a mission and the joy of life was living in the moment. I disagreed. And I cried.

I had been abstinent about a month, when I saw a friend perform in a play.

"You should write a book," she said afterward.

It came out of her in such a force, I had to heed its call. I heard this often over the past year from various friends, and had always brushed it aside, because I never had a desire to write a book. That evening, I listened. The book was the mission I had been seeking. Yes. I had a story to tell.

The next day, I bought a legal pad and took it to a coffee shop and wrote the story about David, through streams of tears, and the stories of some, but not all, of the women and men with whom I shared my heart, mind, and body. I wrote at night and on weekends. A few days later, I had a text from Jeremy.

How have you been?
Abstinent
You're way too horny to be abstinent

I laughed. Maybe a man like Jeremy who loved a sexual woman would be better for me than a man like David, who wanted an abstinent woman who sat around waiting for a man.

I kept writing. I debated what to include or exclude. Dare I admit I don't orgasm from penetration, or that I preferred fucking over spending time with my children? Should I admit my vicodin addiction? Maybe there was no need for it in a sex memoir. Was it fair to talk about my ex-husband, when he didn't agree to be in a book?

Writing wasn't so difficult, because of the force from deep within that urged me forward. It was a force of creative expression from deep in the pit of my belly. All my sexual repression from my childhood, work, social media, society, and my ex-husband came out in my book. It was the only place I could be free.

WHAT IF I NEVER FIND A MAN?

About six weeks into my abstinence, I was in a women's self-discovery class led by Chelli, the woman who led the course where I met David. In one exercise, Chelli sat across from me. She looked at me a long time and then she smiled sweetly.

"I can feel you are seeking for a man. You have a seeking energy," and she moved both her hands in a grabbing motion to demonstrate.

Damn. How could she tell? I didn't want anyone to see my neediness. I wanted to be independent and strong. Yet she was right. Although I wasn't having sex or dating or talking to men or sexting them, and I was abstinent, I felt unfulfilled and was constantly looking outside of myself. It was my way of being.

"Yes," I admitted.

She looked at me a few seconds. "What would your life be like if you never found a man….if you were single forever?"

Wow. I opened my mouth and stared at her. That could actually happen. In that moment, I became free. Since I could be single forever, I was going to live for <u>me</u>, and not for some potential Mr. Right like David who required a sexless passive woman who deprived herself of sexual pleasure until he came along.

I liked sex and I wanted sex. I would have all the sex I wanted, if that's what I wanted. Any man, who was right for me, would like me the way I was. I got right to it.

    July 13   Jeremy again, no condom since I was his only sex partner, B
    July 17   Rick again, female condom slipped, B
    July 26   Billie again, female condom slipped, B
    July 27   Chris again, could not get hard : "You remind me of my mom", D

In August, Chandi and I went to Aspen for a week long vacation. August looked like this:

    Aug 1   Danny, 20, college hockey player, awesome body, B
    Aug 7   Jeremy again, no condom, 3 rounds, B
    Aug 8   Danny, 19, extremely hard and passionate, A++
    Aug 9   Cory, 24, my first Tinder hookup, A
    Aug 14   Lonny, 32, guaranteed me an orgasm from penetration only if we did not use a condom and I agreed because I trusted him but he totally lied., D
    Aug 18   Joseph, 25, former Marine, A+

Nate texted and asked if he could come over. That time, he wanted to spend the night. Did that mean he was finally ready to date me? I wasn't that interested in young men anymore, because they lacked emotional follow-through, did not know what they wanted, and ghosted me after just one date. And I no longer had a crush on him. But if he wanted to open the doors to dating, I could consider it.

August 30. Nate again (23, former Marine).

Nate and I had dinner, a bottle of wine, and our sleepover. We did not use a condom, because I trusted him on his safe sex status and wanted the closeness, romance, and intimacy. He deserved my bare pussy, because he was so tender with me. He was amazing in bed. He orgasmed in the condom in the missionary position, holding me tight. He slept peacefully, without tossing or turning or snoring and I liked that. When he left the next morning, I did not mind, because I no longer considered him for a relationship.   I was so horny, I texted Jeremy and asked him to come over the next day.

Aug 31   Jeremy again, A

TINDER

I got more responsibilities at work. At night and on weekends, I wrote my book.

I was getting all my hookups on Tinder. I liked Tinder because I could only receive messages from men I had chosen, and each man was presented to me only once. I was so horny, all I could think about was penetration. My panties were constantly damp from being aroused. September looked like this:

Sept 7	Bryce, 21, no condom, 4x, very passionate! A+++
Sept 14, morning	Tyson, 31, best curved cock ever, his house, A+
Sept 14, evening	Joseph, 24, Marine officer, rocked my world in bed, A++++
Sept 15	Jeremy again, no condom, B
Sept 16	Christian, 28, drove 30 miles to his place. I was so horny, B
Sept 16	Justin, 24, Marine, A

Sept 17	Kevin, 35, boring, D
Sept 19	Jake, 23, Marine, hurt me because his cock was too long, C
Sept 22, morning	Jack, 18, Marine, A++
Sept 22, evening	Tyler, 24, Marine, A
Sept 24	Tyler again, A
Sept 25	Robbie again, B
Sept 26	Kevin, met him at a strip club celebrating my birthday and went back to their bachelor party, B

After my hookup with the artillery officer, I was hooked on Marines. For the next 10 months, I limited my hookups to Marines. I met them all on Tinder. Most were ages 19-24. Their passion, sensuality, and fitness excited me. They always went down on me and wanted me to come first. Some wanted to spend the night, more than once. They held me at night, shared their feelings, and made me laugh. I had sex in the barracks at Camp Pendleton, the base at Miramar, and once at the base hotel at Coronado.

LINGERING

I kept looking for men for a relationship, or sex, or both, depending on my mood. I got attached to a few more men, including a Marine with whom I had two sex dates over a three month period because he was out of town. I was puzzled by my attachment. I was not a needy girl. I went out alone all the time, and between the two sex dates, I was happy and satisfied with our texting. I justified my crying over him as healthy, because at least I was feeling something in my heart. I finally realized crying and self-pity had become a comfort zone. It was pathetic.

I noticed a pattern. I got attached to men, even if did not like them that much, because I played back fulfilling affectionate, pleasurable sexual moments in my mind. I was holding onto my thoughts, a process called lingering.

Our minds were not made to hold on to thoughts, and our bodies were not made to hold on to feelings. We were meant to think and feel in in the moment, and flow with life.

Letting go of a man was actually easy to do, once I became committed to letting thoughts go, instead of clutching them tightly.

I was on a roll. The Marines had ignited a zest for dominant passionate men who could fuck me with abandon. The beginning of October looked like this:

Oct 2   Troy, 22, grad student, B
Oct 4   Dale, 24, student, C
Oct 5   Daniel, 23, Mormon, no orgasm in 8 months and didn't want one, C
Oct 6   Wes, 29, musician I met at a music festival, A+++
Oct 8   Josh, 24, auditor, wanted to date me, A++
Oct 14 Tyler again, sleepover

HE HAD A GIRLFRIEND (OCTOBER)

Nate had a girlfriend, but he wanted to come over on Thursday after work. All my life, I had chosen single men for dating and sex. I had to break my rigidity and try sex with a man in a relationship. That time I would use a condom. A man with a girlfriend did not deserve the intimacy of my bare pussy.

October 16, morning. Nate again (24, former Marine).

Nate's strong grip and tender lips aroused me in seconds. His big hard cock slid in easily. He laid me on my stomach and entered me from behind, thrusting slowly and sensually deep inside me, in the same steady rhythm, while I masturbated. I had never orgasmed on my stomach, and I worried he was getting tired. I loved that he knew he needed to keep everything the same: the same thrust, same speed, and same rhythm. Eventually, the comfort of the rhythm helped me let go and after 30 minutes of his thrusting, I came hard on his cock. Then he gave a few more thrusts and had his orgasm.

That time, he didn't want to cuddle. He got his cuddling at home. He quickly got dressed and came back to my bed for a few minutes to talk. He said his girlfriend was beautiful and the sex was good. There was nothing lacking in the relationship. He just liked having sex with other women.

Nate taught me that sex, no matter how passionate, was just sex. I stopped mistaking affection in the bedroom as a gauge of the man's feelings for me. A relationship was decided on whether we enjoyed each other outside the bedroom.

A feeling of appreciation and accomplishment washed over me. All those years, I had wondered if I could make it without Brad, because he earned the money. I had attributed my stability and happiness to him, when in fact it was mine.

The rest of October looked like this:

Oct 16, eve	Matthew, 21, Marine, sleepover, A++
Oct 18	Matthew again, sleepover, A++
Oct 22	Steve again, sex was boring that time, C
Oct 24	William, 21, Marine, was drunk but passionate, no condom, A++
Oct 29	William again, no condom, A++
Oct 31	Jeremy again, no condom, A

THE CLITORIS IS A LARGE ORGAN, MOSTLY INTERNAL

I was reading some sex articles online, when a headline about the clitoris grabbed my attention. A diagram labeled a clitoris showed the tiny button or glans that was usually labeled the clitoris in diagrams was just the tip of the iceberg. The majority of the clitoris was actually hidden from view! That's why it felt good to press on my pubic mound and labia: I was stimulating the hidden parts of my clitoris!

I read more articles to be sure. Indeed, the clitoris is about 4" long. Its tiny glans has 8,000 nerve endings (more than double that of a penis). The clitoris keeps growing, and doubles in size after menopause. The glans, shaft, and hood of the clitoris were made of the same tissue as the corresponding parts in a penis. And like the penis, the clitoris is made of erectile tissue and gets engorged and hard.

How could I be 54 years old and not even know this?

I gained more respect for my body. We women were indeed mysterious.

November looked like this:

Nov 5	Bruce, 24, Marine officer, his place, C
Nov 7	Blake, 19, Marine, B
Nov 8	Ryan, 22, Marine, sleepover, A+
Nov 10	Brett, 35, B
Nov 11	Joseph again (24, Marine), C
Nov 13	Roger, 27, Marine, sleepover, he fell asleep on me, B
Nov 20	Lucas, 20, C
Nov 21	Mark, 33, Marine officer, his place, B
Nov 22	Randy, 22, grad student, sleepover, his place, A+
Nov 23	Zack, 22, Marine, too nervous to get hard, passionate, A+
Nov 24	Greg, 22, C
Nov 25	STD tests – came back negative for everything

Walter, the massage therapist, texted to wish me a happy thanksgiving. He had moved to Washington and got a job working as a physical therapist.

"I DON'T USE LUBE"

I was having sex mostly because I was horny and playful, not because I wanted a relationship. During penetration, I got very wet and I got wetter and wetter, as long as the man was hard, kept the action moving forward, and held me tight. I was surprised by my wetness, because I was not taking any hormones and had expected menopause to cause vaginal dryness.

If the mans' penis got soft or he paused thrusting or did not hold me, I dried out quickly. Sometimes the man would ask for lube or started to put spit on my pussy. I did not allow this. A dry pussy meant I was not ready for fucking. My natural lubrication indicated my readiness for penetration and protected me from pain, germs, and urinary tract infections.

"I don't like spit on my pussy. Spit is water based and drying, and my pussy juices are slippery and feel much better."

"I don't use lube. My pussy is only fuckable if it's wet. I'll tell you what you can do to make me get wetter."

The men listened and then they saw that their actions had an immediate effect on me and I got immediately soaking wet. For some reason, they really liked penetration when I was sloshing wet. I enjoyed it less because I had less friction.

December looked like this:

Dec 1	Barrett, 38, Marine, no condom, only partially hard, considered him for a relationship, C
Dec 3	Brice, 21, C
Dec 5	Gary, 29, professional bull rider, B
Dec 13	Barrett again, no condom, he was only partially hard, B
Dec 21	Craig, 23, Marine, C
Dec 29	Willie, 24, B
Dec 29	William again, he was drunk but so passionate, A++
Dec 30	Brice, 22, Marine, A
	David, 30, B
Dec 31	Randy again, A

MANY OF TODAY'S YOUNG MEN ROCK IN BED

The young men I met were not the same as the young men I fucked in high school and college. Men ages 19-24 were good in bed. They were sensuous and gave me good foreplay. They shared their feelings and held me at night.

I Orgasmed While Masturbating During Penetration
Brad, a 24-year-old Marine officer, was no exception. He had a gorgeous curved cock with a thick mushroom head. The second time we hooked up, he was lovingly patient. He thrusted slowly on top of me, in the missionary position, for about 20 minutes, while I masturbated. I came on his cock while I looked at his handsome face. He did for me, what most men much older could not do.

His First Time Doing Oral And I Had An Orgasm
I was getting fatigued with the random hookups. I agreed to meet Adam, an 18-year-old Marine, anyway for our planned beach walk. A beach walk sounded nice. I had no obligation to hookup.

"I've never gone down on a girl," he said.
"What? Have you had sex?"
"Yes, but I did not go down before. I really want to try it."
That got my attention. I invited Adam over.
At my place, he moved his tongue in the most delicious way and after only ten minutes, I orgasmed on his tongue. That showed me a man's sensuality and attitude, not a book of techniques and instructions, determined whether he could get me off.

CHAPTER 14
FINDING MY GROOVE

MY CAREER (MAY, TWO YEARS SINGLE)

I was not challenged at work. A few times I had thought to quit, because I had a wonderful boss and opportunities, and I was pretending to care.

Sexual Harassment

We had our company Christmas party, and Oliver came as my guest. He sat next to me at lunch. I chatted about my safe sex blowjobs and latest hookups to people who often talked to me about sex, so I was totally blindsided when they filed a complaint against me. My boss called me into his office. He said he was concerned I was talking too much about sex, and it could make associates and clients uncomfortable. He followed up with a formal complaint of sexual harassment.

I couldn't decide whether to laugh, or be furious. I had never heard of a woman being written up for sexual harassment. I used this as a learning opportunity. Not everyone was interested in sex, and I needed to get to a place in my life where I had interests other than sex. But everything other than sex bored me.

I kept writing my book. David, the reason for the book, never called me to say he changed his mind. I had forgot all about him.

If he had not been the reason for my book, I would not even be thinking of him today.

I would have to quit my job when the book came out, because sex memoirs and school districts did not mix. Schools were terrified of women who liked sex. I had worked at my company four years and contributed a great deal. It would be fine, career wise, to leave. I imagined the whole world would want to read a book about a woman who liked sex, and my book royalties would replace my office job income.

I was getting tired of the meaningless hookups, so often when I was horny did not do anything about it. Instead, I worked on my book.

Quitting My Job
That spring, almost two years after moving into my apartment, there was a change in management at work. My former boss was a seasoned leader who gave us freedom to work and make mistakes, because he trusted us as professionals. My new boss micromanaged all our activities, so he could stay updated on everything. His need to control made me furious and I felt trapped. I had to leave. I had planned to quit anyway, because my book was almost done.

"Don't quit your job until you get another job," my brother advised.

"Keep your fear to yourself," I replied, because I was convinced my book would take off.

I met with my boss and gave my one month notice. He thanked me for my loyalty and the good work we had done together, and asked if I could stay part-time to close out my projects.

My Sex Memoir
I self-published my sex memoir, The F-ck List. The title conveyed my right to sexual pleasure. Brad read my book and said I was a good writer and some other sweet things and I was so moved, I

cried. He also said he did not want to be linked to my book. I had to legally change my last name.

I considered going back to my maiden name. I called my dad to ask. He said he had worked his whole life to build his reputation and career, and did not want it destroyed by me and my book. Then he sent an email telling me e he never wanted to speak to me again, because a proper woman keeps her sex life private. I wasn't even sad he said it.

Maybe it was better to have my own name, so I could say what I wanted without anyone getting mad. I wasn't fucking guys or writing a sex memoir to upset anyone. I just wanted to be free.

I went to the courthouse and filed a legal name change to Morgan.

A Nude Strip Club

I applied for a City of San Diego Entertainer's Permit, so I could have fun and work on that relationship with my pussy. I was fingerprinted and paid my permit fees. Our city had strict rules for nude strip clubs. No alcohol could be served. Dancers could only be nude when they were a minimum six feet away from patrons. We were not allowed to touch the patron's genitals. I was sure I could abide by these rules.

I applied at a nude strip club. I was surprised the club hired me, even though I could not pole dance. Did men really want to see a 55-year-old woman in the nude?

I worked part-time in my office by day, and at the strip club at night. The strip club was fun. It did not matter that I could not pole dance. Each girl gave the DJ a playlist. We could choose our songs, clothes, and how we wanted to dance. Each girl danced for two songs, and had to remove her panties for the entire second song, since it was after all a nude club.

I showed my pussy to men on stage. At first, I spread my legs for just one second. I built up to ten seconds. The men were staring at my pussy and smiling. That showed me they liked it.

The men just liked seeing our bodies. I watched the other girls dance and complimented them on their performance. Some women danced fast and hard, others very slowly, barely moving at all. The slow movement was sensuous and erotic. The fun playful dancing was hot. I changed my dancing to copy my favorite styles.

Most of the men came in to see us dance for free. Sometimes they gave us a few $1 bills, thrown on stage or respectfully placed in our G-strings. They probably felt that paying the cover charge earned them the right to see us perform. We did not get any of the cover money. Our money was earned in the lap dances. The girls who made the most money excelled at talking men into these dances. It had nothing to do with looks, personality, or dancing talent.

At the end of each shift, we tipped out the DJ, manager, and bouncers. They deserved it, because all the staff was nice and respectful.

A Ph.D. scientist from Europe, who was in town on business, propositioned me for an encounter. After work, I went to his hotel. He showered and we went to his bed. He marveled at my wetness. He touched me gently with his fingers on my clit like he probably touched his wife, and gave me an orgasm. We had intercourse with a condom After his orgasm, we cuddled..

On the drive home, I wondered why I did not feel slutty or used. I felt happy, appreciated, and valued.

I was afraid to do this again, because a man could be a police officer trying to set me up or get the club into trouble. I just did my dancing, and sometimes I pushed the limits because I was horny and playful. In the lap dances, I kissed men, ground on them, or stuck my breasts in their face. One night, I took my panties off in a lap dance. One of the club bouncers stormed into the private dancing area.

"What do you think you're doing?" he asked.

I fumbled for my panties and put them on. I did not know there were cameras in the private dancing area. I broke the rules. The bouncer was just doing his job. At the end of the shift, the supervisor called me into his office and gave me a 48-hour notice that I was fired. I came in for my two remaining shifts, and then I was done.

Why was I always getting into trouble for liking sex?

I applied at a strip club closer to home, and vowed to follow the rules. In the daytime, I was still going into the office. Professional woman by day, stripper by night.

After a few months at the new club, nude dancing lost its appeal. I did not like the rules forbidding me to touch men, baring my pussy for just a few $1 bills, and hustling for lap dances. A woman should not have to talk a man into a lap dance. A man should pursue a woman when she showed her interest and availability. The energy was all mixed up.

I closed out my projects at work and handed in my office key. I felt free. Right away, my orgasms became more powerful. They lasted longer, and I roared almost every time, just as I had with David.

Escort

I placed an ad in the escort section of a online site. The men followed my rules to get the appointment. I liked that men were pursuing me, which was the opposite of the strip club where I had to chase the man. The energy was finally right.. The men were nice to me and wanted to please me.

I was finally free. I worked for myself. Nobody was telling me what I could or could not do. There was no reason to remain a stripper. After four months, I gave my notice and quit my stripper job.

As an escort, I charged men for my companionship, a legal activity. My rates were higher than those of younger women. Only porn stars traveling through town charged more. I was stunned that men preferred an older woman. Men of all ages, races, and professions clamored to see me. I started a YouTube channel about sex, dating, and relationships, and was inundated with fan mail from all over the world.

"I've been following your videos and your book. I love how open you are."

"You're a fascinating woman."

"I've watched all your videos, and I am intrigued by you. I would like to schedule an appointment."

"I found you on the keyword mature. I like older women."

"I don't want to see a woman my daughter's age or younger, so my minimum age is 32."

In my appointments, they wanted to go down on me and give me orgasms. I was always surprised. I thought, *You don't think I'm dirty? So many men have been down there.*

"You don't mind I'm with so many men?"

"No. You're gorgeous."

Women were equally fascinated when I told them my occupation.

"Oh my God, you're amazing."

"Wow, tell me more."

My children easily adapted. If they were home when I had an appointment, they would go for a coffee or workout.

"Mom, we'll be back in a couple hours."

After I became an escort, I rarely hooked up anymore. I was tired of men just having sex and leaving. Sometimes, when I wanted a hot young hunk or a relationship, I went online.

A Relationship Prospect : He Wore His Pajamas
I still had the belief that relationships were for weak needy people who could not be happy alone, as well as a yearning for the deep intimate relationship I could never get with Brad. Thus, my internal battle was between the independent woman who did not need anyone, and the passionate vulnerable woman who longed to surrender to a man.

I went on Tinder for a relationship that could lead to marriage. Many people said Tinder was just a hookup app, and I had definitely used it for that. However, many of the men I met for hooking up also wanted a relationship. One of my friends met the love of her life on Tinder. Tinder could be whatever people wanted it to be.

Tony was a 43-year-old man mid-level programming manager. I could not fathom how a man who chose the safety of corporate life could excite me, but I wanted to be open to possibilities. I liked his genuine interest in me, and that he stayed away from the topic of sex.

The day after we matched up, Chandi and I visited Oliver at college. I was distracted with my phone instead of paying attention to my kids.

"Mom, are you on your phone again?" Oliver asked.

"Yeah, but this guy is different. He seems like a relationship prospect."

"Ok, Mom, but pay some attention to us."

I put my phone away, and texted him when the kids were not looking. Looking for something on my phone, rather than being present with life in front of me, was a bad habit I intended to break one day.

Texting with Tony put me outside my comfort zone. What was I supposed to talk about, when sex was all I talked about? What would we discuss when we finally met? I had no idea how to start a friendship leading to a relationship. I had only a few familiar ways of being with men. I could work with them, joke with them if they were neighbors or worked behind a counter at a store, smile at them if I saw them in public, or fuck them if I met them online.

If I wanted a relationship, I had to stop seeing men as objects that could give me sex, status, and money. I needed to care about the man, get interested in his dreams and personal life, give him love, and overlook his faults.

All this meant I had to open my heart to him. But that was something I resisted, because opening my heart to men always led to disappointment, and I was done being disappointed by men or crying over them. Was it even possible to open my heart and feel safe? Was my heart a safe place or a scary place? All these questions were too big for me, so I pushed them away and figured it would all work out.

Hopefully he would overlook my faults and ask me to a nice dinner. And then what? Go home and fuck? Was a dinner really any different than coffee, because both lacked a foundation of friendship and were just a short conversation in a public place, followed by sex. What about getting to know each other? Did I want to get to know him? What would we do to get to know each other? Activities? He liked the ocean and I liked forests. Did I have to start loving the ocean? And what about sex? Only 5-10% of men were good in bed and I would never again fall for a man and think the sex was amazing just because of how I felt about him. I wanted the sex to be amazing because it was.

When was I supposed to have sex with my relationship prospect? Was David right, that I should wait 4 – 6 weeks? I did not want to wait that long with my corporate cog-in-a-wheel, just to be let down if the sex was bad. No, I needed to have sex right away to make sure he was good in bed. If he was a real relationship prospect, he could come over without first meeting for coffee or a courtship dinner. I texted him with my decision.

I'll be home by 8pm. You can over at 9.

He came over at 9pm. I would meet him in the guest parking lot to give him an overnight parking pass and because I wanted time to scope him out before I invited him into my home.

Here, he texted me promptly at 9pm.

I walked down the guest parking lot, and looked for a man in a suit or something stylishly casual.

"Schahrzad?" a man called out.

Tony was walking briskly toward me. His clothes were loose. As he got closer, I saw he wore pajamas.

Hmmm, I did not expect my date to arrive in pajamas. Maybe I was too serious. Was his pajama move playful, or was he protecting his heart by showing our date was not worth the bother of a dress shirt and tie.

Tony and I sat on my sofa and talked over a glass of wine. He held my hand and sought sympathy as he recounted his cheating ex-wife, thankless teenage son, and boring job. If I had not been so horny and curious about sex with a man wanting a relationship, I would have asked him to leave.

Since he seemed like a good relationship prospect, we had sex without a condom. He was a C in bed, possibly a B. There was no way I would ever date him. Cuddling was out too.

"Can I get you some water?" I asked as I got up, signaling him it was time to leave.

"I better get going," he said and got his pajamas off the chair.

I sat back on the bed and watched him get dressed.

"Thanks for coming over," I said.

"I waited to leave until my son was asleep," he confessed. " I need to be quiet when I go back home, so my son doesn't wake up and know I went out."

"Really?"

"Yeah, if he wakes up, I'll tell him I was driving around the block because I could not sleep. That's why I'm wearing these pajamas."

"Oh, I see, I was wondering about that."

I wasn't in a position to judge him or what his son could handle, but this man was out, out, out for dating. His whimpiness repulsed me. Why did I have sex with Tony, without a condom? He did not deserve it. I called Chandi the next day and told her all about Tony and his pajamas. She laughed.

"Chandi, going forward, I will always use a condom unless I have been to the man's house. Yes, I need to have been to his house."

"Raising your standards, Mom," and we both laughed.

Tony texted me the next day and asked to see me again. I told him to never contact me again. He texted me again a few times and I stood firm, and then he left me alone.

My unhung pictures seemed out of place on the floor. When Oliver came over, I asked him to help me hang my pictures. My apartment felt more like a home.

Right after Thanksgiving, Chandi called to ask if I could take back our cat, Tabby. I did not want to be bothered with a cat, but I wanted to help her out. She came over with the pet carrier the next day. I took Tabby to the vet for his shots, ran tests for his sniffling, and bought medicine. My apartment felt more like a home.

He Led Me On
Right after New Year, I met a client close to my age who excited me. Chester talked all about himself, in an effort to impress. I overlooked his neediness and insecurity because he was a client. Chester said he was going to leave his selfish adulterous wife as soon as he could afford it. He wanted a relationship, and he seemed interested in me.

I enjoyed him a lot in our appointment, so I debated seeing him privately. I googled him and looked him and his wife up on Facebook. They were not even friends on Facebook. I believed him about the marriage. I couldn't figure out if he stayed for the kids, or because he really could not afford a divorce.

Chester had recently completed some major personal development work, so I overlooked his past pyramid scheme involvement and invited him over.

He came in, closed the door, and pushed me against the door. Hot move. I felt immediately aroused and swollen. I pushed back against him, teasing him to be stronger. He pushed back and we tousled with a sexual lust and then he grabbed me tight and kissed me. I was moaning really hard. He took me to bed and ravaged me with his strength, dominance, and rock hard cock, no condom. I could not physically feel a difference but offering my bare pussy seemed more intimate. I was more aroused, expressed, wild, surrendered, swollen, and wet than with other men. He thrusted for almost half an hour and was dripping in sweat. I liked his energy, endurance, and passion. I gave him an A+.

Two days later, at 10am, Chester texted me. He wanted to come over. I loved morning sex. But I thought he wanted a relationship? Maybe he would want lunch after the sex. Chester was even better in bed that time. When we were done with sex, he said he had to go. He needed to travel for work and would be in touch when he got back. Maybe he would ask me to dinner when he got back?

A week later, he texted and said he was stressed and what would help him most, would be coming over. I agreed because I was horny and loved good sex.

"My wife is the most beautiful woman I have ever seen," he said after we fucked.

It was a odd comment, because he hated his wife. Was he letting me know he would never leave his wife, or was he saying I was not beautiful enough?

I saw Chester only once more and then I ended it, because he led me on. He never asked me out. He just wanted sex and he was dishonest. That was the last time I would offer my bare pussy so easily.

I told Chandi about him the next time we talked.

"Chandi, I am done with no condoms. A man needs to get STD tested, be in a monogamous relationship with me, and have introduced me to his children. Otherwise, he doesn't deserve it."

"Raising your standards, Mom," she smiled.

In the next three months, I only had four hookups. There was nothing appealing anymore about hooking up.

A RELATIONSHIP WITH MYSELF
(MAY, THREE YEARS SINGLE)

It was spring again. Three years had gone by since I left Brad and filed for divorce. Three years of living alone and not a relationship in sight. All I had to show for it was a long fuck list, while my ex husband was married to a wonderful woman. I had to take an honest look at myself.

I started with my feelings. How could I ever be present with a man's feelings, when I could not even be present with my own?

Next, I had to deal with my sexual insecurities. I brought it up to my friends.

"I think I am work in the bedroom and it takes me too long to climax compared to men," I told my friend.

"Who made the man the authority in the bedroom?" she asked.

Wow. I had never considered it like that. It made sense. Men never expected me to be fast. The entire "I am work in the bedroom" theme was in my own mind. My vagina was always wet and ready for penetration,. Women were just as horny as men. Our bodies worked differently, with a long arousal process lasting 20 – 30 minutes, which men did not get to experience. For us, foreplay was crucial not because we were less horny, but because our bodies had the capacity to go to much deeper levels. The quickie guys like Brad were no longer my yardstick. They missed out on the pleasures of opening a woman to surrender and abandon. They needed instruction and compassion.

That May and June, I did not hookup at all. I took my STD tests and they came back negative for everything.

The Softness And Mystery Of Us Women
I met some women my age who were intrigued by my sexual openness. Two of them asked me about having sex with them. It had been a long time since I was with a woman. I did not desire to be with women. Was I was resisting something? I decided to find out. I had my encounters. The women reminded me of the beauty of my feminine essence. Laying on the woman, kissing her, inhaling her scent, seeing her soft curly hair, her vivacious hips, her soft pussy lips that swelled, I saw why men loved us so much. Maybe my feminine softness was not weak, and I could be soft and feminine too.

Public Speaker and Consultant
After that, I showed my feelings of sadness, loneliness, and even crying in my YouTube videos. Male subscribers said they liked to see a woman feel. I did not know they would. I realized men yearned for women to be soft and open and surrender to them. The feminine mystique, and how our feelings flowed through us, were alluring.

My YouTube channel videos reminded me of public speaking I had done as a youth. People said they loved my voice and listening to me talk. I liked it too. All that I had learned about love, sex, dating, and relationships went into my talks. More people subscribed to my channel. I yearned to take my speaking out into a bigger public setting. Most people were afraid of public speaking. I could not wait to do it. Public speaking, consulting, being out with people and getting involved in social causes while wearing my suits and professional clothes, excited me.

People were coming to me for advice. They said I was easy to talk with, like a therapist. I did not tell anyone what to do. I took them within themselves.

I started a self-love meetup group, to practice taking my message out into the world. This required a seating area. I bought an ottoman and a deep red sofa with seating for five. My apartment finally was a home.

A friend took some photos of me and photo shopped them to look like paintings. He had them mounted on 11 x 17 canvas, and shipped to my house. I felt like a queen who had paintings commissioned in her name. This felt loving. This felt good.

Falling In Love

And God said "Love Your Enemy," and I obeyed him and loved myself.

– Khalil Gibran

It finally happened. It was just different from how I thought it would be.

I got weary of looking for something outside of myself, remaining hopeful, having an "available" radar on, checking out men wherever I went, being smart and attractive on my social media, and even loving myself in the hopes a man would find me more attractive. I was tired of looking, waiting, and hoping for someone outside of myself to love me, instead of doing it myself. I had to shatter the Prince Charming fantasy, for it had betrayed me.

I let myself fall in love with myself. I was Prince Charming. I was the source, I was the love.

I let go of the belief that a relationship was for needy people. A healthy relationship required two full people who loved themselves and out of that fullness created a third entity, a partnership. I just had not been taught the right messages.

Relationship Coaches
I hired relationship coaches. On our first call, I got right to the point of what was bothering me.

"All men I see out and about, are with a woman or they are into their careers and don't want to date. They are not available."

"What do you mean by unavailable? Why do men occur as unavailable to you?"

So unavailable men were not a fact of life? It was just how I viewed them?

On our second call, I got to the point.

"Where am I supposed to go to find available men to date?"

"We're not doing that yet. We're laying the foundation…the relationship with yourself."

"I love that!"

They taught me it wasn't my partner's job to love me. My partner's love is a bonus, a gift. In fact, it was impossible to feel loved beyond the love I had for myself. If someone loved me more than I loved myself, I could not accept that love.

On our next call, I brought up my limitations.

"I want to care more about people. I feel selfish."

My coach smiled at me. "Just fill up your love bucket. Fill yourself so full of love, that you overflow with love. You'll automatically give away the overflow of the love you have for yourself."

The woman who had channeled about the relationship with myself had it right all along. The entire basis for any relationship is the relationship with myself. I wish I had learned this in grade school.

I no longer go online to find men. My relationship man, if he ever shows up, will have to be created in the real world. I still have no interest in doing porn, swinging, group sex, or bedroom toys. All I need for passion and surrender is one man.

Two weeks ago, I took Brad off my insurance policy and sold my engagement ring. I get it. I don't owe him anything, and I had to let him go. Soon, I celebrate four years in my apartment. I still have no dating prospect, but I have found something valuable: myself.

Thank you for reading my book. March 30, 2017

EPILOGUE

DREAMS

I dream of falling deep love for myself and life as it is.
I dream of inspiring people.
I dream that you love my book.
I dream of going on town book tour, especially through small towns, to promote my book.
I dream my book is made into a movie.
I dream of a partnership with a masculine man, that will be more magical and nourishing than anything I can imagine, that will blow his heart and mine wide open and from there deepen our ability to serve the world.
I dream that you like me.

ABOUT THE AUTHOR

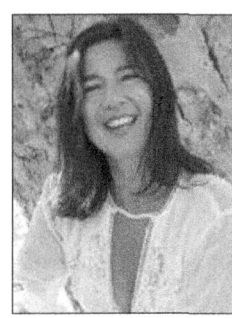

Schahrzad Morgan grew up in small German towns and moved to Nebraska as a child. She acquired a B.S. in Computer Science from the University of Nebraska - Omaha and an MBA from Arizona State University-West. She is fluent in German and speaks Farsi. She loves her three children, Transcendental Meditation, trail runs, playing piano, asking questions, and sex. She lives in San Diego, California.

www.WhatIDidForSex.com

Photography and Cover Design by Bill Gunn

**Printed by CreateSpace, An Amazon.com Company
Available on Kindle and other devices**